# Clinical Genetics and Genomics of Aging

Juan Carlos Gomez-Verjan
Nadia Alejandra Rivero-Segura
Editors

# Clinical Genetics and Genomics of Aging

Springer

*Editors*
Juan Carlos Gomez-Verjan
Basic Sciencies Division
National Institute of Geriatrics
Ciudad de México
Mexico

Nadia Alejandra Rivero-Segura
Instituto Nacional de Geriatría (INGER)
Ciudad de México
Mexico

ISBN 978-3-030-40957-9 ISBN 978-3-030-40955-5 (eBook)
https://doi.org/10.1007/978-3-030-40955-5



This Springer imprint is published by the registered company Springer Nature Switzerland AG
The registered company address is: Gewerbestrasse 11, 6330 Cham, Switzerland

# Foreword

Medical care for older adults has long focused on preventing and treating chronic diseases and the conditions that come with them. But now, researchers and clinicians hope a new understanding can lead to better and more effective interventions by targeting the aging process itself rather than discrete conditions or concerns. Aging is complex and varies from one person to the other, but there's a growing body of evidence that aging itself is driven by interconnected biological factors we call "hallmarks" or "pillars"; disrupting these hallmarks, which cover everything from the stability of our genes to ways our cells communicate, can contribute to chronic disease and frailty, which is why a better understanding of how they work is so important. Besides, how does aging affect the onset and progression of chronic disease? The work of many aging researchers has focused on studying the specific mechanisms that contribute to the aging process, and not so much on its effects on various diseases. However, age represents a major risk factor for several chronic diseases and conditions, including frailty and lack of resilience.

Geroscience's approach seeks to understand the genetic, molecular, and cellular mechanisms that make aging an important risk factor and, sometimes, a determining factor in the diseases and common chronic conditions of older people. This lies at the intersection of basic aging biology, chronic diseases, and health care. This book adopts this perspective, even though it focuses on the specifics of genetics and genomics.

This book is also a significant contribution to support aging research. As more and more people benefit from increased longevity, clinician-investigators will be empowered by this knowledge to contribute to the progress of aging research. Collaboration will be particularly important, and partnering across disciplines previously seen as independent will be important to future progress, which is why the aging research needs a book linking knowledge from different fields for moving forward these discussions.

Since 2013 when the seminal paper by López Otin on the hallmarks of aging was published, significant progress has ensued. And an update of the molecular pillars of aging is needed, which is the focus of the first chapter.

If we feel optimistic about the malleability of aging, nevertheless, neurodegeneration remains the main obstacle to healthspan extension, and a molecular update is urgent as it is a better understanding of its relationship to dysbiosis and the microbiota, a domain of increasing interest. As aging is the main risk factor for Alzheimer's disease, the hippocampus probably harbors the key to understand its relationship; this expanding field of knowledge merits a review of the molecular mechanisms of hippocampal aging.

The key to the understanding of the metabolic regulation as we age probably lies within the mitochondria. There is solid evidence that accumulated DNA damage in mitochondria is a cause directly related to metabolic disorders such as diabetes and neurodegeneration. The central nervous system is particularly susceptible to oxidative damage. Free radicals are generated at many cell sites, and the mitochondrial respiratory chain is one of the main sources. While many studies have been conducted in experimental animal models, the results are relevant because at least some of their interventions suggest a directing aim at reducing the effects of aging.

Reviewing genomic tools used in molecular clinical aging research is a need, particularly next-generation sequencing (NGS), massively parallel or deep sequencing which has revolutionized genomic research. Using NGS an entire human genome can be sequenced within a single day. Although in genome research NGS has mostly superseded conventional Sanger sequencing, it has not yet translated into routine clinical practice; in this chapter, different NGS strategies that have been used in the study of longevity, aging, and age-related diseases are reviewed.

To make significant progress in aging research, we urgently need molecular biomarkers for aging studies, particularly in humans. This chapter focuses on the inflammatory state, the markers of oxidative stress, and the hormonal profile which are the main functions that impact the development of aging and can be influenced by the gene and environmental variables in which human beings develop.

Alternative splicing and aging. Alternative splicing, or differential splicing, is a regulated process during gene expression that results in a single gene coding for multiple proteins. In this process, exons of a gene may be included within or excluded from the final, processed messenger RNA (mRNA) produced from that gene. Aberrant splicing events have been correlated with several diseases including those related to age; most of them lead to aberrant protein formation and therefore to misfolding protein accumulation, a common process in age-related diseases. In this context, AS seems to be a critical process not only for developing therapeutic purposes but also for a better understanding of the pathophysiology of these diseases.

The dynamic interface between genome and environment is covered by the field of epigenetics. Through a lifetime of exposures, this field grows in importance as we age, particularly to better understand the diversity of aging. Besides, DNA methylation is emerging as a biomarker of the aging process itself, and, furthermore, epigenetic modifications being reversible might be preventable, becoming therapeutic targets to promote a healthy aging process. In this chapter, the authors provide an overview of current research.

The human holobiont (commensal microbes and their multicellular eukaryotic host) constitutes a highly integrated system, which undergoes dynamic changes through time as it integrates and responds to signals from the environment. Microbiome research and aging is flourishing as we better understand the bidirectional interactions, and its evolution with a life-course perspective for the gut microbiota undergoes dynamic changes during host aging. Changes in host intestinal cell composition and architecture occurring during aging are matched by a decrease in the microbiota taxonomic diversity. Age-related decrease in taxonomic diversity leads to larger population size for a few age-associated microbial species, increasing the chances for the evolution of novel potentially pathogenic microbial strains, which have been related both to neurodegeneration and frailty. This knowledge positions the microbiome as a promising element for translational research.

Progeroid syndromes provide us with natural human models of accelerated aging. Advances in knowledge about their molecular basis have allowed a better understanding of DNA repair mechanisms and the role of LMNA gene and progerin in Hutchinson's and Gilford disease. The authors of this chapter particularly discuss the perspectives for therapeutic developments, which have been tested so far in vitro (human HGPS fibroblast cultures) and in vivo (HGPS mice models) and in clinical trials, with argumentation of their main limitations.

Genome editing has always been a challenging area to provide more efficient ways to create a meaningful change in the genome. Today, the CRISPR (clustered regularly interspaced short palindromic repeat) restoration system is considered as one of the suitable and promising options for genome editing. Compared to the previous systems, CRISPR can deactivate or eliminate a gene without interfering with intracellular mechanisms. The system could be used in the treatment of diseases and in related research by identifying the performance of defective genes in these diseases. CRISPR seems to have more potential and applications compared to previous systems. Among these applications, we can note the use of CRISPR in understanding complex genetic and epigenetic conditions such as aging or cancer. The complex interactions between several genetic and epigenetic mechanisms that characterize aging pose significant challenges to scientists attempting to understand this phenomenon and its causes and still constitute a barrier to a better understanding of aging and the ability to develop effective application of CRISPR-cas to aging research.

Pharmacological treatment for aging: Are we there yet? Probably not, but significant progress has been made in the development of specific experimental approaches in the field of senolytics, while we wait for the results of the TAME study on the efficacy of metformin to delay noncommunicable disorders onset. Many more drugs will ensue as several targets are being revealed with progress in the understanding of the aging process.

And finally, no doubt this knowledge will contribute to advance the field of personalized medicine. Indeed, advances in human genomics open the way as we understand linkage of genes to disease and develop specifically targeted drugs. This last chapter on molecular clinical aging research focuses on the translational potential of geroscience and its potential to improve healthspan and well-being.

• López-Otín C, Blasco MA, Partridge L, Serrano M, Kroemer G. The hallmarks of aging. Cell. 2013;153(6):1194–217. https://doi.org/10.1016/j.cell.2013.05.039.

General Director, National Institute of Geriatrics, Mexico City, Mexico

Luis Miguel Gutierrez-Robledo

# Acknowledgments

To the National Institute of Geriatrics (INGER) for supporting our academic development as early-career researchers and for allowing us to use their facilities in the preparation of this volume.

To all the chapter authors for their efforts on this project.

Together to Sydney Keen and Sheik Mohideen K for their editorial support.

To Dr. Oscar Salvador Barrera-Vazquez for his academic support.

**Dr. Juan Carlos Gomez-Verjan:**

To my parents for their unconditional support and advice in life.

To my little apple for its support and collaboration.

**Dr. Nadia Alejandra Rivero-Segura:**

To my parents, my sister, and my grandma for their constant support throughout my academic and nonacademic life. Also, I am grateful to my partner, Dr. Juan Carlos Gómez-Verjan, for his kind invitation to contribute to this book as coeditor; for his extensive support throughout many years, especially when I feel frustrated; and for trusting me to develop this volume.

*"Aging is an extraordinary process where you become the person you always should have been."*

*–David Bowie*

# Contents

# Contributors

**Alma Alamillo-Iniesta, BCE, MSc** Department of Genetics and Molecular Biology, Center of Research and Advanced Studies (CINVESTAV-IPN), Mexico City, Mexico

**A. Alarcón-Aguilar, PhD** Departamento de Ciencias de la Salud, Universidad Autónoma Metropolitana-Iztapalapa, Mexico City, Mexico

**Clorinda Arias, MD, PhD** Departamento de Medicina Genómica y Toxicología Ambiental, Instituto de Investigaciones Biomédicas, Universidad Nacional Autónoma de México, Mexico City, Mexico

**O. S. Barrera-Vázquez, PhD** División de Ciencias Básicas, Instituto Nacional de Geriatría (INGER), Mexico City, Mexico

División de Investigación Básica, Instituto Nacional de Geriatría (INGER), Mexico City, Mexico

National Institute of Geriatrics, Mexico City, Mexico

**M. F. Carrillo-Vega, PhD** Department of Clinical Epidemiological Research, Instituto Nacional de Geriatría (INGER), Mexico City, Mexico

**Susana Castro-Obregón, PhD** Department of Neurodevelopment and Physiology, Institute of Cellular Physiology, National Autonomous University of Mexico (UNAM), Mexico City, Mexico

**B. P. Chávez-Elizalde, BSND** Department of Clinical Epidemiological Research, Instituto Nacional de Geriatría (INGER), Mexico City, Mexico

**Bulmaro Cisneros, PhD** Department of Genetics and Molecular Biology, Center of Research and Advanced Studies (CINVESTAV-IPN), Mexico City, Mexico

**E. Delgado-de Anda, MD** National Institute of Geriatrics, Mexico City, Mexico

**Ian García-Aguirre, MSc** Department of Genetics and Molecular Biology, Center of Research and Advanced Studies (CINVESTAV-IPN), Mexico City, Mexico

**C. García-Peña, MD, PhD** National Institute of Geriatrics, Mexico City, Mexico

**Lizbeth García-Velázquez, MSc** Departamento de Medicina Genómica y Toxicología Ambiental, Instituto de Investigaciones Biomédicas, Universidad Nacional Autónoma de México, Mexico City, Mexico

**Alfredo García-Venzor, MSc, PhD** Epigenetics Laboratory, Instituto Nacional de Medicina Genómica, Mexico City, Mexico

**Juan Carlos Gomez-Verjan, Pharm, MSc, PhD** División de Ciencias Básicas, Instituto Nacional de Geriatría (INGER), Mexico City, Mexico

**Jose Mario Gonzalez-Meljem, PhD** Bioengineering Department, School of Engineering and Science, Tecnologico de Monterrey, Mexico City, Mexico

**A. A. Guerrero-Cruz, Biol** División de Investigación Básica, Instituto Nacional de Geriatría (INGER), Mexico City, Mexico

**Scott Haston, PhD** Developmental Biology and Cancer Research Programme, Birth Defects Research Centre, UCL Great Ormond Street Institute of Child Health, London, UK

**M. Königsberg, PhD** División de Ciencias Biológicas y de la Salud, Departamento de Ciencias de la Salud, Universidad Autónoma Metropolitana-Iztapalapa, Mexico City, Mexico

**Luísa V. Lopes, PhD** Instituto de Medicina Molecular João Lobo Antunes, Faculdade de Medicina, Universidade de Lisboa, Lisbon, Portugal

**A. Luna-López, PhD** Departamento de Investigación Básica, Instituto Nacional de Geriatría, Mexico City, Mexico

**Edna Ayerim Mandujano-Tinoco, PhD** Laboratory of Connective Tissue, Instituto Nacional de Rehabilitación "Luis Guillermo Ibarra Ibarra", Mexico City, Mexico

**Raúl Medina-Campos, MD, MSc** National Institute of Geriatrics, Mexico City, Mexico

**Nancy Monroy-Jaramillo, PhD** Departamento de Genética, Instituto Nacional de Neurología y Neurocirugía, Manuel Velasco Suárez, Mexico City, Mexico

**Feliciano Monterrubio-Ledezma, MSc** Department of Genetics and Molecular Biology, Center of Research and Advanced Studies (CINVESTAV-IPN), Mexico City, Mexico

**S. L. Morales-Rosales, MSc** División de Ciencias Biológicas y de la Salud, Departamento de Ciencias de la Salud, Universidad Autónoma Metropolitana-Iztapalapa, Mexico City, Mexico

Posgrado en Biología Experimental, Universidad Autónoma Metropolitana-Iztapalapa, Mexico City, Mexico

**G. Pedraza-Vázquez, MSc** Posgrado en Biología Experimental, Universidad Autónoma Metropolitana-Iztapalapa, Mexico City, Mexico

**Sara Pozzi, PhD** The Novo Nordisk Foundation Center for Stem Cell Biology, University of Copenhagen, Copenhagen, Denmark

**Nadia Alejandra Rivero-Segura, Biol, PhD** División de Investigación Básica, Instituto Nacional de Geriatría, Mexico City, Mexico

**Mariana Temido-Ferreira, PhD** Instituto de Medicina Molecular João Lobo Antunes, Faculdade de Medicina, Universidade de Lisboa, Lisbon, Portugal

**Edgar Ricardo Vázquez-Martínez, PhD** Unidad de Investigación en Reproducción Humana, Instituto Nacional de Perinatología-Facultad de Química, Universidad Nacional Autónoma de México, Mexico City, Mexico

**J. C. Yustis-Rubio, Biol** Departamento de Ecología Funcional, Instituto de Ecología, UNAM, Mexico City, Mexico

# An Update on the Molecular Pillars of Aging

# 1

Lizbeth García-Velázquez and Clorinda Arias

## Abbreviations

| | |
|---|---|
| 53BP1 | Tumor suppressor p53-binding protein 1 |
| 5mC | 5-Methylcytosine |
| AD | Alzheimer's disease |
| ADP | Adenosine diphosphate |
| AICAR | 5-Aminoimidazole-4-carboxamide ribonucleotide |
| AKT | Protein kinase B, also called PKB |
| AMP | Adenosine monophosphate |
| AMPK | AMP-activated protein kinase |
| ANT2 | Adenine nucleotide translocator 2 |
| ARF | ADP-ribosylation factor |
| ATP | Adenosine triphosphate |
| BRASTO | Brain-specific SIRT1-overexpressing transgenic mice |
| CDk | Cyclin-dependent kinase |
| circRNA | Circular RNA |
| CNV | Copy number variant |
| COX | Cyclooxygenase |
| CpG dinucleotide | Cytosine nucleotide followed by a guanine nucleotide in the linear sequence of bases along its 5′ → 3′ direction |
| CR | Calorie restriction |
| DDR | DNA damage response |
| FOXO | Forkhead box O |
| HLA-E | Major histocompatibility complex class I antigen E |
| HP1 | Heterochromatin protein 1 |

L. García-Velázquez (✉) · C. Arias
Departamento de Medicina Genómica y Toxicología Ambiental, Instituto de Investigaciones Biomédicas, Universidad Nacional Autónoma de México, Mexico City, Mexico
e-mail: lizgarvel@comunidad.unam.mx; carias@unam.mx



J. C. Gomez-Verjan, N. A. Rivero-Segura (eds.), *Clinical Genetics and Genomics of Aging*, https://doi.org/10.1007/978-3-030-40955-5_1

| | |
|---|---|
| IGF | Insulin growth factor 1 |
| IL | Interleukin |
| LHON | Leber hereditary optic neuropathy |
| LINE | Long interspersed nuclear element |
| lncRNA | Long noncoding RNA |
| MBD1 | Methyl-CpG-binding domain protein |
| MDC1 | Mediator of DNA damage checkpoint protein 1 |
| MELAS | Mitochondrial encephalomyopathy, lactic acidosis, and stroke-like episodes |
| MFRTA | Mitochondrial free radical theory of aging |
| miRNA | MicroRNA |
| mtDNA | Mitochondrial DNA |
| mTOR | Mammalian target of rapamycin |
| mTORC | Mammalian target of rapamycin complex |
| $NAD^+$ | Nicotinamide adenine dinucleotide |
| NBS1 | Nibrin protein |
| NFkB | Nuclear factor kB |
| NR4A | Nuclear receptor subfamily 4 group A member |
| NRF2 | Transcription factor named nuclear factor E2-related factor 2 |
| PI3K | Phosphatidylinositol 3-kinase |
| POT1 | Protection of telomeres 1 protein |
| ROS | Reactive oxygen species |
| S6K | Ribosome S6 kinase |
| SASP | Senescence-associated secretory phenotype |
| SIRT | Sirtuin |
| SNV | Single-nucleotide variant |
| TERC | Template telomerase RNA component |
| TFRC | Transferrin receptor |
| TGF-β | Transforming growth factor-β |
| TIN2 | TRF1-interaction nuclear factor 2 |
| TOX protein | Thymocyte selection-associated high mobility group box |
| TPE | Telomere position effect |
| TPP1 | Tripeptidyl-peptidase 1 |
| TRF1 | Telomeric repeat binding factor 1 |
| UPS | Ubiquitin-proteasome system |
| VEGF | Vascular endothelial growth factor |

## Introduction

Aging is a multifactorial process characterized by progressive functional decline at the molecular, cellular, tissue, and organismal levels. As an organism ages, it is more susceptible to developing age-associated diseases and has an increased likelihood of dying. In many organisms, including humans, age is the main risk factor for a variety of diseases, including neurodegeneration, cardiovascular diseases, diabetes, osteoporosis, cataracts, and cancer [1, 2]. The abundant research on the aging process across different species, including yeast, *C. elegans*, *D. melanogaster*, mammals, and genetically modified organisms, has enabled the identification of conserved cellular pathways associated with the biology of aging. López-Otín and colleagues have cataloged these alterations into nine hallmarks in their influential review, including genome instability, loss of proteostasis, deregulated nutrient sensing, mitochondrial dysfunction, cellular senescence, and stem cell exhaustion (Fig. 1.1) [1]. Interestingly, these hallmarks interact with each other and have molecular patterns that resemble those commonly found in cancer. The advent of new technologies and the development of the "omics" era have led to important advances in the comprehension and description of age-related processes at the molecular level in spite of the difficulty represented by great interindividual variability. In this chapter, we summarize some recent evidence of the potential mechanisms underlying the mammal aging process and longevity that may provide a rationale for the development of therapeutic tools that improve human health during this stage of life.

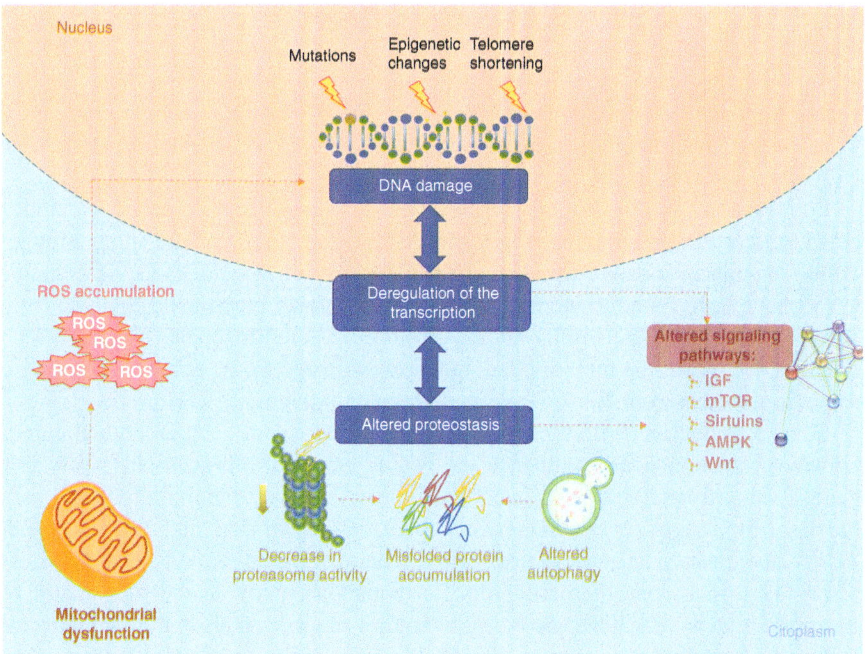


**Fig. 1.1** Molecular processes involved in cellular aging. Altered metabolic and developmental pathways, genomic damage, and mitochondrial dysfunction convey in the expression of the aged phenotype

## DNA: A Central Molecule of the Aging Process

The genome instability associated with cellular aging was proposed in the 1950s. This association was based on the observation that low doses of radiation shortened the life span and resulted in a myriad of mutations in somatic cells [3]. Since then, ample evidence has reinforced the association of accumulative DNA damage with aging. Genomic damage is highly diverse and originates from endogenous and exogenous sources, resulting in chemical reactions of the oxidative metabolism that leads to depurination and depyrimidination, DNA replication and repair errors. DNA is also a target of exogenous biological, physical, and chemical stressors, including viruses, ultraviolet radiation, and alkylating agents, among others [1, 4]. Loss of the capacity for DNA repair and other genomic changes lead to general deregulation of the genomic architecture, genome accessibility and gene expression [2, 5].

## Mutations Accumulate in Nuclear and Mitochondrial DNA During Aging

The human genome is thought to be subject to tens of thousands of lesions per cell per day, and although the vast majority of these are rapidly repaired, somatic mutations accumulate irreversibly and continue to accumulate with age adding to a previously acquired mutation background [6, 7]. Evidence from whole genome sequencing of human-derived organoids suggests that age-somatic mutations increase exponentially, not linearly as previously thought, which is in accordance with other sequencing- and nonsequencing-based assays [6, 8].

Point mutations, insertions and deletions (*indels*), copy number variations (CNVs), telomere shortening and gene disruption caused by the integration of viruses or transposons are frequent alterations found in aged cells [3, 4]. Somatic CNVs have been found to increase with aging in human blood cells obtained from monozygotic twins, and similar findings from microsatellite repeats have also been reported, for which the mutation rate increases with age from approximately 1% to 4% in blood cells from 20- to 70-year-old human individuals [9, 10].

Somatic mutations with the inherited gene variations of each individual cumulatively or synergistically influence the health span and life span [11]. Very few genetic variants have been associated with human longevity, but those found include the transcription factor *FOXO3* gene, the *APOE/TOMM40* and the *CDKN2B/ANRIL* loci, which are associated with Alzheimer's disease and cellular senescence [12–14]. In fact, the heritability for human longevity has been estimated to be approximately 20–30%, according to studies of twins, suggesting that external factors such as diet, environment, physical activity and microbiomes are important factors that influence the health span [14–16]. The increase in the rate of retrotranscription reflects genome deregulation, creating additional mutations, DNA damage, and other forms of genome instability. For instance, the expression of several families of retrotransposable elements increases with age, as observed in mouse skeletal muscle and human fibroblasts, particularly the long interspersed nuclear element-1 (L1 LINE) [17, 18].

Mutations accumulate not only in the nuclear genome but also in the mitochondrial DNA (mtDNA), which accumulates point mutations and deletions as a result of spontaneous errors during the replication or repair process [19]. Point mutations significantly increase with age in the human brain, heart, skeletal muscle and liver, while deletions have been reported in aging mouse models and human skeletal muscle and brain [20–22]. A frequent consequence of these mutations is the deficiency in COX activity, which indicates complex IV defects that compromise the production of ATP and increase the accumulation of ROS [23, 24]. Nevertheless, the strongest association of mtDNA mutations and aging comes from the study of mtDNA-mutated mice that express a deficient version of the proofreading exonuclease activity of mtDNA polymerase γ ($Polg^{mut/mut}$), generating a significant accumulation of mtDNA mutations and exhibiting a premature or accelerated aging phenotype [25]. Nevertheless, each human cell has multiple mtDNA copies, and in healthy aging, the abundance of mutated mtDNA rarely exceeds 1%, which is well below the phenotypic expression threshold (>60%) needed to be responsible for the phenotype [19].

## Telomere Attrition: More Than a Consequence of Cellular Replication

Telomeres are protective structures found at the end of chromosomes that are shortened because of cellular replications. Telomeres are constituted by hexameric (TTAGGG)n repeats associated with the multimeric shelterin complex, which prevents the access of DNA repair proteins to the telomeres, thereby avoiding chromosome fusion [26].

The shelterin complex comprises telomeric repeat binding factors 1 and 2 (TRF1 and TRF2), which bind the hexameric double-stranded repeat. TRF1 interacts with TIN2 (TRF1-interaction nuclear factor 2), while TRF2 interacts with RAP1 (repressor/activator protein 1). Single-stranded TTAGGG repeats bind to POT1 (protection of telomeres 1) and connect with TRF1 and TRF2 through TPP1, which also associates with TIN2 [26]. In this way, 5'C-rich and 3'G-rich overhangs bind to one of the double-stranded telomere regions and form a lariat-like structure, named the telomere-loop (t-loop) [27].

During the common process of lagging-strand synthesis, RNA primers allow DNA polymerases to initiate DNA replication. However, upon removal of the last primer at the 3′ end, the newly synthesized strand is a few nucleotides shorter than the original, resulting in loss of telomere repeats after each replication cycle, which is also known as the "end-replication problem" [27]. Telomere shortening is observed during healthy aging in most mammals and explains the limited proliferative capacity of some types of cells, the so-called replicative senescence [26, 27].

Telomerase, a specialized polymerase, can completely replicate the terminal ends of the telomeres with the help of the template telomerase RNA component (TERC).

Most mammalian somatic cells express the telomerase-coding gene (*TERT*) only for a short period. In humans, it is silenced between 12 and 18 weeks of gestation by the autoregulation of alternative splicing [28]. Interestingly, the phenotype of telomerase-deficient mice can be reversed if telomerase is reactivated [29].

Although cellular replication is a major contributor to telomere shortening, the rate at which telomeres shorten also depends on the presence of reactive oxygen species (ROS) [30]. The high content of guanine triplets in the telomeres is susceptible to oxidative modifications, and evidence suggests that oxidative damage at telomeres displaces shelterin proteins TRF1 and TRF2 [27]. Furthermore, mild oxidative stress is also associated with the accumulation of single-strand breaks and thus accelerates telomere shortening [27, 31]. In vitro studies show that the reduction in the levels of intracellular peroxide with antioxidants also reduces the rate of telomere shortening and extends the replicative life span of human fibroblasts [31]. Similar results were obtained with the overexpression of the antioxidant enzyme superoxide dismutase 3 gene (*SOD3*) [30, 32]. The correlation between ROS and telomere length has also been observed in patients with multiple sclerosis, who have increased markers of oxidative stress (*8-iso-PGF2α*) and shorter telomeres compared to those of healthy controls [33].

The telomere shortening rate is also influenced by mitochondrial function; reduction in mitochondrial superoxide extends the life span of human fibroblasts and decreases the rate of telomere shortening [34]. Furthermore, white blood cells from patients with the mitochondrial diseases MELAS or LHON, characterized by respiratory chain dysfunction, have shorter telomeres than controls [27].

Similar observations have been described for Alzheimer's disease patients, who present shorter telomere length in leukocytes compared to controls, which reinforces the importance of studying telomere-shortening mechanism beyond replication, since this disease is also associated with increased ROS production due to mitochondrial dysfunction, stress, and inflammation [35].

The length of chromosomes has important implications for the expression of proximal genes. The canonical TTAGGG repeats form heterochromatin through their association with the trimethylation of the histones H3K9 and H4K20, induce compaction of nucleosomes and altered spacing such that the potential of silencing proximal genes increases through a process known as telomere position effect (TPE) [36]. The first described human gene to be regulated by TPE was *ISG15* (interferon-stimulated gene 15), which is located 1Mb from the end of chromosome 1p and was shown to be expressed at low levels in young cells with long telomeres and at high levels in the progressively shortened telomeres [37].

## The Epigenome and Its Architectural Importance

DNA is compacted into chromosomes through the formation of chromatin, which has a structure and function that depend on DNA methylation, a variety of histone marks, and nucleosome positioning. These variations control the spatiotemporal expression of genes and provide the proper and functional genome architecture [2].

DNA methylation occurs mainly at the cytosine (5mC) of CpG dinucleotides and is a heritable and conserved regulatory marker generally associated with transcriptional repression. In mammals, the genome-wide pattern of DNA methylation changes during aging [38]. The DNA methylation pattern has been proposed as a biomarker for human chronological age, and the gradual accumulation of differential DNA methylation is thought to act as an "epigenetic clock" [38–40]. Global hypomethylation with age has been commonly described; however, some CpG islands and gene-rich regions become hypermethylated [38, 39]. In this regard, the loci with age-dependent DNA hypermethylation are preferentially close to tissue-specific genes, genes involved in differentiation and development, and genes encoding transcription factors and transcription factor binding sites [38, 39]. It is surprising that there is not a clear correlation between age-dependent differential DNA methylation and altered gene expression [41].

Histone proteins that package DNA to form nucleosomes are subject to a variety of posttranslational modifications, which have been associated with a particular function described in the histone code. Histone marks such as H3K27me3, H3K4me, and H3K27ac help control the expression of genes [2]. Other histones, such as H3K9me or H4K20me2, act as silencers through the formation of heterochromatin and H3K56ac or H3K14ac and regulate genome stability [2]. The pattern of these marks changes during aging [39]. For instance, global H3K27me3 decreases during *C. elegans* aging and in human progeria models [42–44]. Nevertheless, age-associated changes in global H3K27me3 levels could also be context dependent since cultured senescent human lung fibroblasts have large-scale gains and losses of H3K27me3 compared to H3K27me3 in early-passage proliferating cells [2, 45]. On the other hand, H3K4me3 also changes with age in murine hematopoietic stem cells and during cellular senescence of human fibroblasts [45, 46].

Mice with higher levels of the histone demethylase PHF8/JMJD-1.2 live longer, and similar results were observed in *C. elegans*, suggesting that there is a link between longevity and PHF8/JMJD-1.2, and that it might be conserved [47].

Higher levels of chromatin structure create the three-dimensional architecture of the genome through associations among distal genomic regions as well as associations between the nuclear envelope and DNA [48]. Interestingly, the positioning of nucleosomes on DNA and the general chromatin structure changes with age, and these changes have been associated with longevity [2].

The loss of heterochromatin has been suggested to be a common feature of aging because the levels of HP1 and H3K9me3 decline during healthy aging in humans and invertebrates, and DNA damage has been proposed to contribute to this heterochromatin loss [42, 49]. Nucleosome occupancy decreases likely because of a reduction in the number of core histones or a change in the activity of histone chaperones, but ameliorating this loss in yeast increases life span [42, 50]. In mammalian muscle stem cells, the loss of core histones with age appears to be due to the suppressed H3K27me3 mark at the histone genes, which lowers their expression; therefore, altered chromatin states at specific loci, such as those of the histone genes, may precede the reduction in nucleosome occupancy during aging [2, 51]. A more detailed description of the influence of epigenetics in the aging process is presented deeply in Chap. 8.

## Transcriptome Deregulation in Aging

The universe of transcripts in a cell or tissue at a precise time and metabolic conditions is highly variable and dynamic. Since aging is a continuous process, the set of genes that are differentially expressed between young and old cells is highly heterogeneous and depends, among other factors, on the individual's genetic background and life history, making it difficult to analyze or predict. Nevertheless, the study of the transcriptome has brought to light important information that helps us understand the mechanisms that underlie the aging process.

Changes in gene expression can be found when comparing samples from young or old cells; however, the type of change is also variable. While some genes maintain similar expression levels during life, others increase during development, and then, the rate of expression becomes progressively slower in adulthood. Another set of genes shows a peak of expression at middle age and then a declined expression; this is the case for calbindin 1 (*CALB1*), a gene involved in calcium regulation [16, 52]. Furthermore, the patterns of expression of a specific gene during aging can be opposite depending on the tissue, as observed for Wnt signaling components, which may have important implications for preserving tissue homeostasis [53]. Nevertheless, aging has been associated with transcriptional deregulation and aberrant production and maturation of many RNAs, some of which encode key components of inflammatory, mitochondrial, and lysosomal degradation pathways [1, 54]. The changes in the presence and abundance of transcripts can be explained by the abundance and availability of transcriptional factors, transcript stability, RNA splicing, and genome integrity, to name a few [2].

The analysis of gene expression in the prefrontal cerebral cortex of humans and macaques showed a loss of correlation in the expression of developmental pathway components during aging; that is, genes that were significantly increased during fetal development decreased in the aging cortex, whereas the expression of genes that decreased during fetal development was increased during aging. However, there are also examples of genes that are upregulated and downregulated twice [16, 55].

Age-associated changes in transcriptional factors represent a critical aspect of aging [2]. Some conserved pro-longevity factors are FOXO/DAF-16, NRF/SKN-1, HSF-1, XBP-1, REST/SPR-4, and p53/CEP-1. FOXO/DAF-16 promotes longevity in a variety of species from worms to humans, and it is regulated by the insulin/IGF signaling pathway, the nutrient sensor AMPK, and stress [56, 57]. This transcription factor controls the expression of genes involved in stress response, metabolism, immunity, and neuronal function in a variety of organisms, and interestingly, the *FOXO3* locus is associated with extreme longevity in humans (centenarians) [2, 58, 59].

NRF/SKN-1 activates the expression of genes involved in protecting the cell in response to ROS, toxins, and metabolic changes through mTOR and insulin/IGF signaling, and it is also dysregulated later in life [60, 61]. Increasing the levels of active NRF/SKN-1 activity extends the life spans of worms [62]. Additionally, a variety of noncoding RNAs are deregulated during aging, including microRNAs (miRNAs), long noncoding RNAs (lncRNAs), and circular RNAs (circRNAs) [63].

Some important microRNAs that are differentially regulated in aged cells are miR-29, miR-34, miR-212 and miR-132. The expression of miR-29 is induced by iron, which accumulates during aging and targets *IREB2* mRNA, which codes for an upstream translational activator of the transferrin receptor, TFRC. Antagonists of miR-29 induce upregulation of TRFC, iron accumulation, and neurodegeneration [64]. The expression of miR-34 also increases with age in the primate brain; its transcription depends on TP53 and its target is the *MYC* gene. The downregulation of miR-34 prolongs the *C. elegans* life span and prevents age-related cardiac dysfunctions in mice [16, 65]. Interestingly, miR-212 and miR-132 regulate the expression of *SIRT1* and are decreased in lymphoblastic cell lines generated from centenarians compared with those of AD patients, suggesting a protective effect of these miRNAs against neurodegeneration [66].

Long noncoding RNAs are important regulators of transcriptional networks and the closed or opened chromatin state [2]. One interesting example of an lncRNA is that associated with aging, H19. This lncRNA interacts with MBD1 (a methyl-CpG-binding domain protein) to suppress the expression of several genes, including a gene likely to have implications for aging, *Igf2*, which encodes an insulin-like growth factor [67]. The loss of *Igf2* imprinting occurs with aging in histologically normal human prostate tissues, and this epigenetic alteration is more extensive in men with prostate cancer [68].

A variety of noncoding RNAs are involved in the regulation of the senescence-associated secretory phenotype (SASP), including miR-15b, miR-187, miR-9, miR-222, miR-34a, miR-125b, miR152, and miR-199a, which participate in regulating mRNA turnover and translation, whereas miR-146a, miR-335, and miR-21 are associated with factor secretion [69]. Interestingly, a number of miRNAs associated with inflammation and aging (inflammaging) have been found in exosomes [70]. Additionally, several mRNAs responsible for the expression of SASP mediators are regulated by lncRNAs, such as lncRNA-LET, LincRNA-Cox2, NEAT1, lnc-IL7R, Lethe, and THRIL, most of which regulate interleukin-related genes [69].

Recently, thousands of circular RNAs (circRNAs) have been described in mammalian cells. They are generated by backsplicing that joins the 5′ and 3′ ends of transcript sequences. Only a few circRNAs have been associated with SASP, including Circ-Foxo3 and CircPVT1 [69]. Circ-Foxo3 is highly expressed in aged heart, intestines, lung, and skin compared to young organs and enhances the production of SASP factors through indirect mechanisms. On the other hand, CircPVT1, whose function is to sequester let-7, has been found in reduced levels in senescent human fibroblasts [69, 71]. More examples of lncRNAs involved in the aging process are presented in Chap. 8 and the consequences of alternative splicing in the aging process are described in Chap. 7.

## Proteome Findings in Aging Research

Multiple mechanisms that contribute to the loss of functional proteins during aging have been discovered: changes in protein synthesis, degradation, aggregation, post-translational modifications and localization. Studies in replicative and chronological aging have shown that the correlation between transcript levels and protein abundance is progressively reduced during aging (decoupling), which could be due to buffering mechanisms that prevent the transmission of the transcriptional alterations to the protein [16].

Age-dependent changes in translation efficiency but not transcript abundance were detected in 15% of age-dependent transcripts in the rat brain [72]. The decoupling of mRNA and protein expression levels in aging is consistent in different species and organs, such as the prefrontal cortex of human and macaque brains, where the mRNA/protein disparity was evident for genes involved in mammalian target of rapamycin (mTOR) signaling, mitochondrial function, and neurodegeneration [73].

The expression of ribosomal components usually increases with aging; nevertheless, proteasome protein levels and activity decrease with changes in its composition, driving protein accumulation in human liver [74]. This process has important implications for life span, and there is evidence that the reduction in protein synthesis or depletion of the components needed for the protein synthesis machinery has been shown to extend life span of multiple organisms, and similar effects are observed when proteasome activity is enhanced [75, 76].

A number of proteins have altered subcellular localization during aging as a result of impaired trafficking and the presence of protein aggregates, particularly in neurons. Subcellular fractionation and quantitative mass spectrometry studies have shown that complexes involved in molecular transport (COPI, COPII, and the retromer complex) exhibit changes in stoichiometry, and interestingly, these protein complexes are linked to neurodegenerative diseases, highlighting the importance of axonal transport for neurodegeneration [77, 78]. Nucleocytoplasmic trafficking is impaired in aged human fibroblasts and neurons, probably due to the presence of cytosolic protein aggregates that interfere with this transport system by sequestering factors involved in nuclear import and export, and because of the alteration of the nuclear pore complex [79, 80].

## Altered Proteostasis

In general, loss of protein homeostasis (proteostasis) is also a common feature of aging and has been associated with some age-related pathologies, such as Alzheimer's disease, Parkinson's disease, and cataracts, and they have been named *proteinopathies*. They are characterized by the appearance of unfolded, misfolded, or aggregated proteins [81].

Altered protein homeostasis can lead to stoichiometric imbalances in protein complexes and signaling pathways [16]. Protein homeostasis is usually maintained by the proteostasis network, which consists of the integration of a set of proteolytic systems that preserve proteome integrity across subcellular compartments and between tissues through different and complementary mechanisms [82].

The ubiquitin-proteasome system and the autophagy-lysosomal system are two of the principal proteolytic systems implicated in protein quality control, and both of them show decline and or dysfunction during aging, supporting the idea that collapsing proteostasis constitutes a common feature in this stage of life [83, 84]. Interestingly, long-lived species, such as the naked mole rat, show higher proteasome activity and increased levels of a subset of proteasome subunits compared to those of mice [85]. Additionally, overexpression of proteasome components (Psmd11/Rpn6 and Psmd14/Rpn11) and activation of the ubiquitin-proteasome system (UPS) can confer increased stress resistance and lead to extended life spans in lower species [86].

On the other hand, interventions using chemical inducers of macroautophagy, such as rapamycin, an mTOR inhibitor, can increase the life span of middle-aged mice like that induced by spermidine or polyamine-producing gut flora supplementation [87]. In an unexpected finding, aged cells showed an increased accumulation of protein aggregates, suggesting a decline in lysosome functionality during aging even though the number of lysosomes increased [72, 88]. This disparity could be due to changes in the pH, as suggested by the fact that the vacuolar V-type ATPase complex, which is responsible for maintaining vacuolar pH, decreased during aging, suggesting a mechanistic link between altered protein complex composition and lysosome dysfunction [72, 88]. The stress-induced synthesis of cytosolic and organelle-specific chaperones was also impaired in aging. Mutant mice that were deficient in a co-chaperone of the heat-shock family exhibited accelerated aging phenotypes, whereas long-lived mouse strains showed a marked upregulation of some heat-shock proteins [89].

## Conserved Metabolic Pathways Offer Clues to the Factors of Aging and Longevity

Evolutionarily conserved pathways, from yeast to mammals, robustly correlate with aging and longevity, and their deregulation has been implied with the development of cellular aging and include the mechanistic target of rapamycin (mTOR), insulin/insulin growth factor 1 signaling (IIS), AMPK sensing, and sirtuin (SIRT) pathways [90]. The harmonized regulation of these metabolic pathways maintains cellular and organismal homeostasis, even in the presence of external perturbations like changes in nutrient availability, temperature, oxygen level, or internal alterations, including protein misfolding and DNA damage [91].

### mTOR

Mammalian or mechanistic target of rapamycin, mTOR is a serine/threonine kinase in the family of phosphatidylinositol 3-kinase (PI3K)-related kinases [92]. It is involved in processes such as cell proliferation and growth, regulation of metabolism, protein synthesis, transcription, autophagy and synaptic plasticity [93, 94]. This protein is included in complexes called mTORC1 (mTOR, mLST8, deptor, TTI1-TEL2, PRAS40, and raptor) and mTORC2 (mTOR, mLST8, deptor, TTI1-TEL2, proctor, rictor, and mSIN1) [92]. A compound that acts as an mTOR inhibitor, rapamycin (a macrolide used as an immunosuppressant), was found to have an antiaging potential. In mammals, ribosome S6 kinase (S6K) is known to inhibit autophagy, which can be prevented by rapamycin [90].

mTOR activates the kinase S6K, which phosphorylates S6, inhibiting autophagy [92]. Rapamycin can extend the life span of organisms from yeast to mammals in a dose-dependent manner [95]. However, some data suggest that rapamycin has unwanted metabolic effects, including insulin resistance, hyperlipidemia, glucose intolerance, and hypophosphatemia; however, whether rapamycin is responsible for these effects remains controversial, and some of the effects are reversible [96, 97]. The mTOR pathway integrates different signals from insulin, cytokines, nutrients, oxygen, and mitogenic stimuli, and its regulation has important implications for longevity and against the negative effects of aging [92].

## Sirtuins

Sirtuins (SIRTs) belong to a family of seven essential enzymes responsible for the deacetylation of several transcription factors and residues in histone tails that leads to either the activation or repression of genes [98]. SIRTs constitute a highly conserved family of proteins that connect metabolic status to the regulation of aging and age-related phenotypes [99, 100]. SIRTs were identified as genetic silencing factors and are capable of extending the yeast life span by 50% when they are overexpressed [101]. Mammals express seven forms of SIRTs, which belong to class III histone deacetylases; the mechanism of action of SIRTs depends on nicotinamide adenine dinucleotide ($NAD^+$), with which they interact through a highly conserved binding site. SIRTs have a specific subcellular distribution, being found in the nucleus (SIRT 1, 6, and 7), the cytosol (SIRT2), and mitochondria (SIRT3–5) [102].

SIRT1 deacetylates a diverse array of cellular proteins, such as histones and transcription factors that drive metabolism, stress, and a host of other cellular functions. SIRT1 favors healthy aging and decreases metabolic syndrome-associated cancers [103]. SIRT1 is linked to cellular energy metabolism and cell senescence, and a recent report showed that mitochondrial SIRT4 regulates mitochondrial ATP homeostasis by the adenine nucleotide translocator 2 (ANT2) and AMPK [103, 104]. Male and female brain-specific SIRT1-overexpressing (BRASTO) transgenic mice have a significantly extended life span, and aged BRASTO mice exhibit phenotypes consistent with a delay in aging [103]. In the kidney, SIRT1 has been shown to inhibit renal cell apoptosis, inflammation, and fibrosis [104].

The *SIRT3* gene correlates with increased survival in centenarians [105, 106]. A genetic variant in the *SIRT3* gene was found to be a biomarker for longevity in some elderly populations [105, 106]. SIRT3 is also important in the regulation of mitochondrial functions, including ATP production, ROS generation, and cell death [102]. This protein also partially reverses the aging-associated functional decline of hematopoietic stem cells [107]. SIRT3-deficient mice present a variety of defects associated with impaired mitochondrial function, especially under stress conditions or during the aging process [90].

The overexpression of *Sirt6* extends the median life span by 14.6% in mice, but only in males. SIRT6 plays an essential role in metabolic homeostasis, inflammation, stress response, and genomic stability [108]. On the other hand, SIRT1 is considered a metabolic sensor that delays cellular senescence and extends the organismal life span through the regulation of diverse cellular processes. The suppression of cellular senescence by SIRTs is mainly mediated by delaying age-related telomere attrition, sustaining genome integrity and promoting DNA damage repair [100]. In addition, SIRTs modulate the organismal life span by interacting with several pathways including the insulin/IGF-1, AMP-activated protein kinase, and forkhead box O (FOXO) pathways [109]. Although still controversial, it is suggested that the pro-longevity effect of Sirt1 depends on the level it is expressed in the cell and the availability of the substrate $NAD^+$. Since SIRT1 is also believed to mediate the pro-longevity effect of calorie restriction, activators of this deacetylase have attracted the attention of researchers as a therapeutic target for age-related diseases [109]. Resveratrol, a phytochemical enriched in the skin of red grapes and wine, has been actively investigated to determine whether it promotes SIRTs activity with consequent beneficial effects on aging [110].

## IGF

Because insulin/IGF-1 function through signaling as a nutrient sensor and controls the transcription of stress response genes, the insulin/IGF-1 pathway provides a molecular connection between dietary intake and cellular stress response pathways [111]. Indeed, experimental data support the idea that insulin/IGF-1 pathways mediate at least part of the beneficial effect of calorie restriction (CR) [112]. CR decreases the levels of insulin/IGF-1 in mammals, which may be perceived by an organism as a mild type of stress, providing hormetic benefits. Recent genetic studies have found inherited SNVs in genes of the insulin/IGF-1 signaling pathway that correlate with longevity. Genetic variants in the *IGF1* receptor gene have been identified in Ashkenazi Jewish centenarians [113]. SNVs have also been identified in the insulin signaling genes *AKT1*, *FOXO1*, and *FOXO3a* in multiple centenarian cohorts [114]. The regulation of aging by insulin-like factors involves downstream signaling through phosphatidylinositol 3-kinase (PI3K), AKT, and FOXOs. Furthermore, life span extension requires signaling through the transcription factors DAF-16, HSF-1 (heat-shock factor-1), and SKN-1, which induce the expression of a broad network of genes involved in antioxidant defense, mitochondrial function, proteostasis, and autophagy [115]. Thus, signaling through insulin/IGF-1 modulates cellular and organismal stress responses by controlling key transcriptional programs.

## AMPK

The AMP-activated kinase (AMPK) is a conserved sensor of AMP and ADP production in response to ATP depletion, and this kinase can serve as a rheostat for cellular energy status. Some stressors such as glucose deprivation, ischemia, hypoxia, and exercise that depletes cellular ATP induces AMPK activation, which results in transcriptional and posttranslational signaling responses that increase catabolic pathways [116]. AMPK activity promotes fatty acid oxidation through phosphorylation and inhibition of ACC, an enzyme that synthesizes malonyl CoA from acetyl CoA. Thus, during periods of nutrient stress resulting in low ATP, the switch from fatty acid synthesis to oxidation is mediated in large part by increased AMPK activity [91, 117]. Declining AMPK activity during aging may contribute to insulin resistance and metabolic syndrome [118]. The decline in AMPK activity in aging skeletal muscle is deemed partially responsible for insulin resistance because it can be reversed by treatment with AICAR, an AMP analog that activates this kinase [119]. In this sense, compelling evidence suggests that compounds such as metformin and resveratrol are mild mitochondrial poisons that induce a low energy state characterized by increased AMP levels and activation of AMPK [120]. Importantly, metformin extends the life span of *C. elegans* through the induction of a compensatory stress response mediated by AMPK and the master antioxidant regulator NRF2 [121]. In a mammalian example, metformin can increase the mouse life span when administered from early life [122]. A more detailed description of the metabolic alterations in the aging process is presented in Chap. 4.

## The Role of Mitochondria in the Aging Process

For decades, mitochondria have been the center of attention in many studies of aging, which have led to theories based on their dysfunction as the origin of the aging phenotype, such as the Mitochondrial Free Radical Theory of Aging (MFRTA), and although these theories have been recently confronted, the role of mitochondria in the aging process is undeniable because of their versatile roles and implications for cellular function. MFRTA suggests that the oxidative damage of mtDNA is the key event disturbing the respiratory chain proteins to induce its dysfunction and increase ROS production in a vicious cycle [123]. However, alterations in mitochondrial function originate not only from oxidative damage but also from mtDNA damage, altered mitogenesis, deregulated mitochondrial dynamics (fusion/fission), and impaired communication with other organelles [1, 123].

During the aging process, the number and density of mitochondria are reduced in human and mouse organs, although the role of the mitochondrial dynamics remains controversial [123–125]. Mitochondrial bioenergetics can be impaired in the human brain and skeletal muscle in terms of ATP production and respiratory chain capacity and activity [126, 127]. Defective bioenergetics can result from the accumulation of mutated mtDNA, oxidation of mitochondrial proteins, destabilization of respiratory chain complexes, alterations in mitochondrial membranes, imbalance of fission and fusion events, and combination of increased damage and reduced turnover in mitochondria [1]. Although severe mitochondrial dysfunction is pathogenic, mild respiratory deficiencies may increase the life span of *C. elegans*, which could be due to a hormetic response [111].

Mitochondrial function is controlled by a number of signaling pathways and molecules that sense energetic conditions and contribute to life span regulation, including the SIRT, mTOR, and AMPK signaling pathways [128]. These pathways enable the cell to adjust energy consumption and mitochondrial number. The mitochondrial dysfunction associated with aging can be blocked by restricting the calorie intake due to the interplay between the signaling pathways described herein that converge to the transcriptional coactivator PGC-1α, a central regulator of mitochondrial biogenesis [128, 129]. Calorie restriction partially prevents the age-related decline of mitochondrial gene expression in mouse heart, brain, and skeletal muscle [130, 131]. A more detailed description of the relationship between mitochondrial function and the aging process is presented in Chap. 4.

## Major Features of Cellular Aging

Cellular aging occurs heterogeneously across different groups of cells, regardless of whether they are terminally differentiated or are stem or progenitor cells. For example, neurons, cardiac myocytes, and renal podocytes are postmitotic, and the specific hallmarks of their aging differ from those observed in epithelial cells, which are highly replicative throughout life [132].

Some of the age-associated phenotypes in postmitotic cells are closely linked to two phenomena: an increase in cell mass or cell hypertrophy and re-entry into the cell cycle without completing mitosis, which causes cell death. Terminally differentiated postmitotic cells permanently withdraw from the cell cycle, and the response to external or internal damage reactivates the expression of cell cycle-related proteins that are necessary to initiate and execute cell death programs. The cause of neuronal death in Alzheimer's disease is rooted in an ectopic entrance into the cell cycle [133, 134].

In contrast, proliferative cells undergo cellular senescence, which is characterized by permanent cell cycle arrest and a hyperfunctional phenotype that is associated with the overproduction and secretion of growth factors, proteases, and inflammatory mediators. This particular phenotype is termed the senescence-associated secretory phenotype (SASP). Replicative cellular aging includes biochemical, morphological, and functional modifications that lead to the irreversible impairment of cell proliferation associated with DNA damage, shortening of the telomeres, and changes in chromatin architecture, as previously described [135, 136].

The molecular mechanisms that drive cellular senescence in proliferative and nonproliferative cells are being discovered. One of the metabolic pathways associated with aging is the growth-promoting mitogen/nutrient-sensing pathway, in which the target of rapamycin (mTOR) is considered a central signaling molecule that affects multiple cellular pathways associated with aging [137]. In particular, mTOR participates in the transition of cells from quiescence to senescence [138].

## Cellular Senescence

Senescence at the cellular level is induced by several factors such as telomere attrition, oncogene activation, and molecular damage, which mediate p38 MAPK- and NFκB-stimulated signaling [139, 140]. The main feature of cellular senescence is the loss of proliferative capacity without loss of metabolic activity; in fact, the phenotype of senescence is characterized by the expressed markers of DNA damage, autophagy, and, through an increase in inflammatory molecules, senescence-associated β-galactosidase activity and lipofuscin accumulation [141].

During several cycles of chromosomal replication, the chromosomal ends are progressively shortened. When telomeres reach a minimal critical length, their protective structure is disrupted. This disrupted protection triggers the DNA damage response (DDR), which is associated with the appearance of DNA foci that stain positive for γ-H2AX (a phosphorylated form of the histone variant H2AX) and other proteins, such as 53BP1, NBS1, and MDC1; these proteins activate mechanisms that control cell cycle progression through the phosphorylation and activation of factors such as the tumor suppressor protein p53; the *CDKN2A* locus, which encodes p16Ink4a; and ARF proteins [142, 143]. These proteins induce cell-cycle arrest, enabling cells to repair their DNA. However, if the DDR is intense, then the cell-cycle progression is permanently arrested, and the cells become senescent [141].

The kinase inhibitor Ink4a enforces growth arrest, which contributes to the decline in the replicative potential of self-renewing cells during aging. This effect is mediated by the inhibition of the cyclin-dependent kinases CDk4 and CDk5, which in turn enable the hyperphosphorylation and activation of the retinoblastoma protein (p-Rb), causing cell cycle arrest [143]. The role of p16Ink4a in cellular senescence was explored by molecularly removing the p16Ink4a-positive cells, which delayed the appearance of the aging phenotype and aging-associated disorders [144]. Activating the promoter of p16Ink4a through Ras oncogene signaling has also been shown to be a useful technique for in vivo studies of the aging process [145]. As another feature, senescent cells can transform their metabolic patterns to excessively produce and secrete proinflammatory cytokines, growth factors, and proteases.

## The Senescence-Associated Secretory Phenotype (SASP)

SASP is one of the most representative features of senescent cells and may explain the organismal expression of aging and age-related diseases. Senescent cells produce a deleterious microenvironment through the production and secretion of proliferative and proinflammatory molecules such as IL-1α and -1β, IL-6, IL-8, the chemotactic cytokine GROα, IGBP-7, growth factors, VEGF, TGF-β, serine proteases, and matrix remodeling enzymes [146]. It has been determined that the activation of the *RAS* oncogene and loss of p53 function markedly amplify and accelerate SASP development in senescent human fibroblasts [147].

The activation of two transcription factors, NFκB and CEBPβ, mediates the expression of several SASP-related proteins, including IL-1α, which is one of the most important because of its ability to interact with surface receptors at the same senescent cell to induce a positive loop of NFκB activation [148, 149]. On the other hand, mRNA translation of the SASP-related proteins, particularly involved in protein synthesis of IL-1α, depends on mTORC1, which is sustainably activated in senescent cells [150]. SASP factors exert their functions in either an autocrine or a paracrine manner and are responsible for the induction of the chronic inflammation and cell proliferation that contributes to cell dysfunction and cancer. Thus, the accumulation of senescent cells in tissue is closely associated with aging-related diseases. Recently, it was determined that senescent fibroblasts significantly increase the expression of HLA-E, which inhibits the receptor NKG2A in killer cells, and CD8+ T cells evading the immune response [151]. The expression of HLA-E is induced by proinflammatory cytokines and regulated by p38 signaling in vitro by senescent cells with a SASP-related phenotype, suggesting a vicious cycle by which SASP contributes to the accumulation of senescent cells that block the immune response.

## Cellular Exhaustion

Continuous DDR activation and cellular stress signaling may result in the loss of tissue renewal capability due to cellular replicative exhaustion, particularly in T lymphocytes and somatic stem cells. Exhaustion is also characterized by cellular hypofunction resulting from growth arrest after prolonged antigen stimulation, as occurs in immune T cells after chronic viral infections or after excessive proliferation in the case of somatic stem cells [152]. In CD8+ T cells, exhaustion is defined as a condition characterized by hypo-responsiveness with reduced production of cytokines and excessive production of inhibitory receptors. It has been shown that TOX and NR4A transcription factors are critical for the transcriptional program of CD8+ T cell senescence and exhaustion and may contribute to the antitumor responses and immunosenescence associated with aging [153]. Stem cell renewal is essential to maintain tissue homeostasis. Stem cells undergoing senescence exhibit diminished proliferative capacity as well as reduced differentiation properties that compromise tissue integrity. The causes of stem cell exhaustion during aging are not completely understood, but the role of several transcription factors, such as Sox2, which is crucial for the regulation and maintenance of self-renewal and pluripotency in embryonic stem cells, has been studied [154, 155]. In this case, it has been found that aging is accompanied by a reduction of *Sox2* expression [156]. Although stem cell exhaustion is associated with diminished capacity for self-renewal and reduced capability for generating progeny, it is a different condition than senescence, which is characterized by cell cycle arrest and secretory phenotype.

The Wnt pathway has recently emerged as a key potential regulator of cellular senescence, particularly in the maintenance and repair of stem cells and progenitor cells [53]. It has also been shown that the genes of the Wnt ligands *WNT4* and

*WNT5a* are upregulated in senile human lungs, where increased myofibroblast differentiation was found to depend on these two ligands [157].

## Conclusions and Perspectives

The advent of new technologies has allowed the identification of conserved pathways involved in the aging process, as well as the association of genomic variants with human longevity. Nevertheless, heritability of human longevity has been estimated from 20% to 30%, reinforcing the fact that external factors such as diet, environment, and physical activity play a critical role in the human life span.

The several lines of evidence support the hypothesis that essential metabolic pathways interconnected with environmental factors and genetic background are involved in the appearance of different markers of cellular senescence. They have emerged as potential regulators of cellular senescence, particularly through those pathways involved in the maintenance and repair of stem cells and progenitor cells: mitochondrial integrity, mitotic competence, and eradication of senescent cells. The complexity of events that are under the control of the genetic programs induced in response to environmental challenges creates the need for further studies that must be performed to unravel the biological roles of the highly dynamic aging process through different tissues and different stages of cell life. The increasing research across different species has allowed the identification of conserved processes associated with the biology of aging. However, it is essential to consider that information from lower organisms cannot be generalized, since worms do not develop age-associated diseases such as osteoporosis, arthritis, or Alzheimer's disease.

A greater understanding of the relationship between human aging and external and internal stressors would be valuable in the study of age-associated diseases, of which neurological diseases are among the most disabling conditions. Thus, changes in the balance of protective and damaging mechanisms in different tissues have been explored leading to the development of recent therapeutic strategies aimed to promote healthy aging and extend human longevity.

**Acknowledgments** Our apologies to the authors whose work we could not cite due to space constraints.

This work was supported by CONACYT, A1-S-9559.

## References

1. López-Otín C, Blasco MA, Partridge L, Serrano M, Kroemer G. The hallmarks of aging. Cell. 2013;153:1194–217.
2. Booth LN, Brunet A. The aging epigenome. Mol Cell. 2016;62:728–44.
3. Vijg J, Suh Y. Genome instability and aging. Annu Rev Physiol. 2013;75:645–68.
4. Hoeijmakers JHJ. DNA damage, aging, and cancer. N Engl J Med. 2009;361:1475–85.
5. Veitia RA, Govindaraju DR, Bottani S, Birchler JA. Aging: somatic mutations, epigenetic drift and gene dosage imbalance. Trends Cell Biol. 2017;27:299–310.

6. Milholland B, Suh Y, Vijg J. Mutation and catastrophe in the aging genome. Exp Gerontol. 2017;94:34–40.
7. Maslov AY, Ganapathi S, Westerhof M, Quispe-Tintaya W, White RR, Van Houten B, et al. DNA damage in normally and prematurely aged mice. Aging Cell. 2013;12:467–77.
8. Blokzijl F, de Ligt J, Jager M, Sasselli V, Roerink S, Sasaki N, et al. Tissue-specific mutation accumulation in human adult stem cells during life. Nature. 2016;538:260–4.
9. Coolbaugh-Murphy MI, Xu J, Ramagli LS, Brown BW, Siciliano MJ. Microsatellite instability (MSI) increases with age in normal somatic cells. Mech Ageing Dev. 2005;126:1051–9.
10. Forsberg LA, Rasi C, Razzaghian HR, Pakalapati G, Waite L, Thilbeault KS, et al. Age-related somatic structural changes in the nuclear genome of human blood cells. Am J Hum Genet. 2012;90:217–28.
11. Vijg J. Somatic mutations, genome mosaicism, cancer and aging. Curr Opin Genet Dev. 2014;26:141–9.
12. Morris BJ, Willcox BJ, Donlon TA. Genetic and epigenetic regulation of human aging and longevity. Biochim Biophys Acta Mol basis Dis. 2019;1865(7):1718–44.
13. Sanese P, Forte G, Disciglio V, Grossi V, Simone C. FOXO3 on the road to longevity: lessons from SNPs and chromatin hubs. Comput Struct Biotechnol J. 2019;17:737–45.
14. Fortney K, Dobriban E, Garagnani P, Pirazzini C, Monti D, Mari D, et al. Genome-wide scan informed by age-related disease identifies loci for exceptional human longevity. Li H, editor. PLoS Genet. 2015. https://doi.org/10.1371/journal.pgen.
15. Polderman TJC, Benyamin B, de Leeuw CA, Sullivan PF, van Bochoven A, Visscher PM, et al. Meta-analysis of the heritability of human traits based on fifty years of twin studies. Nat Genet. 2015;47:702–9.
16. Cellerino A, Ori A. What have we learned on aging from omics studies? Semin Cell Dev Biol. 2017;70:177–89.
17. Maxwell PH. What might retrotransposons teach us about aging? Curr Genet. 2016;62:277–82.
18. De Cecco M, Criscione SW, Peterson AL, Neretti N, Sedivy JM, Kreiling JA. Transposable elements become active and mobile in the genomes of aging mammalian somatic tissues. Aging (Albany NY). 2013;5:867–83.
19. Srivastava S. The mitochondrial basis of aging and age-related disorders. Genes (Basel). 2017;8(12) https://doi.org/10.3390/genes8120398.
20. Kraytsberg Y, Kudryavtseva E, McKee AC, Geula C, Kowall NW, Khrapko K. Mitochondrial DNA deletions are abundant and cause functional impairment in aged human substantia nigra neurons. Nat Genet. 2006;38:518–20.
21. Bua E, Johnson J, Herbst A, Delong B, McKenzie D, Salamat S, et al. Mitochondrial DNA–deletion mutations accumulate intracellularly to detrimental levels in aged human skeletal muscle fibers. Am J Hum Genet. 2006;79:469–80.
22. Cortopassi GA, Arnheim N. Detection of a specific mitochondrial DNA deletion in tissues of older humans. Nucleic Acids Res. 1990;18:6927–33.
23. Wanagat J, Cao Z, Pathare P, Aiken JM. Mitochondrial DNA deletion mutations colocalize with segmental electron transport system abnormalities, muscle fiber atrophy, fiber splitting, and oxidative damage in sarcopenia. FASEB J. 2001;15:322–32.
24. Cottrell DA, Blakely EL, Johnson MA, Ince PG, Borthwick GM, Turnbull DM. Cytochrome c oxidase deficient cells accumulate in the hippocampus and choroid plexus with age. Neurobiol Aging. 2001;22:265–72.
25. Trifunovic A, Wredenberg A, Falkenberg M, Spelbrink JN, Rovio AT, Bruder CE, et al. Premature ageing in mice expressing defective mitochondrial DNA polymerase. Nature. 2004;429:417–23.
26. Shay JW. Telomeres and aging. Curr Opin Cell Biol. 2018;52:1–7.
27. Victorelli S, Passos JF. Telomeres and cell senescence – size matters not. EBioMedicine. 2017;21:14–20.
28. Ulaner GA, Hu JF, Vu TH, Giudice LC, Hoffman AR. Tissue-specific alternate splicing of human telomerase reverse transcriptase (hTERT) influences telomere lengths during human development. Int J Cancer. 2001;9:644–9.

29. Jaskelioff M, Muller FL, Paik J-H, Thomas E, Jiang S, Adams AC, et al. Telomerase reactivation reverses tissue degeneration in aged telomerase-deficient mice. Nature. 2011;469:102–6.
30. Von Zglinicki T. Role of oxidative stress in telomere length regulation and replicative senescence. Ann N Y Acad Sci. 2006;908:99–110.
31. von Zglinicki T, Pilger R, Sitte N. Accumulation of single-strand breaks is the major cause of telomere shortening in human fibroblasts. Free Radic Biol Med. 2000;28:64–74.
32. Serra V, von Zglinicki T, Lorenz M, Saretzki G. Extracellular superoxide dismutase is a major antioxidant in human fibroblasts and slows telomere shortening. J Biol Chem. 2003;278:6824–30.
33. Guan J-Z, Guan W-P, Maeda T, Guoqing X, GuangZhi W, Makino N. Patients with multiple sclerosis show increased oxidative stress markers and somatic telomere length shortening. Mol Cell Biochem. 2015;400:183–7.
34. Passos JF, Saretzki G, Ahmed S, Nelson G, Richter T, Peters H, et al. Mitochondrial dysfunction accounts for the stochastic heterogeneity in telomere-dependent senescence. De Lange T, editor. PLoS Biol. 2007. https://doi.org/10.1371/journal.pbio.0050110.
35. Forero DA, González-Giraldo Y, López-Quintero C, Castro-Vega LJ, Barreto GE, Perry G. Meta-analysis of telomere length in Alzheimer's disease. J Gerontol A Biol Sci Med Sci. 2016;71:1069–73.
36. Blasco MA. The epigenetic regulation of mammalian telomeres. Nat Rev Genet. 2007;8:299–309.
37. Lou Z, Wei J, Riethman H, Baur JA, Voglauer R, Shay JW, et al. Telomere length regulates ISG15 expression in human cells. Aging (Albany NY). 2009;1:608–21.
38. Zampieri M, Ciccarone F, Calabrese R, Franceschi C, Bürkle A, Caiafa P. Reconfiguration of DNA methylation in aging. Mech Ageing Dev. 2015;151:60–70.
39. Benayoun BA, Pollina EA, Brunet A. Epigenetic regulation of ageing: linking environmental inputs to genomic stability. Nat Rev Mol Cell Biol. 2015;16:593–610.
40. Horvath S. DNA methylation age of human tissues and cell types. Genome Biol. 2013;14:R115.
41. Yuan T, Jiao Y, de Jong S, Ophoff RA, Beck S, Teschendorff AE. An integrative multi-scale analysis of the dynamic DNA methylation landscape in aging. Greally JM, editor. PLOS Genet. 2015. https://doi.org/10.1371/journal.pgen.1004996.
42. Ni Z, Ebata A, Alipanahiramandi E, Lee SS. Two SET domain containing genes link epigenetic changes and aging in *Caenorhabditis elegans*. Aging Cell. 2012;11:315–25.
43. Shumaker DK, Dechat T, Kohlmaier A, Adam SA, Bozovsky MR, Erdos MR, et al. Mutant nuclear lamin A leads to progressive alterations of epigenetic control in premature aging. Proc Natl Acad Sci U S A. 2006;103:8703–8.
44. Zhang W, Li J, Suzuki K, Qu J, Wang P, Zhou J, et al. A Werner syndrome stem cell model unveils heterochromatin alterations as a driver of human aging. Science. 2015;348:1160–3.
45. Shah PP, Donahue G, Otte GL, Capell BC, Nelson DM, Cao K, et al. Lamin B1 depletion in senescent cells triggers large-scale changes in gene expression and the chromatin landscape. Genes Dev. 2013;27:1787–99.
46. Sun D, Luo M, Jeong M, Rodriguez B, Xia Z, Hannah R, et al. Epigenomic profiling of young and aged HSCs reveals concerted changes during aging that reinforce self-renewal. Cell Stem Cell. 2014;14:673–88.
47. Merkwirth C, Jovaisaite V, Durieux J, Matilainen O, Jordan SD, Quiros PM, et al. Two conserved histone demethylases regulate mitochondrial stress-induced longevity. Cell. 2016;165:1209–23.
48. Pombo A, Dillon N. Three-dimensional genome architecture: players and mechanisms. Nat Rev Mol Cell Biol. 2015;16:245–57.
49. Oberdoerffer P, Sinclair DA. The role of nuclear architecture in genomic instability and ageing. Nat Rev Mol Cell Biol. 2007;8:692–702.
50. Feser J, Truong D, Das C, Carson JJ, Kieft J, Harkness T, et al. Elevated histone expression promotes life span extension. Mol Cell. 2010;39:724–35.

51. Liu L, Cheung TH, Charville GW, Hurgo BMC, Leavitt T, Shih J, et al. Chromatin modifications as determinants of muscle stem cell quiescence and chronological aging. Cell Rep. 2013;4:189–204.
52. Geng Y, Lin HT, Chen W, Liu ZC, Xiang W, Chen WR. Age-related reduction in calbindin-D28K expression in the Sprague-Dawley rat lens. Mol Med Rep. 2015;11:422–6.
53. García-Velázquez L, Arias C. The emerging role of Wnt signaling dysregulation in the understanding and modification of age-associated diseases. Ageing Res Rev. 2017;37:135–45.
54. de Magalhães JP, Curado J, Church GM. Meta-analysis of age-related gene expression profiles identifies common signatures of aging. Bioinformatics. 2009;25:875–81.
55. Somel M, Guo S, Fu N, Yan Z, Hu HY, Xu Y, et al. MicroRNA, mRNA, and protein expression link development and aging in human and macaque brain. Genome Res. 2010;20:1207–18.
56. Eijkelenboom A, Burgering BMT. FOXOs: signalling integrators for homeostasis maintenance. Nat Rev Mol Cell Biol. 2013;14:83–97.
57. Salih DA, Brunet A. FoxO transcription factors in the maintenance of cellular homeostasis during aging. Curr Opin Cell Biol. 2008;20:126–36.
58. Webb AE, Kundaje A, Brunet A. Characterization of the direct targets of FOXO transcription factors throughout evolution. Aging Cell. 2016;15:673–85.
59. Willcox BJ, Donlon TA, He Q, Chen R, Grove JS, Yano K, et al. FOXO3A genotype is strongly associated with human longevity. Proc Natl Acad Sci. 2008;105:13987–92.
60. Tebay LE, Robertson H, Durant ST, Vitale SR, Penning TM, Dinkova-Kostova AT. Mechanisms of activation of the transcription factor Nrf2 by redox stressors, nutrient cues, and energy status and the pathways through which it attenuates degenerative disease. Free Radic Biol Med. 2015;88:108–46.
61. Rahman MM, Sykiotis GP, Nishimura M, Bodmer R, Bohmann D. Declining signal dependence of Nrf2-MafS-regulated gene expression correlates with aging phenotypes. Aging Cell. 2013;12:554–62.
62. Tullet JMA, Hertweck M, An JH, Baker J, Hwang JY, Liu S, et al. Direct inhibition of the longevity-promoting factor SKN-1 by insulin-like signaling in C. elegans. Cell. 2008;132:1025–38.
63. Gomez-Verjan JC, Vazquez-Martinez ER, Rivero-Segura NA, Medina-Campos RH. The RNA world of human ageing. Hum Genet. 2018;137:865–79.
64. Ripa R, Dolfi L, Terrigno M, Pandolfini L, Savino A, Arcucci V, et al. MicroRNA miR-29 controls a compensatory response to limit neuronal iron accumulation during adult life and aging. BMC Biol. 2017;15:9.
65. Boon RA, Iekushi K, Lechner S, Seeger T, Fischer A, Heydt S, et al. MicroRNA-34a regulates cardiac ageing and function. Nature. 2013;495:107–10.
66. Hadar A, Milanesi E, Walczak M, Puzianowska-Kuźnicka M, Kuźnicki J, Squassina A, et al. SIRT1, miR-132 and miR-212 link human longevity to Alzheimer's disease. Sci Rep. 2018;8:8465.
67. Monnier P, Martinet C, Pontis J, Stancheva I, Ait-Si-Ali S, Dandolo L. H19 lncRNA controls gene expression of the imprinted gene network by recruiting MBD1. Proc Natl Acad Sci U S A. 2013;110:20693–8.
68. Fu VX, Dobosy JR, Desotelle JA, Almassi N, Ewald JA, Srinivasan R, et al. Aging and cancer-related loss of insulin-like growth factor 2 imprinting in the mouse and human prostate. Cancer Res. 2008;68:6797–802.
69. Panda AC, Abdelmohsen K, Gorospe M. SASP regulation by noncoding RNA. Mech Ageing Dev. 2017;168:37–43.
70. Prattichizzo F, Micolucci L, Cricca M, De Carolis S, Mensà E, Ceriello A, et al. Exosome-based immunomodulation during aging: a nano-perspective on inflamm-aging. Mech Ageing Dev. 2017;168:44–53.
71. Panda AC, Grammatikakis I, Kim KM, De S, Martindale JL, Munk R, et al. Identification of senescence-associated circular RNAs (SAC-RNAs) reveals senescence suppressor CircPVT1. Nucleic Acids Res. 2017;45:4021–35.

72. Ori A, Toyama BH, Harris MS, Bock T, Iskar M, Bork P, et al. Integrated transcriptome and proteome analyses reveal organ-specific proteome deterioration in old rats. Cell Syst. 2015;1:224–37.
73. Wei Y-N, Hu H-Y, Xie G-C, Fu N, Ning Z-B, Zeng R, et al. Transcript and protein expression decoupling reveals RNA binding proteins and miRNAs as potential modulators of human aging. Genome Biol. 2015;16:41.
74. Bellavista E, Martucci M, Vasuri F, Santoro A, Mishto M, Kloss A, et al. Lifelong maintenance of composition, function and cellular/subcellular distribution of proteasomes in human liver. Mech Ageing Dev. 2014;141–142:26–34.
75. Charmpilas N, Daskalaki I, Papandreou ME, Tavernarakis N. Protein synthesis as an integral quality control mechanism during ageing. Ageing Res Rev. 2015;23:75–89.
76. Steffen KK, Dillin A. A ribosomal perspective on proteostasis and aging. Cell Metab. 2016;23:1004–12.
77. Bettayeb K, Hooli BV, Parrado AR, Randolph L, Varotsis D, Aryal S, et al. Relevance of the COPI complex for Alzheimer's disease progression in vivo. Proc Natl Acad Sci U S A. 2016;113:5418–23.
78. Li C, Shah SZA, Zhao D, Yang L. Role of the retromer complex in neurodegenerative diseases. Front Aging Neurosci. 2016;8:42.
79. D'Angelo MA, Raices M, Panowski SH, Hetzer MW. Age-dependent deterioration of nuclear pore complexes causes a loss of nuclear integrity in postmitotic cells. Cell. 2009;136:284–95.
80. Woerner AC, Frottin F, Hornburg D, Feng LR, Meissner F, Patra M, et al. Cytoplasmic protein aggregates interfere with nucleocytoplasmic transport of protein and RNA. Science. 2016;351:173–6.
81. Koga H, Kaushik S, Cuervo AM. Protein homeostasis and aging: the importance of exquisite quality control. Ageing Res Rev. 2011;10:205–15.
82. Labbadia J, Morimoto RI. The biology of proteostasis in aging and disease. Annu Rev Biochem. 2015;84:435–64.
83. Rubinsztein DC, Mariño G, Kroemer G. Autophagy and aging. Cell. 2011;146:682–95.
84. Tomaru U, Takahashi S, Ishizu A, Miyatake Y, Gohda A, Suzuki S, et al. Decreased proteasomal activity causes age-related phenotypes and promotes the development of metabolic abnormalities. Am J Pathol. 2012;180:963–72.
85. Rodriguez KA, Edrey YH, Osmulski P, Gaczynska M, Buffenstein R. Altered composition of liver proteasome assemblies contributes to enhanced proteasome activity in the exceptionally long-lived naked mole-rat. Brodsky JL, editor. PLoS One. 2012. https://doi.org/10.1371/journal.pone.0035890.
86. Chondrogianni N, Georgila K, Kourtis N, Tavernarakis N, Gonos ES. Enhanced proteasome degradation extends Caenorhabditis elegans lifespan and alleviates aggregation-related pathologies. Free Radic Biol Med. 2014;75:S18. https://doi.org/10.1016/j.freeradbiomed.2014.10.632.
87. Harrison DE, Strong R, Sharp ZD, Nelson JF, Astle CM, Flurkey K, et al. Rapamycin fed late in life extends lifespan in genetically heterogeneous mice. Nature. 2009;460:392–5.
88. Janssens GE, Meinema AC, González J, Wolters JC, Schmidt A, Guryev V, et al. Protein biogenesis machinery is a driver of replicative aging in yeast. Elife 2015. https://doi.org/10.7554/eLife.08527.
89. Min J-N, Whaley RA, Sharpless NE, Lockyer P, Portbury AL, Patterson C. CHIP deficiency decreases longevity, with accelerated aging phenotypes accompanied by altered protein quality control. Mol Cell Biol. 2008;28:4018–25.
90. Mazucanti CH, Cabral-Costa JV, Vasconcelos AR, Andreotti DZ, Scavone C, Kawamoto EM. Longevity pathways (mTOR, SIRT, insulin/IGF-1) as key modulatory targets on aging and neurodegeneration. Curr Top Med Chem. 2015;15:2116–38.
91. Haigis MC, Yankner BA. The aging stress response. Mol Cell. 2010;40:333–44.
92. Johnson SC, Rabinovitch PS, Kaeberlein M. mTOR is a key modulator of ageing and age-related disease. Nature. 2013 Jan 16;493:338–45.
93. Lamming DW, Ye L, Astle CM, Baur JA, Sabatini DM, Harrison DE. Young and old genetically heterogeneous HET3 mice on a rapamycin diet are glucose intolerant but insulin sensitive. Aging Cell. 2013;12:712–8.

94. Chakrabarti P, English T, Shi J, Smas CM, Kandror KV. Mammalian target of rapamycin complex 1 suppresses lipolysis, stimulates lipogenesis, and promotes fat storage. Diabetes. 2010;59:775–81.
95. Miller RA, Harrison DE, Astle CM, Fernandez E, Flurkey K, Han M, et al. Rapamycin-mediated lifespan increase in mice is dose and sex dependent and metabolically distinct from dietary restriction. Aging Cell. 2014;13:468–77.
96. Lamming DW, Ye L, Katajisto P, Goncalves MD, Saitoh M, Stevens DM, et al. Rapamycin-induced insulin resistance is mediated by mTORC2 loss and uncoupled from longevity. Science. 2012;335:1638–43.
97. Tataranni T, Biondi G, Cariello M, Mangino M, Colucci G, Rutigliano M, et al. Rapamycin-induced hypophosphatemia and insulin resistance are associated with mTORC2 activation and klotho expression. Am J Transplant. 2011;11(8):1656–64.
98. Haigis MC, Sinclair DA. Mammalian Sirtuins: biological insights and disease relevance. Annu Rev Pathol Mech Dis. 2010;5:253–95.
99. Giblin W, Skinner ME, Lombard DB. Sirtuins: guardians of mammalian healthspan. Trends Genet. 2014;30:271–86.
100. Lee S-H, Lee J-H, Lee H-Y, Min K-J. Sirtuin signaling in cellular senescence and aging. BMB Rep. 2019;52:24–34.
101. Kaeberlein M, McVey M, Guarente L. The SIR2/3/4 complex and SIR2 alone promote longevity in Saccharomyces cerevisiae by two different mechanisms. Genes Dev. 1999;13(19):2570–80.
102. Verdin E, Hirschey MD, Finley LWS, Haigis MC. Sirtuin regulation of mitochondria: energy production, apoptosis, and signaling. Trends Biochem Sci. 2010;35:669–75.
103. Satoh A, Brace CS, Rensing N, Cliften P, Wozniak DF, Herzog ED, et al. Sirt1 extends life span and delays aging in mice through the regulation of Nk2 homeobox 1 in the DMH and LH. Cell Metab. 2013;18:416–30.
104. Dong Y, Liu N, Xiao Z, Sun T, Wu S, Sun W, et al. Renal protective effect of Sirtuin 1. J Diabetes Res. 2014;2014:1–8.
105. Halaschek-Wiener J, Amirabbasi-Beik M, Monfared N, Pieczyk M, Sailer C, Kollar A, et al. Genetic variation in healthy oldest-old. Mary Bridger J, editor. PLoS One. 2009. https://doi.org/10.1371/journal.pone.0006641.
106. Rose G, Dato S, Altomare K, Bellizzi D, Garasto S, Greco V, et al. Variability of the SIRT3 gene, human silent information regulator Sir2 homologue, and survivorship in the elderly. Exp Gerontol. 2003;38:1065–70.
107. Brown K, Xie S, Qiu X, Mohrin M, Shin J, Liu Y, et al. SIRT3 reverses aging-associated degeneration. Cell Rep. 2013;3:319–27.
108. Beauharnois JM, Bolívar BE, Welch JT. Sirtuin 6: a review of biological effects and potential therapeutic properties. Mol BioSyst. 2013;9:1789.
109. Ghosh HS. The anti-aging, metabolism potential of SIRT1. Curr Opin Investig Drugs. 2008;9:1095–102.
110. Lee S-H, Lee J-H, Lee H-Y, Min K-J. Sirtuin signaling in cellular senescence and aging. BMB Rep. 2019;52:24–34.
111. Haigis MC, Yankner BA. The aging stress response. Mol Cell. 2010;40:333–44.
112. López-Lluch G, Navas P. Calorie restriction as an intervention in ageing. J Physiol. 2016;594:2043–60.
113. Suh Y, Atzmon G, Cho M-O, Hwang D, Liu B, Leahy DJ, et al. Functionally significant insulin-like growth factor I receptor mutations in centenarians. Proc Natl Acad Sci. 2008;105:3438–42.
114. Pawlikowska L, Hu D, Huntsman S, Sung A, Chu C, Chen J, et al. Association of common genetic variation in the insulin/IGF1 signaling pathway with human longevity. Aging Cell. 2009;8:460–72.
115. Kenyon CJ. The genetics of ageing. Nature. 2010;464:504–12.
116. Kahn BB, Alquier T, Carling D, Hardie DG. AMP-activated protein kinase: ancient energy gauge provides clues to modern understanding of metabolism. Cell Metab. 2005;1:15–25.
117. Osler ME, Zierath JR. Minireview: adenosine 5′-monophosphate-activated protein kinase regulation of fatty acid oxidation in skeletal muscle. Endocrinology. 2008;149:935–41.

118. Qiang W, Weiqiang K, Qing Z, Pengju Z, Yi L. Aging impairs insulin-stimulated glucose uptake in rat skeletal muscle via suppressing AMPKalpha. Exp Mol Med. 2007;39:535–43.
119. Kjøbsted R, Treebak JT, Fentz J, Lantier L, Viollet B, Birk JB, et al. Prior AICAR stimulation increases insulin sensitivity in mouse skeletal muscle in an AMPK-dependent manner. Diabetes. 2015;64:2042–55.
120. Hawley SA, Ross FA, Chevtzoff C, Green KA, Evans A, Fogarty S, et al. Use of cells expressing gamma subunit variants to identify diverse mechanisms of AMPK activation. Cell Metab. 2010;11:554–65.
121. Onken B, Driscoll M. Metformin induces a dietary restriction-like state and the oxidative stress response to extend C. elegans Healthspan via AMPK, LKB1, and SKN-1. Hart AC, editor. PLoS One. 2010. https://doi.org/10.1371/journal.pone.0008758.
122. Anisimov VN, Berstein LM, Popovich IG, Zabezhinski MA, Egormin PA, Piskunova TS, et al. If started early in life, metformin treatment increases life span and postpones tumors in female SHR mice. Aging (Albany NY). 2011;3:148–57.
123. Theurey P, Pizzo P. The aging mitochondria. Genes (Basel). 2018;9:22.
124. Tauchi H, Sato T. Age changes in size and number of mitochondria of human hepatic cells. J Gerontol. 1968;23:454–61.
125. Herbener GH. A morphometric study of age-dependent changes in mitochondrial population of mouse liver and heart. J Gerontol. 1976;31:8–12.
126. Short KR, Bigelow ML, Kahl J, Singh R, Coenen-Schimke J, Raghavakaimal S, et al. Decline in skeletal muscle mitochondrial function with aging in humans. Proc Natl Acad Sci. 2005;102:5618–23.
127. Preston CC, Oberlin AS, Holmuhamedov EL, Gupta A, Sagar S, Syed RHK, et al. Aging-induced alterations in gene transcripts and functional activity of mitochondrial oxidative phosphorylation complexes in the heart. Mech Ageing Dev. 2008;129:304–12.
128. Hunt ND, Hyun D-H, Allard JS, Minor RK, Mattson MP, Ingram DK, et al. Bioenergetics of aging and calorie restriction. Ageing Res Rev. 2006;5:125–43.
129. Kelly DP, Scarpulla RC. Transcriptional regulatory circuits controlling mitochondrial biogenesis and function. Genes Dev. 2004;18:357–68.
130. Lee C-K, Allison DB, Brand J, Weindruch R, Prolla TA. Transcriptional profiles associated with aging and middle age-onset caloric restriction in mouse hearts. Proc Natl Acad Sci. 2002;99:14988–93.
131. López-Lluch G, Hunt N, Jones B, Zhu M, Jamieson H, Hilmer S, et al. Calorie restriction induces mitochondrial biogenesis and bioenergetic efficiency. Proc Natl Acad Sci. 2006;103:1768–73.
132. Campisi J, Warner HR. Aging in mitotic and post-mitotic cells. Adv Cell Aging Gerontol. 2001;4:1–16.
133. Raina AK, Zhu X, Smith MA. Alzheimer's disease and the cell cycle. Acta Neurobiol Exp (Wars). 2004;64:107–12.
134. Yang Y, Mufson EJ, Herrup K. Neuronal cell death is preceded by cell cycle events at all stages of Alzheimer's disease. J Neurosci. 2003;23:2557–63.
135. Taylor RC, Dillin A. XBP-1 is a cell-nonautonomous regulator of stress resistance and longevity. Cell. 2013;153:1435–47.
136. Armanios M. Telomeres and age-related disease: how telomere biology informs clinical paradigms. J Clin Invest. 2013;123:996–1002.
137. Maiese K. Erythropoietin and mTOR: a "One-Two Punch"; for aging-related disorders accompanied by enhanced life expectancy. Curr Neurovasc Res. 2016;13:329–40.
138. Galluzzi L, Kepp O, Kroemer G. TP53 and MTOR crosstalk to regulate cellular senescence. Aging (Albany NY). 2010;2:535–7.
139. Muñoz-Espín D, Serrano M. Cellular senescence: from physiology to pathology. Nat Rev Mol Cell Biol. 2014;15:482–96.
140. Sharpless NE, Sherr CJ. Forging a signature of in vivo senescence. Nat Rev Cancer. 2015;15:397–408.

141. Kuilman T, Michaloglou C, Mooi WJ, Peeper DS. The essence of senescence. Genes Dev. 2010;24:2463–79.
142. Krishnamurthy J, Torrice C, Ramsey MR, Kovalev GI, Al-Regaiey K, Su L, et al. Ink4a/Arf expression is a biomarker of aging. J Clin Invest. 2004;114:1299–307.
143. Diekman BO, Sessions GA, Collins JA, Knecht AK, Strum SL, Mitin NK, et al. Expression of p16 INK 4a is a biomarker of chondrocyte aging but does not cause osteoarthritis. Aging Cell. 2018. https://doi.org/10.1111/acel.12771.
144. Baker DJ, Wijshake T, Tchkonia T, LeBrasseur NK, Childs BG, van de Sluis B, et al. Clearance of p16Ink4a-positive senescent cells delays ageing-associated disorders. Nature. 2011;479:232–6.
145. Yamakoshi K, Takahashi A, Hirota F, Nakayama R, Ishimaru N, Kubo Y, et al. Real-time in vivo imaging of p16Ink4a reveals cross talk with p53. J Cell Biol. 2009;186:393–407.
146. Kuilman T, Michaloglou C, Vredeveld LCW, Douma S, van Doorn R, Desmet CJ, et al. Oncogene-induced senescence relayed by an interleukin-dependent inflammatory network. Cell. 2008;133:1019–31.
147. Coppé J-P, Patil CK, Rodier F, Sun Y, Muñoz DP, Goldstein J, et al. Senescence-associated secretory phenotypes reveal cell-nonautonomous functions of oncogenic RAS and the p53 tumor suppressor. Downward J, editor. PLoS Biol. 2008;6:2853–68.
148. Orjalo AV, Bhaumik D, Gengler BK, Scott GK, Campisi J. Cell surface-bound IL-1alpha is an upstream regulator of the senescence-associated IL-6/IL-8 cytokine network. Proc Natl Acad Sci U S A. 2009;106:17031–6.
149. Su Y, Xu C, Sun Z, Liang Y, Li G, Tong T, et al. S100A13 promotes senescence-associated secretory phenotype and cellular senescence via modulation of non-classical secretion of IL-1α. Aging (Albany NY). 2019;11:549–72.
150. Laberge R-M, Sun Y, Orjalo AV, Patil CK, Freund A, Zhou L, et al. MTOR regulates the pro-tumorigenic senescence-associated secretory phenotype by promoting IL1A translation. Nat Cell Biol. 2015;17:1049–61.
151. Pereira BI, Devine OP, Vukmanovic-Stejic M, Chambers ES, Subramanian P, Patel N, et al. Senescent cells evade immune clearance via HLA-E-mediated NK and CD8+ T cell inhibition. Nat Commun. 2019;10:2387.
152. Ruzankina Y, Brown EJ. Relationships between stem cell exhaustion, tumour suppression and ageing. Br J Cancer. 2007;97:1189–93.
153. Seo H, Chen J, González-Avalos E, Samaniego-Castruita D, Das A, Wang YH, et al. TOX and TOX2 transcription factors cooperate with NR4A transcription factors to impose CD8+ T cell exhaustion. Proc Natl Acad Sci U S A. 2019;116:12410–5.
154. Rizzino A. Concise review: the Sox2-Oct4 connection: critical players in a much larger interdependent network integrated at multiple levels. Stem Cells. 2013;31:1033–9.
155. Vilas JM, Carneiro C, Da Silva-Álvarez S, Ferreirós A, González P, Gómez M, et al. Adult Sox2+ stem cell exhaustion in mice results in cellular senescence and premature aging. Aging Cell. 2018. https://doi.org/10.1111/acel.12834.
156. Carrasco-Garcia E, Moreno-Cugnon L, Garcia I, Borras C, Revuelta M, Izeta A, et al. SOX2 expression diminishes with ageing in several tissues in mice and humans. Mech Ageing Dev. 2019;177:30–6.
157. Kovacs T, Csongei V, Feller D, Ernszt D, Smuk G, Sarosi V, et al. Alteration in the Wnt microenvironment directly regulates molecular events leading to pulmonary senescence. Aging Cell. 2014;13:838–49.

# Age-Related Neurodegenerative Diseases: An Update

2

Nadia Alejandra Rivero-Segura, A. A. Guerrero-Cruz, and O. S. Barrera-Vázquez

## Abbreviations

| | |
|---|---|
| AD | Alzheimer's disease |
| ALS | Amyotrophic lateral sclerosis |
| APOE | Apolipoprotein E |
| APP | Amyloid precursor protein |
| ARND | Age-related neurodegenerative diseases |
| Aβ | Beta-amyloid peptide |
| CDK5 | Cyclin-dependent kinase |
| CNS | Central nervous system |
| ER | Endoplasmic reticulum |
| FTD | Frontotemporal dementia |
| GLT1 | Glutamate transport-1 |
| GSK-3 | Glycogen synthase kinase-3β |
| iPSC | Induced pluripotent stem cell |
| LPS | Lipopolysaccharide |
| *MAPT* | Microtubule-associated protein tau gene |
| ND | Neurodegenerative diseases |
| NFTs | Neurofibrillary tangles |
| OMIM | Online Mendelian Inheritance in Man |
| PD | Parkinson's disease |
| *PGRN* | Progranulin gene |
| PHFs | Paired helical filaments |
| PolyQ | Polyglutamine |

Rivero-Segura NA and Guerrero-Cruz AA contributed equally to this work.

N. A. Rivero-Segura (✉) · A. A. Guerrero-Cruz · O. S. Barrera-Vázquez
División de Investigación Básica, Instituto Nacional de Geriatría, Mexico City, Mexico
e-mail: nrivero@inger.gob.mx





J. C. Gomez-Verjan, N. A. Rivero-Segura (eds.), *Clinical Genetics and Genomics of Aging*, https://doi.org/10.1007/978-3-030-40955-5_2

| | |
|---|---|
| PSEN1 | Presenilin 1 |
| PSEN2 | Presenilin 2 |
| P-tau | Phosphorylated tau |
| PTMs | Posttranslational modifications |
| SCAs | Spinocerebellar ataxias |
| SNpc | Substantia nigra pars compacta |
| *SOD1* | *Superoxide dismutase 1* |
| Spp | Species |
| T-tau | Total tau |
| UPR | Unfolded protein response |
| UPS | Ubiquitin-proteasome system |
| α-Syn | Alpha-synuclein |

## Introduction

Aging has been widely studied from the philosophical to the scientific perspectives. The biology of aging recognizes this process as the cells, tissues, and organs function decline. In this sense, as we age, the brain becomes more vulnerable to develop some neurological diseases. Matilla-Dueñas et al. mentioned that the central nervous system (CNS) is the target for 600 diseases at least [1]. Among these, neurodegenerative diseases (ND) stand out from the rest. ND is a group of progressive neurological disorders that affect specific brain areas, and until now, they are incurable [2]. These have various factors beyond their pathogenesis, such as genetic factors, environmental factors, and nutritional habits, and recent evidence also suggests the role of microbiota dysbiosis in the ND development.

Interestingly, age appears as the common risk factor for the development of these [3]. Therefore, this chapter only focuses on the most prevalent ND in the elderly population, such as Alzheimer's disease (AD), Parkinson's disease (PD), Frontotemporal dementia (FTD), Amyotrophic lateral sclerosis (ALS), and the Spinocerebellar ataxias (SCAs), that we set as age-related neurodegenerative diseases (ARND). Moreover, since the knowledge of ARND increases exponentially daily, we summarize the most recent and relevant genetic biomarkers that have been reported in the last decade, as depicted in Fig. 2.1. Moreover, we highlight the lack of efficient strategies that might help in the treatment of ARND and question where we are standing up in this field since the knowledge are quite far from the treatment of these conditions.

## Alzheimer's Disease (AD)

AD is defined as the progressive loss of neurons, and formation of intraneuronal neurofibrillary tangles (NFTs) in the presence of extracellular senile plaques that are predominately composed of beta-amyloid (Aβ) peptide in a fibrillar form that is made up for the form hyperphosphorylated tau protein [6–9]. The most studied theories in AD are the Aβ cascade theory and family inheritance by gene mutation and tau theory.

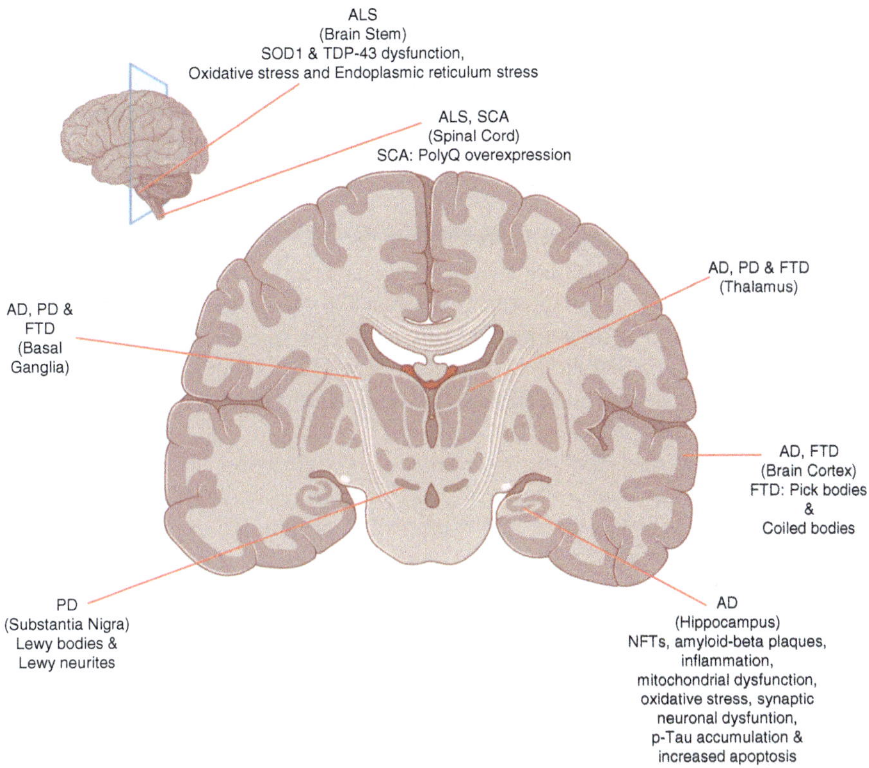


**Fig. 2.1** This figure summarizes the main areas affected in ARND and their most relevant biomarkers reported in the last decade. In Alzheimer's disease (AD), basal ganglia, hippocampus and brain cortex, and thalamus are the main affected areas; in Parkinson's disease (PD), basal ganglia, substantia nigra, and thalamus show to be affected in this condition and is characterised by Lewy bodies and Lewy neurites; in Frontotemporal dementia (FTD), basal ganglia, thalamus, and brain cortex is affected and characterised by pick bodies and coiled bodies; in ALS, Amyotrophic lateral sclerosis is affected spinal cord; TAR DNA-binding protein 43 (TDP-43) is the scaffold of nuclear bodies through of interaction with nuclear protein [4] and is involved in the regulation of gene expression and has also been shown to be involved in the exon splicing of many genes [5]; Spinocerebellar ataxias (SCAs) affect spinal cord and show overexpression of polyglutamine (polyQ), affecting transcriptional deregulation, RNA toxicity, and toxicity caused by repeat-associated non-ATG translational peptides, dysregulation of ubiquitin-proteasome system (UPS), and autophagy

## Beta-Amyloid (Aβ) Cascade Theory

The nuclear genes associated with the autosomal dominant inherited in AD are the Amyloid precursor protein (APP), Presenilin 1 (PSEN1), and Presenilin 2 (PSEN2) [9–11]. The mutation in the gene APP increases the production of Aβ and leads its extracellular aggregation and accumulation that manifesting as plaques in the brain. Aβ oligomers formation is caused by proteolysis of APP, given different lengths of Aβ peptides. The two dominant Aβ species are Aβ1–40 and Aβ1–42, but the isoform that caused neurotoxic effects when aggregated is Aβ1–42. Presenilins mutations cause the formation of these species. Also, the signalling pathways such as glycogen synthase kinase-3β (GSK-3), fyn kinase, and cyclin-dependent kinase (CDK5) can be altered [10, 11]. Leading to an inflammatory response and the formation of amyloid plaques, causing progressive neuronal damage, and affecting homeostasis, which induces tau hyperphosphorylation, lastly, causes neural dysfunction and cell death [6].

Another critical component in this hypothesis is Apolipoprotein E (APOE), a cholesterol transporter in the brain which plays an essential role in the metabolism of amyloid. APOE has three isoforms (ε2, ε3, and ε4), but APOE ε4 has been linked to AD; actually, it is a known genetic risk factor for sporadic AD. Heterozygote has a 20–30% to risk, and homozygote has a 50% [12]. Besides, other biomarkers such as Aβ, phosphorylated tau (P-tau), and total tau (T-tau) are used to support the diagnosis of this disease [13].

Bonham et al. analysed the microglial gene expression in both aging and AD by CellMapper tool, which allows identifying co-expressed gene networks, and TMEM119 as a specific marker of microglia. To explore what genes are implicated in risk for AD, three cohorts were used for differential expression analysis from different brain banks, each cohort is classified in tissue type (Cerebellum, Dorsolateral Prefrontal Cortex, Frontal pole, Inferior Frontal Gyrus, Parahippocampal Gyrus, Superior Temporal Gyrus, and Temporal Cortex) and grouped by diagnosis and sex, the total number of participants included were around 500 individuals (male and female). This study demonstrated that the heterogeneity expression of microglial genes is found overexpressed in the region vulnerable in AD and dysregulated in AD. Thus, this evidence suggests that microglia is presented in vulnerable regions in this disease. Also, it is consistent with other studies which implicated microglia and myeloid expression that may help to understand the relevance of microglia genes mutations in development in AD and neurodegeneration [14].

## Tau Theory

Tau is a protein encoded by the microtubule-associated protein Tau (*MAPT*) gene found on chromosome 17q21. Six isoforms have been found in the adult human brain [7, 14]. It is in the axons of mature neurons. Also, in healthy neurons is present in the synaptic compartments, and it is crucial to synapse physiology. In AD, tau accumulates and folds hyperphosphorylated tau in axons, dendrites, and somas [15]. However, under pathological conditions, it also has other types of posttranslational modifications (PTMs) such as glycosylation, acetylation, oxidation, nitration, glycation, ubiquitination, and SUMOylation [16, 17]. Aβ oligomers can activate the phosphorylation of tau as a part of the mechanism of c-Jun kinase or AKT-GSK-3 beta signalling pathway. Tau can be phosphorylated by three different kinds of kinases: (a) GSK-3, CDK5, and MAPK, these proteins are proline-directed serine/threonine; (b) serine/threonine non-directed

**Table 2.1** Other posttranslational modifications of tau protein

| Posttranslational modifications | Ptm site(s) | Related function(s) |
|---|---|---|
| Glycosylation | 11 putative O-glycosylation sites | Reduces tau-phosphorylation by PKA, CDK5, and GSK-3β |
| Glycation | 12 sites | Contributes to tau accumulation and cell death |
| Nitration | 4 sites | Tau aggregation |
| Ubiquitination | 3 sites | Increases PHFs (paired helical filaments) maturate |
| SUMOylation | K340 | Counteracts ubiquitination in AD |
| Oxidation | C322 | Allows the assembly of PHFs |
| Acetylation | Multiple sites and 3 putative lysines (163, 174, and 180) residues | Tau aggregation by hyperphosphorylation [16] |

For more detailed information, review Ludovic Martin et al. (2010)

by proline such as TTBK1/2, CK1, DYRK1A, MARK, Akt, PKA, PKC, AMPK, and CaMKII; and (c) Src, Fyn, Abl, and Syk (tyrosine kinases). GSK-3β and PP2 play an essential role in the regulation of tau phosphorylation [18]. The hyperphosphorylation of tau reduces the affinity for microtubules and lose stability and affects axoplasmic transport [19]. Additionally, in the literature, other posttranslational modifications (PTMs) in protein tau have been reported to contribute to AD, as described in Table 2.1.

## Parkinson's Disease (PD)

PD is the second most common dementia after Alzheimer's disease; about 1% of people over 60 years are affected. The main clinical manifestations included bradykinesia, postural instability, rigidity, asymmetric onset, and behavioural alterations [20, 21]. This condition is characterised by a continuous loss of dopaminergic neurons in the substantia nigra pars compacta (SNpc) in the midbrain region, decreasing the levels of the dopamine neurotransmitter in the presence of Lewy bodies comprised of insoluble alpha-synuclein (α-Syn) [22]. PD is a non-genetic disease since 90% of the cases are sporadic. Although, mutations in genes with autosomal inheritance have been identified, included *SNCA*, *LRRK2*, *VPS35*, *Parkin*, *PINK1*, and *DJ-1* (see Table 2.2) [27, 30].

Mutations in *PINK1* are involved in mitochondrial homeostasis and early onset PD. The group of Azkona et al. examined the linked between *PINK1* and *LRRK2*. They obtained dermal fibroblasts from five control subjects and seven subjects with mutations in *PINK1* from two Spanish kindreds. Also, generated induced pluripotent stem cells (iPSC) from two Parkinson's patients, carrier and control fibroblasts using lentiviral vectors. This group found dysregulation of *LRRK2* in fibroblasts with mutations in *PINK1*, which suggests that both act in a convergent pathway, in which PINK1 modulate the levels of LRRK2 [25].

**Table 2.2** Main genes involved in the development of PD

| Gene | Map location | Encode protein | Related processes | References |
|---|---|---|---|---|
| *LRRK2* | 12q12 | Leucine-rich repeat serine/threonine-protein kinase 2 | Lysosomal pathway and autophagy regulation | [23, 24] |
| *SNCA* | 4q22.1 | Alpha-synuclein (α-Syn) | α-Syn oligomerization or fibrillization (formation of Lewy bodies and Lewy neurites). Also, this protein is involved in SNARE complex assembly and synaptic vesicle trafficking. | [25, 26] |
| *VPS35* | 16q11.2 | Vacuolar protein sorting-associated protein 35 | Synaptic endocytosis and synaptic vesicle regeneration | [27] |
| *Parkin (PRKN)* | 6q26 | E3 ubiquitin-protein ligase parkin | Regulates different types of ubiquitylation and promote degradation-independent ubiquitylation | [28, 29] |
| *PINK1* | 1p36.12 | PTEN-induced putative kinase 1 | Cellular protection from stress-induced mitochondrial dysfunction | [25] |
| *DJ-1 (PARK7)* | 1p36.23 | Protein/nucleic acid deglycase DJ-1 | Protects neurons against oxidative stress and cell death | [23] |

Frontotemporal dementia (FTD) and Amyotrophic lateral sclerosis (ALS) have been linked clinically and pathologically by *C9orf72* gene that has an expansion of a hexanucleotide-repeat (GGGGCC) unit on chromosome 9, is located between two five prime non-coding exons. Subjects with this kind of condition have been showed that repeat expansion mutation is hundreds of thousands of these repeat units affected the expression of *C9orf72* transcripts causing the loss of protein function and accumulation of RNA foci in the frontal cortex and spinal cord [28, 29, 31].

## Frontotemporal Dementia (FTD)

FTD is characterised by atrophy in the frontotemporal lobes, which encompasses changes in behaviour, language, and executive control of the movements. The prevalence of FTD increases around 65–69 years. The diagnosis of this disease is very difficult due to the similarities it has with a broad range of psychiatric disorders [32].

From the genetic perspective, FTD exhibits the microtubule-associated protein Tau (*MAPT*) gene, progranulin gene (*PGRN*), and the *C9orf72* gene-altered mainly [33]. However, the literature reports less common genes implicated with FTD, such as *VCP*, *CHMP2B*, *TARDBP*, *FUS*, *EXT2*, *TBK1*, and *SQSTM1*, which are out of the scope of this chapter but can be reviewed in Olney, Spina, and Miller [34].

The *PGRN* mutations are related to truncated isoform and hyperphosphorylated TAR DNA-binding protein 43 (TDP-43). In pathological conditions, TDP-43 loss its nuclear function by a modification in cellular location (neuronal nucleus to the cytoplasm) [35]. *MAPT* mutation has been involved in behavioural changes, dementia, and parkinsonism mainly. *MAPT* mutation, located in exons 1, 9 and 11-13 on chromosome 17, has been involved in behavioural changes, dementia and parkinsonism mainly. Moreover, this mutation has been linked woth the disruption of tau binding to microtubles, resunting on the filaments-hyperphosphorylated tau accumulation [36]. Mutations in *TBK1* impact negatively on cellular processes such as inflammation and autophagy; and recently these mutationes have been described as the most common cause if familial FTD. Also, *TBK1* have been found to be implicated in progressive supranuclear palsy and progressive cerebellar ataxia syndromes [37].

## Amyotrophic Lateral Sclerosis (ALS)

ALS is an autosomal dominant disorder characterised by neurodegeneration of the upper and lower motor neurons, for more information consult the database Online Mendelian Inheritance in Man (OMIM) reference #60027. The sporadic form of this condition appears around age 65 and in familial ALS appears on overage at 46 years [33]. The nuclear genes involved in ALS are *superoxide dismutase 1 (SOD1)*, *C9orf72*, *TARDBP*, and *FUS*. The mutation in *SOD1* causes endoplasmic reticulum (ER) stress by exposed to N-terminal short region and the derlin-1-binding region; this conformational change produces motor toxicity. The neurotoxicity can be mediated by glutamate transport-1 (GLT1) for different mechanisms such as cleavage caspase-3, and alternative RNA editing. Resulting in the loss of neuronal calcium homeostasis that produces oxidative stress by mitochondrial dysfunction. Because it has a decrease in the production of ATP and increases the oxidative stressors, leading a motor neuron loss. All this have an impact in ionic Na+/K+ pumps, impacting in the polarization by reverse potentials, the intracellular calcium increases and actives apoptosis pathways [29]. Have been observed in vitro, for all genes implicated in this condition, the self-propagation along corticospinal pathways and transmits misfolding proteins causing toxic aggregation [38].

## Spinocerebellar Ataxias (SCAs)

SCAs are a group of autosomal-dominant and neurodegenerative disorders. The spinal cord and the cerebellum are affected by progressive ataxia and degeneration and is associated with dysarthria, ophthalmoplegia, and dementia. The polyglutamine (polyQ) is the most common SCAs, caused by a CAG repeat expansion in its coding sequence. However, for each type of SCAs, there is a gene. The CAG repeat is translated into a glutamine amino acids sequence in ataxin proteins (polyQ) [39, 40]. Usually appears during the 40s but can be onset in childhood or aging. However, exist a negative correlation between the CAG repeat and age at onset [41]. The polyglutamine localization seems to be essential to induce neurodegeneration. In pathological condition, ataxins are transported into the nuclei.

## Molecular Mechanisms of Neurodegeneration in Spinocerebellar Ataxias

The transcription of specific genes that contain the expansion of a CAG-repeat sequence encodes proteins named ataxins with a large polyglutamine tract. The mutants have a more extended number of glutamines, and it is inversely correlated with the age onset and severity of the symptoms. These proteins lose its native state and misfolded, leading the accumulation and formation of polyglutamine inclusions in nuclei and cytoplasm, which contain cellular components such as transcription factors, ubiquitin, and the proteasome. Ataxins have difficulties to be recognised and degraded by the ubiquitin-proteasome system (UPS), may be by polyQ-expansions, and aggregates that disrupted its function.

On the other hand, caspases cleavage to proteasome subunits by a reduction of proteasome activity inducing apoptosis. This failure in the UPS leads to accumulation of toxic proteins producing neuronal dysfunction and cell death. However, the neurons accurate to restore the homeostasis activated mechanism of cell survival by endoplasmic reticulum (ER) stress pathway, mediated for unfolded protein response (UPR) that encodes chaperones genes. This response can be affected by a change in the calcium ions levels in Purkinje cells. The disruption in calcium channel function can serve as a target for transaminases or bind to nuclear proteins. Also, the mutant proteins can be degraded by the phagosome-lysosome system (autophagy). The mechanism is unclear yet, but the inhibition of mTOR seems to be a negative regulator, inducing autophagy and reduces the toxicity of polyQ in animal models. Suggest that autophagy degrades insoluble cytoplasmic aggregates. Alternately, the mitochondria is affected by toxic proteins, increases free radicals and caused oxidative damage, and inducing apoptosis [42].

## Ischemic Stroke

In elderly, cardiovascular diseases are the leading cause of death worldwide, this set of diseases leads to stroke that could be ischemic or hemorrhagic; however, both have in common that age is the most critical risk factor [43]. Since as we age the risk of stroke increases in both men and women over 65 years [44]. Since in aged patients, the ischemic stroke represents the significant amount of stroke cases (90%), we only focus on this pathology. Ischemic stroke characterised by hypoxia (low levels of oxygen in the body or tissue) and ischemia (lack of blood flow to tissues), leads to the dysfunction of a specific part of the brain tissue. At cellular and molecular levels, the ischemic stroke includes progressive damage of the blood–brain barrier, neuronal death, glial overactivation, inflammation due to the infiltration of immune cells to the brain, excitotoxicity due to the increase in the glutamate transporter GLT-1, and enhanced ROS production. Besides, the mitochondrial function and antioxidant systems decline also contribute to the injury during the ischemic stroke [45, 46].

Among the canonical biomarkers of ischemic stroke damage, recent studies report others that could help to anticipate to the ischemic event in elderly individuals. For instance, in Han population, Wei and collaborators report that patients with ischemic stroke possess an increase CC frequency in the PPARG C161T allele that confers susceptibility and turns the aged individuals more vulnerable to an ischemic stroke event [47]. Following this line that is looking at the prevention and prediction of the outcome of ischemic stroke patients, a study performed in old patients from the Middelheim's Interdisciplinary Stroke study (71 ± 14 years, $n = 50$), reveal that tau concentrations in the cerebrospinal fluid are proportionately directly to stroke severity and outcome, and could be used as a biomarker for this condition [48]. Interestingly, in the pursuit of new non-invasive procedures to find new biomarkers in this neurodegenerative condition, miRNAs become promising biomarkers that not require invasive procedures to obtain samples since they are stable in the blood and recently [49]; in this sense, a study performed in patients with suspected ischemic stroke (74.7 ± 9.7, $n = 20$) showed an increased expression in miR-125a-5p, miR-125b-5p, and miR-143-3p in comparison with the healthy subjects of the study, interestingly these miRNA were validated in 40 patients with ischemic stroke [50], suggesting that these markers might be useful for the early treatment of ischemic stroke.

## Microbiome and Age-Related Neurodegenerative Diseases

Different microorganisms such as bacteria, fungi, archaea, and viruses compose the human intestinal microbiota that represents, in physiologic conditions, a perfect commensalism association with their host [51, 52]. In general, the human intestinal microbiota is shaped by the healthy microbiota (bacteria that normally colonize the intestine) and opportunistic bacteria (which are the agents responsible for infections). Among the billions of symbiotic microorganisms that compose the intestinal microbiome, four bacteria phyla are mainly reported in adults, i.e. Firmicutes (~51%), Bacteroidetes (~48%), Proteobacteria, and Actinobacteria, (1%) [53]. Lactobacteria species stand out among the normal microbiome (*Lactobacillus rhamnosus, Lactobacillus acidophilus, and Lactobacillus plantarum*), *Bifidobacterium* (*B. bifidum*), *Enterococci, Propionobacteria*, and *Peptostreptococci*. In the same way, opportunistic bacteria include the *Bacteriodes* spp. *Bacilli, Clostridia, Enterobacteria, Actinobacteria, Peptococci, Staphylococci*, and *Streptococcus* [54]. Several factors, such as diet, hygiene, antibiotic exposure, and modify the intestinal microbiota [55, 56]. Interestingly, age also contributes significantly to the microbiome modification; in fact a recent publication highlights the vital role that represents the host aging in the microbial evolution since as the host get aged the organism experiments molecular and functional changes that induce shifts to the microbial niche [57], nevertheless, for detailed information about changes in microbiome during aging, please refer to the Chap. 9 in this book. In the following paragraphs, we discuss the recent data about the relationship between the pathogenesis of the two most prevalent ND and the microbiome, which represents a new field of research.

It is well known that aging is a risk factor for neurodegeneration and dementia [58]; nevertheless, recent studies support the idea that gut microbiota may have an effect on the brain and the behaviour of patients, since the evidence suggests that some metabolites secreted by the intestinal microbiota can affect in a certain way, the cognitive capacity of patients diagnosed with ND [59–63]. This hypothesis is not entirely new since several decades ago, the concept that bidirectional communication between the CNS and the intestinal organs plays a role in emotional regulation [64, 65]. Four decades later, the hypothesis that the brain has a regulation of the gastrointestinal tract arose and with the help of the murine model, the existence of the brain-gut axis was reported [66]. This axis is carried out through the neuroendocrine and neuroimmune system, working together with the sympathetic and parasympathetic arms of the autonomic nervous system and the enteric nervous system.

There is a close relationship between the intestines and the CNS, which consists of bidirectional communication. Additionally, the evidence reveals how gut bacteria are responsible for the synthesis of neuroactive molecules and metabolites that can modulate the pathogenesis of many ND and conditions like PD, AD, multiple sclerosis, and amyotrophic lateral sclerosis, as follows.

In PD patients with severe postural instability and gait difficulty, *Prevotellaceace* spp. population is lower than the *Enterobacteria* genus (opportunistic bacteria), suggesting that the intestinal microbiota dysbiosis has a role in the aggravation of this condition [62, 65]. Moreover, is well known that *Enterobacteria* genus increases the amount of lipopolysaccharide (LPS) in blood serum of PD patients, which in combination with proinflammatory cytokines (TNF-a, IL-1b, and IL6) interrupt the blood–brain barrier and promote the deposition of α-synuclein plaques and eliminate the dopaminergic neurons in the substancia nigra [65, 67]. In agreement with this study, another report that PD patients have an increase in proinflammatory cytokine-producing bacteria such as *Ralstonia* spp., *Proteobacteria* spp., and *Enterococcaceae* spp., while the anti-inflammatory butyrate producing-bacteria such as *Blautia* spp., *Coprococcus* spp., *Roseburia* spp., and *Faecalibacterium* spp. is low [68]. Finally, *Helicobacter pylori* has been also proposed as a trigger in the pathogenesis of PD [69]; however, the study is inconclusive and require further investigation.

AD is one of the most studied ND, and as mentioned in the previous section, this is characterized by the deposition of beta-amyloid peptide and other mechanisms that previously were mentioned [59]. On the other hand, there are several controversies about the relation between microbiota dysbiosis and the development of AD; however, other reports suggest that products derived from mycobiome and inflammatory mediators reach the brain, trigger neuroinflammation and also promote the accumulation of amyloid, contributing to AD pathogenesis and progression [70, 71]. Another study shows that AD patients exhibit an increasing population of *Escherichia* spp. *Shigella* spp., which are known to be pro-inflammatory bacteria and decrease in the concentration of anti-inflammatory bacteria such as *Eubacterium rectale* spp. found in faecal microbiome of patients with AD. This dysbiosis can also increase the deposition of amyloid in the brain, accompanied by peripheral inflammation [65].

ALS is another ARND that exhibits a relation with microbiome dysbiosis, for example in ALS patients the concentration of LPS and β-N-methylamino-L-alanine, derived from *Chlamydia pneumoniae,* these molecules contribute to ALS pathogenesis via neuroinflammation and BBB function decline. This study is following by other performed in human faeces from ALS patients that exhibit low levels of butyrate-producing bacteria such as *Oscillibacter*, *Anaerostipes*, and *Lachnospira*, compared with high levels of *Dorea,* opportunistic harmful ethanol-producing bacteria [65]. Despite these studies, we highlight that the relationship between ALS pathogenesis and microbiota dysbiosis remains unclear and is a quite promising research field that requires further study.

Finally, probiotics are beneficial agents that maintain the immunologic equilibrium in the gastrointestinal tract and inhibits the attachment and growth of opportunistic organisms to the intestinal mucosa, improve neuronal plasticity, induce neurogenesis and participate normalizing the hippocampus response in the hypothalamic–pituitary–adrenal axis via BDNF [72, 73]. Due to this, few studies focus on the potential benefits that probiotics might induce on the CNS. Little is known about this relationship; despite this, a study performed in PD patients show that *Lactobacillus casei* Shirota improves bowel movement by decreasing the number of faecal Staphylococci [74]. In vivo studies found that treatment with the combination of probiotics *Lactobacillus rhamnosus* (R0011) and *Lactobacillus helveticus* (R0052) restored memory impairment induced by dysbiosis stress caused by infection with *Citrobacter rodentium* in mice [75], however, in humans this is inconclusive.

On the other hand, a controlled clinical trial demonstrated that the probiotic combination of *Lactobacillus acidophilus*, *Lactobacillus casei*, *Lactobacillus bifidum*, and *Lactobacillus fermentum* improves cognitive function in patients with AD [76]. Also, the administration of *Bifidobacterium* spp. induced in the elderly the reduction of lower levels of proinflammatory cytokines TNF-α, IL-5, IL-6, IL-1β, and IL-8 in serum [77]. While the results in animals are encouraging, further clinical research studies regarding probiotics role preventing ND development, as well as the identification of their origins are highly required.

## Conclusions

In the last decades, aging has become the keystone for several age-related diseases, such as cancer, osteoporosis, cardiovascular disease, and ND. Moreover, around the world, the aged population is increasing quickly, and the treatment of any these diseases represents an enormous cost for the health state departments. For this reason, the research on the main factors or causes that lead to the development of the ARND requires to be carefully analysed. In this sense, the present chapter summarizes the canonical and the most recent genetic markers derived from human genomic studies and highlight the necessity of augmenting the interest of the researchers to delve non-invasive strategies to obtain the human samples for the study of the ARND since one of the main limitations of this field is the acquisition of human living samples.

Moreover, it is essential to mention that the literature reports a vast number of ARND genetics biomarkers; however, the mechanisms that underlie these are not entirely understood. Their study could clarify the genesis of the ARND. Finally, in the last section, we delve into the microbiota dysbiosis role in the ARND, since recently this appears associated with the development of AD, PD, and ALS. However, the evidence results inconclusive and highlights the importance to performed further studies in order to establish the microbiota role in both the modulation of neurotransmitters and the maintenance of the BBB permeability that appears compromised in ARND.

## References

1. Matilla-Dueñas A, Corral-Juan M, Rodríguez-Palmero Seuma A, et al. Rare neurodegenerative diseases: clinical and genetic update. Adv Exp Med Biol. 2017;1031:443–96.
2. Golpich M, Amini E, Mohamed Z, Ali RA, Ibrahim NM, Ahmadiani A. Mitochondrial dysfunction and biogenesis in neurodegenerative diseases: pathogenesis and treatment. CNS Neurosci Ther. 2017;23:5–22.
3. Gitler AD, Dhillon P, Shorter J. Neurodegenerative disease: models, mechanisms, and a new hope. Dis Model Mech. 2017;10:499–502.
4. Mackenzie, Rademakers. The role of transactive response DNA-binding protein-43 in amyotrophic lateral sclerosis and frontotemporal dementia. Curr Opin Neurol. 2008;21(6):693.
5. Buijsen RAM, Toonen LJA, Gardiner SL, van Roon-Mom WMC. Genetics, mechanisms, and therapeutic progress in polyglutamine spinocerebellar ataxias. Neurotherapeutics. 2019;16:263–86.
6. Van Cauwenberghe C, Van Broeckhoven C, Sleegers K. The genetic landscape of Alzheimer disease: clinical implications and perspectives. Genet Med. 2016;18:421–30.
7. Götz J, Halliday G, Nisbet RM. Molecular pathogenesis of the tauopathies. Ann Rev Pathol: Mech Dis. 2019;14:239–61.
8. Barage SH, Sonawane KD. Amyloid cascade hypothesis: pathogenesis and therapeutic strategies in Alzheimer's disease. Neuropeptides. 2015;52:1–18.
9. Alonso Vilatela ME, López-López M, Yescas-Gómez P. Genetics of Alzheimer's disease. Arch Med Res. 2012;43:622–31.
10. Crews L, Masliah E. Molecular mechanisms of neurodegeneration in Alzheimer's disease. Hum Mol Genet. 2010;19:R12–20.
11. Tan SH, Karri V, Tay NWR, Chang KH, Ah HY, Ng PQ, Ho HS, Keh HW, Candasamy M. Emerging pathways to neurodegeneration: dissecting the critical molecular mechanisms in Alzheimer's disease, Parkinson's disease. Biomed Pharmacother. 2019;111:765–77.
12. Genin E, Hannequin D, Wallon D, et al. APOE and Alzheimer disease: a major gene with semi-dominant inheritance. Mol Psychiatry. 2011;16:903–7.
13. Knapskog A-B, Eldholm RS, Braekhus A, Engedal K, Saltvedt I. Factors that influence the levels of cerebrospinal fluid biomarkers in memory clinic patients. BMC Geriatr. 2017;17:210.
14. Tapia-Rojas C, Cabezas-Opazo F, Deaton CA, Vergara EH, Johnson GVW, Quintanilla RA. It's all about tau. Prog Neurobiol. 2019;175:54–76.
15. Tai H-C, Serrano-Pozo A, Hashimoto T, Frosch MP, Spires-Jones TL, Hyman BT. The synaptic accumulation of hyperphosphorylated tau oligomers in Alzheimer disease is associated with dysfunction of the ubiquitin-proteasome system. Am J Pathol. 2012;181:1426–35.

16. Martin L, Latypova X, Terro F. Post-translational modifications of tau protein: implications for Alzheimer's disease. Neurochem Int. 2011;58:458–71.
17. Saha P, Sen N. Tauopathy: a common mechanism for neurodegeneration and brain aging. Mech Ageing Dev. 2019;178:72–9.
18. Jouanne M, Rault S, Voisin-Chiret A-S. Tau protein aggregation in Alzheimer's disease: an attractive target for the development of novel therapeutic agents. Eur J Med Chem. 2017;139:153–67.
19. Spires-Jones TL, Hyman BT. The intersection of amyloid beta and tau at synapses in Alzheimer's disease. Neuron. 2014;82:756–71.
20. Savitt JM. Diagnosis and treatment of Parkinson disease: molecules to medicine. J Clin Investig. 2006;116:1744–54.
21. Hatano Y, Sato K, Elibol B, et al. PARK6-linked autosomal recessive early-onset parkinsonism in Asian populations. Neurology. 2004;63:1482–5.
22. Stojkovska I, Krainc D, Mazzulli JR. Molecular mechanisms of α-synuclein and GBA1 in Parkinson's disease. Cell Tissue Res. 2018;373:51–60.
23. Pilsl A, Winklhofer KF. Parkin, PINK1 and mitochondrial integrity: emerging concepts of mitochondrial dysfunction in Parkinson's disease. Acta Neuropathol. 2012;123:173–88.
24. Schlehe JS, Lutz AK, Pilsl A, Lämmermann K, Grgur K, Henn IH, Tatzelt J, Winklhofer KF. Aberrant folding of pathogenic Parkin mutants: aggregation versus degradation. J Biol Chem. 2008;283:13771–9.
25. Azkona G, López de Maturana R, Del Rio P, et al. LRRK2 expression is deregulated in fibroblasts and neurons from Parkinson patients with mutations in PINK1. Mol Neurobiol. 2018;55:506–16.
26. La CV, Cognata LV, Cavallaro S. PRKN (arkin RBR E3 ubiquitin protein ligase). Atlas Genet Cytogenet Oncol Haematol. 2018; https://doi.org/10.4267/2042/66065.
27. Lunati A, Lesage S, Brice A. The genetic landscape of Parkinson's disease. Rev Neurol. 2018;174:628–43.
28. Valente EM. Hereditary early-onset Parkinson's disease caused by mutations in PINK1. Science. 2004;304:1158–60.
29. Iyer S, Subramanian V, Acharya KR. C9orf72, a protein associated with amyotrophic lateral sclerosis (ALS) is a guanine nucleotide exchange factor. PeerJ. 2018;6:e5815.
30. Scott L, Dawson VL, Dawson TM. Trumping neurodegeneration: targeting common pathways regulated by autosomal recessive Parkinson's disease genes. Exp Neurol. 2017;298:191–201.
31. Mathis S, Goizet C, Soulages A, Vallat J-M, Masson GL. Genetics of amyotrophic lateral sclerosis: a review. J Neurol Sci. 2019;399:217–26.
32. Couratier P, Corcia P, Lautrette G, Nicol M, Marin B. ALS and frontotemporal dementia belong to a common disease spectrum. Rev Neurol. 2017;173:273–9.
33. Lamb R, Rohrer JD, Real R, et al. A novel TBK1 mutation in a family with diverse frontotemporal dementia spectrum disorders. Mol Case Stud. 2019;5:a003913.
34. Lanata SC, Miller BL. The behavioural variant frontotemporal dementia (bvFTD) syndrome in psychiatry. J Neurol Neurosurg Psychiatry. 2016;87:501–11.
35. Olney NT, Spina S, Miller BL. Frontotemporal dementia. Neurol Clin. 2017;35:339–74.
36. Mohandas E, Rajmohan V. Frontotemporal dementia: an updated overview. Indian J Psychiatry. 2009;51(Suppl 1):S65–9.
37. Rademakers R, Cruts M, van Broeckhoven C. The role of tau (MAPT) in frontotemporal dementia and related tauopathies. Hum Mutat. 2004;24:277–95.
38. Siddique N, Siddique T. Amyotrophic Lateral Sclerosis Overview. 2001 Mar 23 [Updated 2019 Oct 3]. In: Adam MP, Ardinger HH, Pagon RA, et al., editors. GeneReviews® [Internet]. Seattle (WA): University of Washington, Seattle; 1993–2020. Available from: https://www.ncbi.nlm.nih.gov/books/NBK1450/.
39. Polymenidou M, Cleveland DW. The seeds of neurodegeneration: prion-like spreading in ALS. Cell. 2011;147:498–508.
40. Buijsen RAM, Toonen LJA, Gardiner SL, van WMC R-M. Genetics, mechanisms, and therapeutic progress in polyglutamine spinocerebellar ataxias. Neurotherapeutics. 2019;16:263–86.

41. Paulson HL, Shakkottai VG, Brent Clark H, Orr HT. Polyglutamine spinocerebellar ataxias – from genes to potential treatments. Nat Rev Neurosci. 2017;18:613–26.
42. Durr A. Autosomal dominant cerebellar ataxias: polyglutamine expansions and beyond. Lancet Neurol. 2010;9:885–94.
43. Dueñas AM, Goold R, Giunti P. Molecular pathogenesis of spinocerebellar ataxias. Brain. 2006;129:1357–70.
44. Kowalska M, Owecki M, Prendecki M, Wize K, Nowakowska J, Kozubski W, Lianeri M, Dorszewska J. Aging and neurological diseases. Senescence Physiol Pathol. 2017; https://doi.org/10.5772/intechopen.69499.
45. Hirtz D, Thurman DJ, Gwinn-Hardy K, Mohamed M, Chaudhuri AR, Zalutsky R. How common are the "common" neurologic disorders? Neurology. 2007;68:326–37.
46. Sohrabji F, Bake S, Lewis DK. Age-related changes in brain support cells: implications for stroke severity. Neurochem Int. 2013;63:291–301.
47. Liu H, Yang Y, Xia Y, Zhu W, Leak RK, Wei Z, Wang J, Hu X. Aging of cerebral white matter. Ageing Res Rev. 2017;34:64–76.
48. Wei W-M, Wu X-Y, Li S-T, Shen Q. PPARG gene C161T CT/TT associated with lower blood lipid levels and ischemic stroke from large-artery atherosclerosis in a Han population in Guangdong. Neurol Res. 2016;38:620–4.
49. De Vos A, Bjerke M, Brouns R, et al. Neurogranin and tau in cerebrospinal fluid and plasma of patients with acute ischemic stroke. BMC Neurol. 2017;17:170.
50. Dewdney B, Trollope A, Moxon J, Thomas Manapurathe D, Biros E, Golledge J. Circulating MicroRNAs as biomarkers for acute ischemic stroke: a systematic review. J Stroke Cerebrovasc Dis. 2018;27:522–30.
51. Tiedt S, Prestel M, Malik R, et al. RNA-Seq identifies circulating miR-125a-5p, miR-125b-5p, and miR-143-3p as potential biomarkers for acute ischemic stroke. Circ Res. 2017;121:970–80.
52. Guarner F, Malagelada J-R. Gut flora in health and disease. Lancet. 2003;361:512–9.
53. Quigley EMM. Gut microbiome as a clinical tool in gastrointestinal disease management: are we there yet? Nat Rev Gastroenterol Hepatol. 2017;14:315–20.
54. Villarán RF, Espinosa-Oliva AM, Sarmiento M, et al. Ulcerative colitis exacerbates lipopolysaccharide-induced damage to the nigral dopaminergic system: potential risk factor in Parkinson's disease. J Neurochem. 2010;114:1687–700.
55. Joshi, D., Roy, S., Banerjee, S., 2018. Chapter 19 - Prebiotics: A Functional Food in Health and Disease, in: Mandal, S.C., Mandal, V., Konishi, T. (Eds.), Natural Products and Drug Discovery. Elsevier, pp. 507–23.
56. Marques TM, Wall R, Ross RP, Fitzgerald GF, Ryan CA, Stanton C. Programming infant gut microbiota: influence of dietary and environmental factors. Curr Opin Biotechnol. 2010;21:149–56.
57. Fouhy F, Ross RP, Fitzgerald GF, Stanton C, Cotter PD. Composition of the early intestinal microbiota: knowledge, knowledge gaps and the use of high-throughput sequencing to address these gaps. Gut Microbes. 2012;3:203–20.
58. Aleman FDD, Valenzano DR. Microbiome evolution during host aging. PLoS Pathog. 2019;15:e1007727.
59. Wyss-Coray T. Ageing, neurodegeneration and brain rejuvenation. Nature. 2016;539:180–6.
60. O'Hara AM, Shanahan F. The gut flora as a forgotten organ. EMBO Rep. 2006;7:688–93.
61. Morais GCP, Arruda MM, de Aguiar Bonadia JC, Pozzan G. Cardiac amyloidosis: a challenging diagnosis. Autopsy Case Rep. 2014;4:9–17.
62. Sperry BW, Tang WHW. Amyloid heart disease: genetics translated into disease-modifying therapy. Heart. 2017;103:812–7.
63. Rogers GB, Keating DJ, Young RL, Wong M-L, Licinio J, Wesselingh S. From gut dysbiosis to altered brain function and mental illness: mechanisms and pathways. Mol Psychiatry. 2016;21:738–48.
64. Giau V, Wu S, Jamerlan A, An S, Kim S, Hulme J. Gut microbiota and their neuroinflammatory implications in Alzheimer's disease. Nutrients. 2018;10:1765.

65. Stilling RM, Dinan TG, Cryan JF. Microbial genes, brain and behaviour – epigenetic regulation of the gut-brain axis. Genes Brain Behav. 2014;13:69–86.
66. Roy Sarkar S, Banerjee S. Gut microbiota in neurodegenerative disorders. J Neuroimmunol. 2019;328:98–104.
67. Dinan TG, Cryan JF. Gut instincts: microbiota as a key regulator of brain development, ageing and neurodegeneration. J Physiol. 2017;595:489–503.
68. Rite I, Machado A, Cano J, Venero JL. Blood-brain barrier disruption induces in vivo degeneration of nigral dopaminergic neurons. J Neurochem. 2007;101:1567–82.
69. Keshavarzian A, Green SJ, Engen PA, Voigt RM, Naqib A, Forsyth CB, Mutlu E, Shannon KM. Colonic bacterial composition in Parkinson's disease. Mov Disord. 2015;30:1351–60.
70. Çamci G, Oğuz S. Association between Parkinson's disease and helicobacter pylori. J Clin Neurol. 2016;12:147–50.
71. Bostanciklioğlu M. Intestinal bacterial Flora and Alzheimer's disease. Neurophysiology. 2018;50:140–8.
72. Morris G, Berk M, Maes M, Puri BK. Could Alzheimer's disease originate in the periphery and if so how so? Mol Neurobiol. 2019;56:406–34.
73. O'Shea EF, Cotter PD, Stanton C, Paul Ross R, Hill C. Production of bioactive substances by intestinal bacteria as a basis for explaining probiotic mechanisms: bacteriocins and conjugated linoleic acid. Int J Food Microbiol. 2012;152:189–205.
74. He B, Hoang TK, Wang T, et al. Resetting microbiota by Lactobacillus reuteri inhibits T reg deficiency–induced autoimmunity via adenosine A2A receptors. J Exp Med. 2017;214:107–23.
75. Cassani E, Privitera G, Pezzoli G, Pusani C, Madio C, Iorio L, Barichella M. Use of probiotics for the treatment of constipation in Parkinson's disease patients. Minerva Gastroenterol Dietol. 2011;57:117–21.
76. Gareau MG, Wine E, Rodrigues DM, Cho JH, Whary MT, Philpott DJ, Macqueen G, Sherman PM. Bacterial infection causes stress-induced memory dysfunction in mice. Gut. 2011;60:307–17.
77. Akbari E, Asemi Z, Daneshvar Kakhaki R, Bahmani F, Kouchaki E, Tamtaji OR, Hamidi GA, Salami M. Effect of probiotic supplementation on cognitive function and metabolic status in Alzheimer's disease: a randomized, double-blind and controlled trial. Front Aging Neurosci. 2016;8:256.

# Molecular Aspects of Hippocampal Aging

3

Mariana Temido-Ferreira and Luísa V. Lopes

## Abbreviations

| | |
|---|---|
| $A_{2A}R$ | Adenosine $A_{2A}R$ receptors |
| AHP | Afterhyperpolarization |
| AMPAR | α-Amino-3-hydroxy-5-methyl-4-isoxazolepropionic acid receptor |
| APP/PS1 | Amyloid precursor protein/presenilin 1 |
| BBB | Blood–brain barrier |
| CA | Cornu ammonis |
| $Ca^{2+}$ | Calcium |
| CaMKII | Calcium/calmodulin-dependent protein kinase II |
| cAMP | Cyclic adenosine monophosphate |
| CaN | Calcineurin |
| CNS | Central nervous system |
| CREB | cAMP response element-binding |
| DNA | Deoxyribonucleic acid |
| EPSP | Excitatory postsynaptic potential |
| FKBP1b | FK506-binding protein 12.6/1b |
| GABA | Gamma-aminobutyric acid |
| GFAP | Glial fibrillary acidic protein |
| hAPP | Human amyloid precursor protein |
| $IP_3$ | Inositol trisphosphate 3 |
| LTD | Long-term depression |
| LTP | Long-term potentiation |
| $Mg^{2+}$ | Magnesium |
| mGluR5 | Metabotropic glutamate receptor 5 |

M. Temido-Ferreira · L. V. Lopes (✉)
Instituto de Medicina Molecular João Lobo Antunes, Faculdade de Medicina, Universidade de Lisboa, Lisbon, Portugal
e-mail: lvlopes@medicina.ulisboa.pt



J. C. Gomez-Verjan, N. A. Rivero-Segura (eds.), *Clinical Genetics and Genomics of Aging*, https://doi.org/10.1007/978-3-030-40955-5_3

| | |
|---|---|
| MTL | Medial temporal lobe |
| NMDAR | N-methyl-D-aspartate receptor |
| NSC | Neural stem cells |
| PKA | Protein kinase A |
| PKC | Protein kinase C |
| PP1 | Protein phosphatase 1 |
| PSD | Postsynaptic density |
| RNA | Ribonucleic acid |
| SNP | Single-nucleotide polymorphism |
| SNV | Single-nucleotide variant |
| TIMP2 | Tissue inhibitor of metalloproteinases 2 |
| TL | Telomere length |
| VDCC | Voltage-dependent calcium channels |
| WHO | World Health Organization |
| WT | Wild type |

## Introduction

According to the World Health Organization (WHO), the proportion of the world's population over 60 years will nearly double from 12% to 22% between 2015 and 2050. Aging is, in fact, the main risk factor for Alzheimer's disease (AD) [1]. These profound demographic changes place "the aging process" as one of the big challenges for scientific research nowadays. Understanding brain aging has the potential to produce a hugely beneficial impact on human welfare and the quality of later life, as age-related decline in performance dependent on this region is consistently found across species and tasks [2–6]. Therefore, much work has been done in the hippocampus.

Recently, new disruptive discoveries have emerged in this context, namely, the ability of umbilical cord plasma treatment in improving cognitive function in aged mice, possibly through the action of tissue inhibitor of metalloproteinases 2 (TIMP2) and other plasticity-promoting proteins [7]. Other discoveries have emerged in this context, opening new avenues to unravel the synaptic mechanisms that drive aging and putative therapies to prevent or at least deaccelerate this physiopathological process.

We guide you through the classical features of the aged hippocampus, focusing on alterations in neuronal morphology, calcium dynamics, and plasticity induced by aging. We provide state-of-the-art knowledge on hippocampal glutamatergic transmission and immune alterations upon aging and discuss the putative therapeutic impact of manipulating these novel players.

## Neuronal Loss

For a long time, aging had been associated with neuronal loss independently of the brain region [8–11]. However, the accuracy of such results is questioned by the methods used [12, 13], and subsequent studies have undoubtedly shown that the cell number is maintained in aging in several brain areas, including the hippocampus [14–19]. These data highlight the differences between aging itself, characterized by structural preservation in the medial temporal lobe (MTL), versus AD, which is associated with neuronal and synaptic loss in the MTL and in the hippocampus in particular [20].

Although there is a preservation of the number of hippocampal neurons, there is a well-documented age-related decline in hippocampal volume, as a result of synaptic dysfunction and atrophy [21], which is significantly associated with cognitive decline in humans, including episodic memory, working memory, processing speed, and executive function [22]. In humans, the hippocampal volume is associated with telomerase activity and leukocyte telomere length (TL) [23]. Telomerase adds telomeric repeats to terminal DNA. When telomeres shorten to a critical length, telomerase activity stalls genomic instability and apoptotic events. Therefore, TL provides an index of cellular age that predicts the incidence of age-related diseases and early mortality in older adults [24]. Remarkably, reactivation of endogenous telomerase activity reversed age-related degenerative phenotypes observed in a telomerase-deficient mouse model [25].

Telomere length has received great attention given the potential of using as an aging marker. However, a recent review of six types of potential biological age estimators – epigenetic clocks; telomere length; transcriptomic-, proteomic-, and metabolomic-based estimators; and composite biomarkers – concluded that the epigenetic clock is the most promising molecular estimator of biological age [26]. Epigenetic "age estimators" are sets of CpGs (also known as "clock CpGs") that are coupled with a mathematical algorithm to estimate the age of a DNA source, such as cells, tissues, or organs. This estimated age, also referred to as epigenetic age or more precisely as DNA methylation-based (DNAm) age, is not only a reflection of chronological age but also of the biological age of the DNA source. Accordingly, evidence from human and mouse studies pinpointed DNAm biomarkers as a molecular biomarker of aging, since they satisfy the following criteria: they apply to all sources of DNA (sorted cells, tissues, and organs) and to the entire age spectrum (from prenatal to centenarians) [27]. Interestingly, many of the CpGs that are being used in the algorithm have, on their own, only negligible correlation with chronological age, which illustrates that the whole is greater than the sum of its parts when it comes to composite biomarkers of aging [28].

Few accurate age estimators have been characterized so far: the Horvath's clock, a multi-tissue 353 CpG methylation-based age estimator, stands out in terms of its correlation with chronological age across multiple tissue types, its high accuracy in children, its strong correlation with gestational age (differentiation day) in neuronal cell culture models, and the homogeneity of its age estimates across tissues. The Hannum's clock is a highly accurate age estimator on the basis of 71 CpGs from DNA of blood. Although some biased estimates in non-blood tissue and children, it gives extremely accurate predictions of life expectancy (reviewed in [28]).

Aging is also associated with a decrease in the amplitude of the Schaffer collaterals-induced field excitatory postsynaptic potentials (fEPSP) recorded in CA1 [29–31]. Furthermore, the postsynaptic density (PSD) area of axospinous synapses is significantly reduced in aged learning-impaired rats [32]. Since at this synapse, the size of the unitary EPSP remains constant during aging [33], these data suggest that aging might not be associated with alterations in the strength of individual synaptic connections but instead with an increase in nonfunctional or silent synapses in the hippocampus [12, 34].

## Gene Expression and Regulation

Aging correlates with alterations in several gene expression and regulation mechanisms. Recently, transcriptomic analysis of the human aged brain revealed robust negative associations of genes encoding pre- and postsynaptic proteins with age, likely related to functional changes in synaptic integrity seen with aging (for a complete review see [12, 34]). Interestingly, these changes occur across inhibitory and excitatory synapses, and some of the strongest effects were observed in the hippocampus, consistent with the increased vulnerability of this structure to the aging process [35].

Circular RNAs (circRNAs) are transcripts most commonly generated by back-splicing events from exons of protein-coding genes. Interestingly, they are enriched in neural tissues, suggesting putative neural functions [36, 37]. Total RNA-seq profiling of young (1 m.o.) and aged (22 m.o.) cortex, hippocampus, and heart showed that circRNAs are upregulated in neural tissues upon aging, which was independent of linear RNA expression of host genes [38]. These findings suggest that circRNAs might play biological roles somehow relevant to the aging nervous system.

Aging was also recently associated with the frequency of single-nucleotide variants (SNV). Single-cell whole-genome sequencing of DNA from 161 single neurons from the prefrontal cortex and hippocampus of 15 healthy individuals (aged 4 months to 82 years) revealed that SNV increase approximately linearly with age in both areas (with a higher rate in the hippocampus) [39]. However, further studies need to address the relationship between SNV frequency and age-mediated pathological processes.

Cells have DNA repair mechanisms to correct DNA damage processes, which accumulate throughout life and are one of the triggers to the aging process itself. Since neurons are postmitotic and do not have many forms of DNA repair, they are particularly vulnerable to neurodegenerative diseases [40]. This notion raises the real possibility that there is a feed-forward relationship between DNA damage and the initiation and progression of neurological disease [40]. As one possible response to accumulating DNA damage, neurons may reenter the cell cycle or become prematurely senescent or undergo apoptosis. Also, such changes can accelerate harmful alterations in the neuronal genome, further disturbing patterns of gene expression [40]. These alterations can ultimately lead to loss of synapses or dendritic arborization, chronic inflammation, or the accumulation and aggregation of misfolded proteins [40], a hallmark of neurodegenerative diseases such as Alzheimer's and Parkinson's disease.

## Electrophysiological Alterations Upon Aging

In rodents, one of the well-characterized electrophysiological markers of physiological aging is a decrease in action potential firing rates of CA1 pyramidal cells, with a concomitant decrease in the amplitude of the postburst afterhyperpolarization (AHP), responsible for spike frequency adaptation [41] (reviewed by [42]). Accordingly, increased AHP may limit excitability by increasing the refractory period of neurons [42].

Electrophysiological recordings coupled with cell-type-specific imaging in the medial temporal lobe of cognitively assessed, aged rhesus macaques showed that neuron excitability in the hippocampal CA3 region is negatively correlated with the density of somatostatin-expressing inhibitory interneurons, showing that disruption of normal interactions between excitatory and inhibitory neurons contribute to age-related memory impairments [43].

The alterations observed at individual synapses have a significant impact on synaptic plasticity. Age-associated memory deficits correlate with impairments in either long-term potentiation (LTP) or long-term depression (LTD) [44, 45]. In aged animals, LTP has been found to be reduced [2, 46–48], not altered [47, 49–52] or even strengthened [53–56]. The latter is inconsistent with the classical correlation between increased LTP magnitude and better performance on hippocampal-dependent memory tasks. Differences in the stimulation protocol [12, 53] or in the synaptic circuit that is being potentiated [47] may then account for the observed discrepancies in LTP magnitude.

Given the involvement of α-amino-3-hydroxy-5-methyl-4-isoxazolepropionic acid receptor (AMPAR) in the expression and maintenance of LTP and LTD, alterations in AMPAR expression and function may be related to age-associated changes in synaptic plasticity. Accordingly, the administration of AMPAR positive allosteric modulators restores age-related memory and synaptic potentiation deficits [57, 58], suggesting an increase in silent AMPAR rather than alterations in the expression of synaptic AMPAR [59].

The transcription factor cAMP response element-binding protein (CREB) has been shown to have fundamental roles in cognition and cellular excitability [60, 61]. Treatment with compounds that activate the cyclic adenosine monophosphate (cAMP)/protein kinase A (PKA) pathway reversed LTP and Barnes test deficits observed in aged animals, possibly by increasing CREB activity [62]. Levels of phosphorylated CREB are decreased in aged versus young animals after training in the Morris water maze, and strongly correlated with individual learning performance, whereas CREB expression itself does not change [63]. These results suggest that alterations of activation rather than expression contribute to the age-related changes in cognition.

The study of LTD upon aging generated controversial results: some authors report increased susceptibility to LTD during aging [52], whereas others failed to observe alterations in LTD magnitude [49, 64]. These differences can be explained by differences in animal strain, stimulation pattern, or $Ca^{2+}/Mg^{2+}$ ratio. Accordingly, age-related differences in LTD induction could be rescued by manipulating the extracellular $Ca^{2+}/Mg^{2+}$ ratio. Indeed, the fact that induction of LTD depends both on age and $Ca^{2+}$ levels in the recording medium strongly supports an age-related $Ca^{2+}$ dysregulation and a shift in $Ca^{2+}$-dependent induction mechanisms rather than in the LTD intrinsic capacity [49, 64]. Consistent with this hypothesis, we showed that aging is associated with a shift in the form of plasticity induced by a weak stimulus (LFS elicited LTP instead of LTD), as a consequence of increased N-methyl-D-aspartate receptor (NMDAR) activation and $Ca^{2+}$ influx [65].

## Calcium Dynamics and Homeostasis

To avoid excessive intracellular levels of calcium ($[Ca^{2+}]_i$) elevations, neurons are equipped with complex machinery that permanently modulates the temporal and spatial patterns of $Ca^{2+}$ signaling [66, 67]. Brief elevations of $[Ca^{2+}]_i$ are essential in controlling membrane excitability, gene transcription, and other major cellular functions [66, 67]. Postsynaptic intracellular levels of $Ca^{2+}$ are also involved in setting a synaptic modification curve by determining the probability that a synapse will be depressed or potentiated for a given pattern of input [68, 69]. Accordingly, since $Ca^{2+}$ homeostasis is disrupted in aged animals [70, 71], we can expect alterations in the probability for a given synapse to undergo potentiation or depression. All these observations support the *calcium hypothesis* of aging, which implicates raised intracellular $Ca^{2+}$ as the major source of functional impairment and degeneration in aged neurons [72–74].

Several studies reported an age-associated increase in basal $[Ca^{2+}]_i$ levels [75, 76] as a result of increased voltage-dependent $Ca^{2+}$ influx [71, 77, 78], aberrant buffering [79–81], extrusion [76, 82–84], and uptake capacity [85]. There is compelling evidence of an age-associated increase in L-type $Ca^{2+}$ channels expression [71, 77, 78] that can be further correlated with performance in hippocampus-dependent memory tests [71]. Furthermore, a significant increase in voltage-gated $Ca^{2+}$ currents in CA1 hippocampal neurons was found in aged rats [86]. Accordingly, treatment with the L-type $Ca^{2+}$ channel blocker nimodipine improved spatial working memory in aged rats [87].

Given the key role of NMDAR in synaptic plasticity and memory [88], putative alterations in NMDAR may also account for $Ca^{2+}$ dysregulation. In aged CA1 pyramidal neurons, there is an increased duration of NMDAR-mediated responses [89] and an NMDAR overactivation upon glutamate or glycine stimulation, despite a decrease in the density of these receptors [90]. However, such alteration in NMDAR-mediated responses may be due to the previously described increase in nonfunctional synapses with aging. The fact that there is an increased binding of the NMDAR antagonist MK-801 in animals with learning and retention deficits [91, 92] suggests that an increase in NMDAR channel open-time happens as a compensatory mechanism for the apparent decrease in receptor number [93], since MK-801 only binds open channels.

Another strong candidate mechanism underlying aging-related $Ca^{2+}$ dysregulation is the disruption of FK506-binding protein 12.6/1b (FKBP1b). In neurons, FKBP1b negatively regulates $Ca^{2+}$ release [94–96]. Hippocampal FKBP1b protein and gene expression declines with normal aging in rats [96], and, most importantly, short-term virally mediated overexpression of FKBP1b in rat hippocampus reverses aging-related elevation of $Ca^{2+}$ transients and spatial memory deficits [96]. Interestingly, the therapeutic effects of FKBP1b overexpression also include transcription regulation, since FKBP1b selectively counteracted aging-induced expression changes in 37% of aging-dependent genes [97].

Besides age-associated alterations in sources of $Ca^{2+}$ dysregulation, previous studies focused on putative impairments in signaling pathways that translate changes in $Ca^{2+}$ regulation into altered neuronal function and cognition [98]. Concretely, several studies described alterations in the activity of protein kinases and phosphatases involved in the expression of synaptic plasticity [98–100]. These kinases and phosphatases are thought to act on AMPAR to mediate the expression of LTP and LTD, respectively. Although in most cases the expression of a particular kinase or phosphatase is unaltered, their basal activity is decreased, localization is shifted, or stimulation-induced activation is impaired upon aging [101].

CaMKII is an enzyme crucial for synaptic plasticity [102]. Aged rats display impairments in activity-dependent regulation of CaMKII transcription [99] and a decrease in the activation/translocation of CaMKII [103–105]. Postsynaptic inhibition of protein phosphatase 1 (PP1) increased synaptic transmission in aged animals, supporting the hypothesis that increased PP1 activity may underlie the age-related decrease in synaptic transmission [106]. PP1 activity is not directly regulated by $Ca^{2+}$ but by calcineurin (CaN), the unique phosphatase that is directly regulated by the level of intracellular $Ca^{2+}$[98]. Hippocampal CaN and PP1 activity increases with aging and is associated with L-type calcium channels function [98]. Furthermore, this impaired CaN activity drives dephosphorylation of CaN substrate proteins, such as CREB, which is associated with decreased cell viability, susceptibility to neurotoxicity [107], and impairments in terms of maintenance of LTP and memory [108, 109]. Consistently, performance in hippocampus-dependent memory tasks can be correlated with CaN activity in aged animals, further linking aberrant CaN activity and $Ca^{2+}$ homeostasis disruption with memory impairments [98].

Altogether, these data support a shift in the balance of activity of $Ca^{2+}$-dependent kinase/phosphatase enzymes as an important marker for age-associated changes in neuronal function and cognition.

## Adenosine $A_{2A}$ Receptors ($A_{2A}R$)

Adenosine influences many functions in the central nervous system. Besides the neuromodulatory actions, adenosine acts as a fine-tuner of synaptic communication, as it is a relevant player in neuron–glia communication and can affect the release and action of many neurotransmitters and other neuromodulators [110–114]. Accordingly, the neuromodulatory role of adenosine is mediated by a balance between the inhibitory and excitatory actions via $A_1R$ (usually coupled to adenylate cyclase inhibitory proteins, Gi/Go) and $A_{2A}R$ (coupled to adenylate cyclase inhibitory proteins Gs), the most relevant adenosine receptors in the central nervous system (CNS) [115]. The effects of adenosine depend on the receptors' expression pattern and signaling, the brain region, and pathophysiological conditions. $A_1R$ are widely distributed, being more abundant in the cortex, cerebellum, and hippocampus [116]. On the opposite, $A_{2A}R$ display a more restricted expression pattern: $A_{2A}R$ are highly expressed in the olfactory bulb and striatum [117], whereas in the neocortex and hippocampus, they are present at residual levels [118, 119]. $A_{2A}R$ are mostly located in glutamatergic synapses [120], although they have been shown in other synapses, such as GABAergic [113, 121, 122], dopaminergic [123, 124], cholinergic [125, 126], serotoninergic [127, 128], or noradrenergic synapses [129].

$A_{2A}R$ expression and signaling are profoundly altered in the hippocampus upon aging. $A_{2A}R$ density and coupling to G protein are increased [65, 111, 130–133], probably enhancing the action of this receptor to facilitate neurotransmitters release in glutamatergic synapses by a presynaptic mechanism [130]. This age-related enhanced $A_{2A}R$-mediated facilitation of synaptic transmission is dependent on PKA and is associated with an increase in cAMP accumulation [111].

Compelling evidence points out an age-related decrease in $A_1R$ expression in both mice and rats [133–135], albeit at a low extent. However, any attempts to treat rodents chronically with either $A_1R$ selective agonists or antagonists have resulted in diminished cognitive performance in both healthy and amyloid precursor protein/presenilin 1 (APP/PS1) mice [136, 137], which argues against an age-related potential of manipulating $A_1R$ in the hippocampus as therapeutics.

$A_{2A}R$ overexpression, in a similar magnitude to the one observed in human aging, is sufficient to trigger synaptic and cognitive deficits. This effect involves a metabotropic glutamate receptor 5 (mGluR5)-dependent NMDAR overactivation, leading to enhanced $Ca^{2+}$ influx [65], which recapitulates the main synaptic alterations observed upon aging. This NMDAR overactivation is associated with a plasticity shift: a low-frequency protocol triggered a significant LTP in these animals, whereas it generated a typical LTD in wild type (WT) animals [65]. The way mGluR5 activates NMDAR is still unclear, and several alternatives are plausible. mGluR5 interacts with NMDAR via the Homer/Shank/PSD-95 protein complex [138–140], and several studies have unraveled a mGluR5-dependent enhancement of NMDAR currents through a protein kinase C (PKC)/inositol trisphosphate 3 ($IP_3$)-calcium-dependent mechanism [141–144]. $A_{2A}R$ activation mediates mGluR5-dependent NMDAR2B phosphorylation at the residue Tyr1472 by Fyn kinases activation in a PD model [145] and in physiological conditions [146]. Whether the mechanisms by which mGluR5 activates NMDAR coexist or are region-specific is still unclear.

Importantly, a 3-week treatment with the selective $A_{2A}R$ antagonist KW6002 restored synaptic and memory impairments [65]. This suggests that $A_{2A}R$ blockade reestablishes the physiological signaling of adenosine, rather than the receptor expression, which is unlikely to occur at such a short time frame. Accordingly, we have prior data showing that chronic KW6002 treatment rescues cognitive and synaptic impairments induced by stress, without altering $A_{2A}R$ levels [147].

The therapeutic effects of $A_{2A}R$ blockade are extended to AD models, some of which exhibit aberrant $A_{2A}R$ expression and signalling [148, 149]. Importantly, chronic treatment with the $A_{2A}R$ antagonist MSX-3 rescued hippocampal-dependent memory even after the onset of the pathology in a mouse model of tauopathy, Thy-Tau22 [148]. Consistent with the central role of $A_{2A}R$ in synaptic and memory dysfunction, $A_{2A}R$ deletion is sufficient to prevent memory defects, LTD impairments, and tau hyperphosphorylation observed in these animals [148].

Since $A_{2A}R$ are expressed in neurons and astrocytes, whether this pathological role is due to astrocytic or neuronal $A_{2A}R$ remains inconclusive. Chemogenetic activation of Gs-coupled signaling in astrocytes increases cAMP and CREB, and reduces long-term memory in mice [150]. An astrocytic contribution is further highlighted by the decreased astrogliosis observed in Thy-Tau22-$A_{2A}R^{-/-}$ mice [148]. In 15–18 m.o. human amyloid precursor protein (hAPP) animals, astrocytic-specific $A_{2A}R$ genetic deletion reduces memory deficits [150]. Immunohistochemistry and correlation between *ADORA2A* and *GFAP* mRNA levels, revealed suggested an astrocytic $A_{2A}R$ overexpression in AD human samples [150]. However, these results do not discard a putative neuronal role, since neuronal expression was not addressed.

Multiple rodent models point out a neuronal $A_{2A}R$ role in synaptic and memory dysfunction observed upon aging and AD. Neuronal $A_{2A}R$ overexpression is sufficient to trigger CREB-dependent synaptic and memory dysfunction [65, 151]. Pharmacological and viral $A_{2A}R$ blockade in neurons rescued lack of associative NMDAR-independent LTP in an early stage and cognitive impairments in the Y-maze test in the AD mouse model APP/PS1 animals (double transgenic mice expressing a chimeric mouse/human amyloid precursor protein (Mo/HuAPP695swe) and a mutant human presenilin 1 (PS1-dE9)) [149]. mGluR5 antagonism also rescued LTP, suggesting that $A_{2A}R$ and mGluR5 operated through a common pathway to impair LTP, as our group also observed [65, 145]. We described that $A_{2A}R$ staining observed in aged humans and AD patients' hippocampus was specific for neurons [65], consistent with previous data, in which single-cell PCR of laser-dissected cells of young rats revealed no $A_{2A}R$ transcripts in glial fibrillary acidic protein (GFAP) positive cells [120].

Overall, this combined evidence suggests a synergism between astrocytic and neuronal $A_{2A}R$-mediated effects that defines its robust ability to control synaptic and memory dysfunction: synaptic dysfunction in aging and early AD may be predominantly triggered by a neuronal $A_{2A}R$ progressive dysfunction, whereas at later Braak stages of AD, astrocytic AD and inflammation may become more relevant.

In humans, an increase in $A_{2A}R$ expression was observed in pathologies associated with cognitive deficits, such as Alzheimer's [65, 150] and Pick's disease [152]. Recently, a single-nucleotide polymorphism (SNP) in a noncoding region of *ADORA2A* was associated with episodic memory performance, hippocampal volume, and total tau in cerebrospinal fluid (CSF) in mild cognitive impairment and AD patients [153], suggesting that this variation may affect $A_{2A}R$ production, although this was not assessed. Importantly, caffeine intake, a nonselective adenosine receptor antagonist, has been consistently shown to slow down cognitive decline in the aged population and reduces the risk of developing Alzheimer's disease (further discussed in the following text).

## Caffeine Effects in Aging and Alzheimer's Disease

Multiple studies showed that coffee intake was inversely associated with cognitive decline, and there was also an inverse association between the number of cups of coffee consumed per day and 10-year cognitive decline, with the least decline for men consuming three cups per day [154]. In a sample of subjects aged 65 years and over, consumption of at least three cups of coffee per day was associated with less decline in verbal memory in women [155]. On the contrary, coffee had no significant protective effect in women with under two daily units [155].

Importantly, other studies support a role for caffeine in the prevention of AD. Both retrospective and prospective studies showed that coffee consumption inversely correlated with disease onset and decreased the risk of AD by 31% during a 5-year follow-up [156, 157]. Furthermore, another prospective study showed that plasma caffeine levels at study onset were substantially lower (−51%) in mild cognitive impairment (MCI) subjects who later progressed to dementia compared to levels in stable MCI subjects. Also, plasma caffeine levels greater than 1200 ng/ml (≈6 μM) in MCI subjects were associated with no conversion to dementia during the ensuing 2/4-year follow-up period [158].

The beneficial effects of caffeine in humans are not confined to aging and Alzheimer's disease. Epidemiological studies also show an inverse relationship between the consumption of caffeine and the risk of developing Parkinson's disease [159, 160], likely via $A_{2A}R$ blockade [161, 162]. Also, two polymorphisms in the gene that encodes for $A_{2A}R$, *ADORA2A* (r71651683 and rs5996696) were inversely associated with risk of developing the disease [163]. In the brain, $A_{2A}R$ activation has an important role in stimulating and reinforcing properties of caffeine [164, 165], and a mutation in the *ADORA2A* gene (C1083T) was associated with caffeine-induced anxiety among non-habitual caffeine consumers [166]. Accordingly, the probability of having such mutation is inversely correlated with caffeine intake, and people with that genotype are more likely to limit their caffeine intake [167].

In aged rodents, caffeine perfusion has a clear therapeutic effect in rescuing neuronal $A_{2A}R$-driven synaptic plasticity shift in the hippocampus [65], while having no effects in excitatory CA1 currents in young animals [168], and caffeine intake for 12 months prevents age-associated recognition memory decline [169].

Memory deficits were prevented by caffeine in both amyloid and tau-based transgenic mouse models of Alzheimer's disease [148, 170–172], including a decrease in several pro-inflammatory (CD68, CD45, TLR2, CCL4, TNFα) and oxidative stress (Nrf2, MnSOD, EAAT3) markers found upregulated in the hippocampus of THY-Tau22 animals [173]. Interestingly, caffeine effects seem to be broader that inhibition of $A_{2A}R$ function itself, since caffeine reduces tau phosphorylation in different residues from the ones observed with $A_{2A}R$ antagonist and genetic deletion [148,

173] and decreases the amount of Tau proteolytic fragments [173], which is not influenced by genetic deletion [148].

## The Neuroimmune System Upon Aging

The age-associated synaptic dysfunction can also be a consequence of alterations in astrocytes and microglia, as the aging process has also been described as *inflammaging*, a status of chronic inflammation that contributes to the pathogenesis of neurodegenerative diseases [174]. Recent data further suggest an important role of the immune system in regulating the progression of brain aging and neurodegenerative disease. This can be seen as a cause-or-consequence dilemma: do immune and inflammatory pathways become hyperactivated with age and promote degeneration or, instead, immune responses fail to cope with age-related stress and may contribute to disease [175]?

Microglia have a crucial role in surveilling and maintaining homeostasis: in minor disturbances, microglia may secrete anti-inflammatory cytokines and supportive growth factors, whereas in major threats, such as pathogen invasion, microglia release toxic factors to kill the pathogen and recruit help by releasing pro-inflammatory cytokines [175].

Microarrays of aged human and mouse brains showed that aging is associated with an increase in genes related to cellular stress and inflammation and a decrease in genes related to synaptic function/transport, growth factors, and trophic support decrease [176, 177]. These age-associated alterations suggest that neurons face increased challenges with age but receive reduced support. Age-dependent microglia activation was found in aged rodents, nonhuman primates, and humans [178–180], characterized by increased expression of MHCII, CD68, TLRs, and pro-inflammatory cytokines such as TNF$\alpha$, IL1$\beta$, and IL6 [181–185]. However, other studies unravel a microglial dystrophic/senescent phenotype in aged individuals [186, 187], thus supporting the hypothesis that, rather than induction of microglial activation, progressive microglial degeneration and loss of microglial neuroprotection, coupled with increased secretion of inflammatory mediators, are associated with aging and lead to neuronal loss and inefficient clearance of toxic protein aggregates, further contributing to the onset and progression of neurodegenerative diseases such as AD [175].

Although the number of astrocytes remains unaffected in aged humans [188–190], in rats there seems to be an increase in the astrocytic size in the hippocampus [190]. In mice, age decreases the expression of ionotropic and purinergic receptors [191] and neurotransmitter-induced $Ca^{2+}$ signaling [192]. Importantly, age is also associated with reduced expression of water channels (aquaporin 4) in astroglial perivascular processes and markedly diminished clearance of the brain parenchyma through the glymphatic pathway [193], a key process in the prevention of the accumulation of misfolded protein aggregates.

Although neurovascular alterations were described in the context of aging and neurodegenerative diseases, the relationship between vascular dysfunction and synaptic and cognitive impairments still remains controversial [194, 195]. The hippocampus is particularly susceptible to changes in oxygen and blood supply [196], which may explain, in part, the vulnerability of this brain structure to the aging and neurodegeneration processes. Using magnetic resonance imaging (MRI) techniques, including cerebral blood volume (CBV)-functional MRI (fMRI) with gadolinium contrast, aging was found to be associated with blood–brain barrier (BBB) disruption in the human hippocampus [197]. Concretely, cognitive impairment in elderly individuals and early stages of AD was significantly associated with hypometabolism and decreased CBV in the hippocampus [197].

BBB integrity loss is constantly associated with immune cells infiltration [198–200]. Infiltrating monocytes are important for the neurodegenerative process [201, 202], and various other peripheral immune cells are clearly present during neurodegenerative disease. T cells, albeit in small numbers, were recently shown to infiltrate the brain in the context of neurodegenerative diseases [203–205] and during aging [206, 207]. Recently, single-cell RNA sequencing in young and aged neurogenic niches in mice revealed an infiltration of T cells in aged neurogenic niches, clonally expanded and generally distinct from those in aged blood, suggesting that they may recognize a specific antigen in the aged brain [208]. Although the exact role of T cells in neural stem cells (NSC) remains to be established, T cells can inhibit the proliferation of neural stem cells in cocultures and in vivo, in part by secreting interferon-$\gamma$, providing a possible cause for the age-mediated decline in NSC suggesting new players in the aging brain [208].

## Conclusion

In summary, age-related memory impairments are explained by changes in neuronal and synaptic morphology and function, driven by genomic, transcriptomic, and proteomic alterations. Importantly, impairments in calcium buffering and influx mechanisms, such as via NMDAR and L-type voltage-dependent calcium channels (VDCC) [71, 77, 78, 89, 90], support the calcium hypothesis of aging, which implicates raised intracellular $Ca^{2+}$ as the major source of functional impairment and degeneration in aged neurons [72–74].

Also, growing evidence pinpoints $A_{2A}R$ as a key mediator in glutamatergic dysfunction upon aging. $A_{2A}R$ expression and signaling are profoundly altered in the hippocampus upon aging. Overexpression of neuronal $A_{2A}R$ in the same magnitude to the one observed in human aging is sufficient to trigger synaptic and cognitive deficits, due to a mGluR5-dependent NMDAR overactivation and linked to enhanced $Ca^{2+}$ influx [65], which recapitulates the main synaptic alterations observed upon aging. Multiple prospective and retrospective studies emphasize the role of caffeine in slowing down cognitive decline in the aged population and reducing the risk of developing Alzheimer's disease. Although the mechanism is not yet disclosed, the beneficial effects seem to be achieved via $A_{2A}R$ blockade [161, 162].

Because of the diversity and complexity of all these regulatory mechanisms, a better understanding of the precise processes that drive physiopathological conditions in different brain regions and CNS cell types will allow the development of novel therapeutic strategies for synaptic and memory dysfunction throughout aging.

## References

1. Reitz C, Brayne C, Mayeux R. Epidemiology of Alzheimer disease. Nat Rev Neurol. 2011;7:137–52.
2. Barnes CA. Memory deficits associated with senescence: a neurophysiological and behavioral study in the rat. J Comp Physiol Psychol. 1979;93:74–104.
3. Colombo PJ, Wetsel WC, Gallagher M. Spatial memory is related to hippocampal subcellular concentrations of calcium-dependent protein kinase C isoforms in young and aged rats. Proc Natl Acad Sci U S A. 1997;94:14195–9.
4. Erickson CA, Barnes CA. The neurobiology of memory changes in normal aging. Exp Gerontol. 2003;38:61–9.
5. Oler JA, Markus EJ. Age-related deficits on the radial maze and in fear conditioning: hippocampal processing and consolidation. Hippocampus. 1998;8:402–15.
6. Tanila H, Shapiro M, Gallagher M, Eichenbaum H. Brain aging: changes in the nature of information coding by the hippocampus. J Neurosci. 1997;17:5155–66.
7. Castellano JM, et al. Human umbilical cord plasma proteins revitalize hippocampal function in aged mice. Nature. 2017;544:488–92.
8. Ball MJ. Neuronal loss, neurofibrillary tangles and granulovacuolar degeneration in the hippocampus with ageing and dementia. A quantitative study. Acta Neuropathol (Berl). 1977;37:111–8.
9. Brizzee KR, Ordy JM, Bartus RT. Localization of cellular changes within multimodal sensory regions in aged monkey brain: possible implications for age-related cognitive loss. Neurobiol Aging. 1980;1:45–52.
10. Brody H. Organization of the cerebral cortex. III. A study of aging in the human cerebral cortex. J Comp Neurol. 1955;102:511–6.
11. Coleman PD, Flood DG. Neuron numbers and dendritic extent in normal aging and Alzheimer's disease. Neurobiol Aging. 1987;8:521–45.
12. Burke SN, Barnes CA. Neural plasticity in the ageing brain. Nat Rev Neurosci. 2006;7:30–40.
13. Morrison JH, Hof PR. Life and death of neurons in the aging brain. Science. 1997;278:412–9.
14. Gazzaley AH, Thakker MM, Hof PR, Morrison JH. Preserved number of entorhinal cortex layer II neurons in aged macaque monkeys. Neurobiol Aging. 1997;18:549–53.
15. Keuker JIH, Luiten PGM, Fuchs E. Preservation of hippocampal neuron numbers in aged rhesus monkeys. Neurobiol Aging. 2003;24:157–65.
16. Merrill DA, Roberts JA, Tuszynski MH. Conservation of neuron number and size in entorhinal cortex layers II, III, and V/VI of aged primates. J Comp Neurol. 2000;422:396–401.
17. Pakkenberg B, Gundersen HJ. Neocortical neuron number in humans: effect of sex and age. J Comp Neurol. 1997;384:312–20.
18. Peters A, Leahu D, Moss MB, McNally KJ. The effects of aging on area 46 of the frontal cortex of the rhesus monkey. Cereb Cortex N Y N. 1994;1991(4):621–35.
19. West MJ. New stereological methods for counting neurons. Neurobiol Aging. 1993;14:275–85.
20. Scheff SW, Price DA, Schmitt FA, Mufson EJ. Hippocampal synaptic loss in early Alzheimer's disease and mild cognitive impairment. Neurobiol Aging. 2006;27:1372–84.
21. Raz N, et al. Regional brain changes in aging healthy adults: general trends, individual differences and modifiers. Cereb Cortex N Y N. 2005;1991(15):1676–89.

22. O'Shea A, Cohen RA, Porges EC, Nissim NR, Woods AJ. Cognitive aging and the Hippocampus in older adults. Front Aging Neurosci. 2016;8
23. Jacobs EG, Epel ES, Lin J, Blackburn EH, Rasgon NL. Relationship between leukocyte telomere length, telomerase activity, and hippocampal volume in early aging. JAMA Neurol. 2014;71:921–3.
24. Honig LS, Kang MS, Schupf N, Lee JH, Mayeux R. Association of shorter leukocyte telomere repeat length with dementia and mortality. Arch Neurol. 2012;69:1332–9.
25. Jaskelioff M, et al. Telomerase reactivation reverses tissue degeneration in aged telomerase-deficient mice. Nature. 2011;469:102–6.
26. Jylhävä J, Pedersen NL, Hägg S. Biological age predictors. EBioMedicine. 2017;21:29–36.
27. Horvath S. DNA methylation age of human tissues and cell types. Genome Biol. 2013;14:R115.
28. Horvath S, Raj K. DNA methylation-based biomarkers and the epigenetic clock theory of ageing. Nat Rev Genet. 2018;19:371–84.
29. Barnes CA, Rao G, Foster TC, McNaughton BL. Region-specific age effects on AMPA sensitivity: electrophysiological evidence for loss of synaptic contacts in hippocampal field CA1. Hippocampus. 1992;2:457–68.
30. Landfield PW, Pitler TA, Applegate MD. The effects of high Mg2+–to-Ca2+ ratios on frequency potentiation in hippocampal slices of young and aged rats. J Neurophysiol. 1986;56:797–811.
31. Rosenzweig ES, Rao G, McNaughton BL, Barnes CA. Role of temporal summation in age-related long-term potentiation-induction deficits. Hippocampus. 1997;7:549–58.
32. Nicholson DA, Yoshida R, Berry RW, Gallagher M, Geinisman Y. Reduction in size of perforated postsynaptic densities in hippocampal axospinous synapses and age-related spatial learning impairments. J Neurosci. 2004;24:7648–53.
33. Barnes CA, Rao G, Shen J. Age-related decrease in the N-methyl-D-aspartateR-mediated excitatory postsynaptic potential in hippocampal region CA1. Neurobiol Aging. 1997;18:445–52.
34. Burke SN, Barnes CA. Senescent synapses and hippocampal circuit dynamics. Trends Neurosci. 2010;33:153–61.
35. McEwen BS. Possible mechanisms for atrophy of the human hippocampus. Mol Psychiatry. 1997;2:255–62.
36. Rybak-Wolf A, et al. Circular RNAs in the mammalian brain are highly abundant, conserved, and dynamically expressed. Mol Cell. 2015;58:870–85.
37. Szabo L, et al. Statistically based splicing detection reveals neural enrichment and tissue-specific induction of circular RNA during human fetal development. Genome Biol. 2015;16:126.
38. Gruner H, Cortés-López M, Cooper DA, Bauer M, Miura P. CircRNA accumulation in the aging mouse brain. Sci Rep. 2016;6
39. Lodato MA, et al. Aging and neurodegeneration are associated with increased mutations in single human neurons. Science. 2018;359:555–9.
40. Chow H, Herrup K. Genomic integrity and the ageing brain. Nat Rev Neurosci. 2015;16:672–84.
41. Disterhoft JF, Thompson LT, Moyer JR, Mogul DJ. Calcium-dependent afterhyperpolarization and learning in young and aging hippocampus. Life Sci. 1996;59:413–20.
42. Wu WW, Oh MM, Disterhoft JF. Age-related biophysical alterations of hippocampal pyramidal neurons: implications for learning and memory. Ageing Res Rev. 2002;1:181–207.
43. Thomé A, Gray DT, Erickson CA, Lipa P, Barnes CA. Memory impairment in aged primates is associated with region-specific network dysfunction. Mol Psychiatry. 2016;21:1257–62.
44. Ge Y, et al. Hippocampal long-term depression is required for the consolidation of spatial memory. Proc Natl Acad Sci U S A. 2010;107:16697–702.
45. Tombaugh GC, Rowe WB, Chow AR, Michael TH, Rose GM. Theta-frequency synaptic potentiation in CA1 in vitro distinguishes cognitively impaired from unimpaired aged Fischer 344 rats. J Neurosci. 2002;22:9932–40.
46. Deupree DL, Bradley J, Turner DA. Age-related alterations in potentiation in the CA1 region in F344 rats. Neurobiol Aging. 1993;14:249–58.
47. Rex CS, et al. Long-term potentiation is impaired in middle-aged rats: regional specificity and reversal by adenosine receptor antagonists. J Neurosci. 2005;25:5956–66.

48. Sankar R, et al. Epileptogenesis after status epilepticus reflects age- and model-dependent plasticity. Ann Neurol. 2000;48:580–9.
49. Kumar A, Thinschmidt JS, Foster TC, King MA. Aging effects on the limits and stability of long-term synaptic potentiation and depression in rat hippocampal area CA1. J Neurophysiol. 2007;98:594–601.
50. Landfield PW, Lynch G. Impaired monosynaptic potentiation in in vitro hippocampal slices from aged, memory-deficient rats. J Gerontol. 1977;32:523–33.
51. Landfield PW, McGaugh JL, Lynch G. Impaired synaptic potentiation processes in the hippocampus of aged, memory-deficient rats. Brain Res. 1978;150:85–101.
52. Norris CM, Korol DL, Foster TC. Increased susceptibility to induction of long-term depression and long-term potentiation reversal during aging. J Neurosci. 1996;16:5382–92.
53. Costenla AR, de Mendonça A, Ribeiro JA. Adenosine modulates synaptic plasticity in hippocampal slices from aged rats. Brain Res. 1999;851:228–34.
54. Diógenes MJ, et al. Enhancement of LTP in aged rats is dependent on endogenous BDNF. Neuropsychopharmacol Off Publ Am Coll Neuropsychopharmacol. 2011;36:1823–36.
55. Kumar A, Foster TC. Enhanced long-term potentiation during aging is masked by processes involving intracellular calcium stores. J Neurophysiol. 2004;91:2437–44.
56. Pinho J, et al. Enhanced LTP in aged rats: detrimental or compensatory? Neuropharmacology. 2017;114:12–9.
57. Bloss EB, et al. Behavioral and biological effects of chronic S18986, a positive AMPA receptor modulator, during aging. Exp Neurol. 2008;210:109–17.
58. Radin DP, Zhong S, Purcell R, Lippa A. Acute ampakine treatment ameliorates age-related deficits in long-term potentiation. Biomed Pharmacother. 2016;84:806–9.
59. Jurado S. AMPA receptor trafficking in natural and pathological aging. Front Mol Neurosci. 2017;10:446.
60. Dash PK, Hochner B, Kandel ER. Injection of the cAMP-responsive element into the nucleus of *Aplysia* sensory neurons blocks long-term facilitation. Nature. 1990;345:718–21.
61. Guzowski JF, McGaugh JL. Antisense oligodeoxynucleotide-mediated disruption of hippocampal cAMP response element binding protein levels impairs consolidation of memory for water maze training. Proc Natl Acad Sci U S A. 1997;94:2693–8.
62. Bach ME, et al. Age-related defects in spatial memory are correlated with defects in the late phase of hippocampal long-term potentiation in vitro and are attenuated by drugs that enhance the cAMP signaling pathway. Proc Natl Acad Sci U S A. 1999;96:5280–5.
63. Porte Y, Buhot M-C, Mons N. Alteration of CREB phosphorylation and spatial memory deficits in aged 129T2/Sv mice. Neurobiol Aging. 2008;29:1533–46.
64. Foster TC, Kumar A. Susceptibility to induction of long-term depression is associated with impaired memory in aged Fischer 344 rats. Neurobiol Learn Mem. 2007;87:522–35.
65. Temido-Ferreira M, et al. Age-related shift in LTD is dependent on neuronal adenosine A2A receptors interplay with mGluR5 and NMDA receptors. Mol Psychiatry. 2018; https://doi.org/10.1038/s41380-018-0110-9.
66. Arundine M, Tymianski M. Molecular mechanisms of calcium-dependent neurodegeneration in excitotoxicity. Cell Calcium. 2003;34:325–37.
67. Delorenzo RJ, Sun DA, Deshpande LS. Cellular mechanisms underlying acquired epilepsy: the calcium hypothesis of the induction and maintenance of epilepsy. Pharmacol Ther. 2005;105:229–66.
68. Bear MF, Cooper LN, Ebner FF. A physiological basis for a theory of synapse modification. Science. 1987;237:42–8.
69. Foster TC, Kumar A. Calcium dysregulation in the aging brain. Neuroscientist. 2002;8:297–301.
70. Foster TC, Norris CM. Age-associated changes in ca(2+)-dependent processes: relation to hippocampal synaptic plasticity. Hippocampus. 1997;7:602–12.
71. Thibault O, Landfield PW. Increase in single L-type calcium channels in hippocampal neurons during aging. Science. 1996;272:1017–20.
72. Khachaturian ZS. The role of calcium regulation in brain aging: reexamination of a hypothesis. Aging Milan Italy. 1989;1:17–34.

73. Khachaturian ZS. Calcium hypothesis of Alzheimer's disease and brain aging. Ann N Y Acad Sci. 1994;747:1–11.
74. Verkhratsky A, Toescu EC. Calcium and neuronal ageing. Trends Neurosci. 1998;21:2–7.
75. Hajieva P, Kuhlmann C, Luhmann HJ, Behl C. Impaired calcium homeostasis in aged hippocampal neurons. Neurosci Lett. 2009;451:119–23.
76. Raza M, et al. Aging is associated with elevated intracellular calcium levels and altered calcium homeostatic mechanisms in hippocampal neurons. Neurosci Lett. 2007;418:77–81.
77. Núñez-Santana FL, et al. Surface L-type Ca2+ channel expression levels are increased in aged hippocampus. Aging Cell. 2014;13:111–20.
78. Veng LM, Browning MD. Regionally selective alterations in expression of the alpha(1D) subunit (Ca(v)1.3) of L-type calcium channels in the hippocampus of aged rats. Brain Res Mol Brain Res. 2002;107:120–7.
79. de Jong GI, et al. Age-related loss of calcium binding proteins in rabbit hippocampus. Neurobiol Aging. 1996;17:459–65.
80. Satrústegui J, Villalba M, Pereira R, Bogónez E, Martínez-Serrano A. Cytosolic and mitochondrial calcium in synaptosomes during aging. Life Sci. 1996;59:429–34.
81. Villa A, Meldolesi J. The control of Ca2+ homeostasis: role of intracellular rapidly exchanging Ca2+ stores. Cell Biol Int. 1994;18:301–7.
82. Martinez-Serrano A, Blanco P, Satrústegui J. Calcium binding to the cytosol and calcium extrusion mechanisms in intact synaptosomes and their alterations with aging. J Biol Chem. 1992;267:4672–9.
83. Michaelis ML, Johe K, Kitos TE. Age-dependent alterations in synaptic membrane systems for Ca2+ regulation. Mech Ageing Dev. 1984;25:215–25.
84. Michaelis ML, Foster CT, Jayawickreme C. Regulation of calcium levels in brain tissue from adult and aged rats. Mech Ageing Dev. 1992;62:291–306.
85. Gibson G, Perrino P, Dienel GA. In vivo brain calcium homeostasis during aging. Mech Ageing Dev. 1986;37:1–12.
86. Campbell LW, Hao SY, Thibault O, Blalock EM, Landfield PW. Aging changes in voltage-gated calcium currents in hippocampal CA1 neurons. J Neurosci. 1996;16:6286–95.
87. Veng LM, Mesches MH, Browning MD. Age-related working memory impairment is correlated with increases in the L-type calcium channel protein alpha1D (Cav1.3) in area CA1 of the hippocampus and both are ameliorated by chronic nimodipine treatment. Brain Res Mol Brain Res. 2003;110:193–202.
88. Tsien JZ, Huerta PT, Tonegawa S. The essential role of hippocampal CA1 NMDA receptor-dependent synaptic plasticity in spatial memory. Cell. 1996;87:1327–38.
89. Jouvenceau A, Dutar P, Billard JM. Alteration of NMDA receptor-mediated synaptic responses in CA1 area of the aged rat hippocampus: contribution of GABAergic and cholinergic deficits. Hippocampus. 1998;8:627–37.
90. Serra M, Ghiani CA, Foddi MC, Motzo C, Biggio G. NMDA receptor function is enhanced in the hippocampus of aged rats. Neurochem Res. 1994;19:483–7.
91. Ingram DK, et al. Reduced density of NMDA receptors and increased sensitivity to dizocilpine-induced learning impairment in aged rats. Brain Res. 1992;580:273–80.
92. Topic B, et al. Impaired maze performance in aged rats is accompanied by increased density of NMDA, 5-HT1A, and alpha-adrenoceptor binding in hippocampus. Hippocampus. 2007;17:68–77.
93. Kumar A. NMDA Receptor function during senescence: implication on cognitive performance. Front Neurosci. 2015;9:473.
94. Gant JC, et al. Disrupting function of FK506-binding protein 1b/12.6 induces the $Ca^{2}$+–dysregulation aging phenotype in hippocampal neurons. J Neurosci. 2011;31:1693–703.
95. Gant JC, et al. FK506-binding protein 1b/12.6: a key to aging-related hippocampal Ca2+ dysregulation? Eur J Pharmacol. 2014;739:74–82.
96. Gant JC, et al. Reversal of aging-related neuronal Ca2+ dysregulation and cognitive impairment by delivery of a transgene encoding FK506-binding protein 12.6/1b to the Hippocampus. J Neurosci. 2015;35:10878–87.

97. Gant JC, et al. FK506-binding protein 12.6/1b, a negative regulator of [Ca2+], rescues memory and restores genomic regulation in the hippocampus of aging rats. J Neurosci. 2018;38:1030–41.
98. Foster TC, Sharrow KM, Masse JR, Norris CM, Kumar A. Calcineurin links Ca2+ dysregulation with brain aging. J Neurosci. 2001;21:4066–73.
99. Davis S, et al. Dysfunctional regulation of alphaCaMKII and syntaxin 1B transcription after induction of LTP in the aged rat. Eur J Neurosci. 2000;12:3276–82.
100. Karege F, Lambercy C, Schwald M, Steimer T, Cissé M. Differential changes of cAMP-dependent protein kinase activity and 3H-cAMP binding sites in rat hippocampus during maturation and aging. Neurosci Lett. 2001;315:89–92.
101. Foster, T. C. Age-related changes in synaptic phosphorylation and dephosphorylation. Adv Cell Aging Gerontol 16 133–152 (Elsevier, 2004).
102. Lisman J, Schulman H, Cline H. The molecular basis of CaMKII function in synaptic and behavioural memory. Nat Rev Neurosci. 2002;3:175–90.
103. Eckles KE, Dudek EM, Bickford PC, Browning MD. Amelioration of age-related deficits in the stimulation of synapsin phosphorylation. Neurobiol Aging. 1997;18:213–7.
104. Mullany P, Connolly S, Lynch MA. Ageing is associated with changes in glutamate release, protein tyrosine kinase and Ca2+/calmodulin-dependent protein kinase II in rat hippocampus. Eur J Pharmacol. 1996;309:311–5.
105. Parfitt KD, Hoffer BJ, Browning MD. Norepinephrine and isoproterenol increase the phosphorylation of synapsin I and synapsin II in dentate slices of young but not aged fisher 344 rats. Proc Natl Acad Sci U S A. 1991;88:2361–5.
106. Norris CM, Halpain S, Foster TC. Alterations in the balance of protein kinase/phosphatase activities parallel reduced synaptic strength during aging. J Neurophysiol. 1998;80:1567–70.
107. Walton MR, Dragunow I. Is CREB a key to neuronal survival? Trends Neurosci. 2000;23:48–53.
108. Impey S, et al. Stimulation of cAMP response element (CRE)-mediated transcription during contextual learning. Nat Neurosci. 1998;1:595–601.
109. Silva AJ, Kogan JH, Frankland PW, Kida S. CREB and memory. Annu Rev Neurosci. 1998;21:127–48.
110. Lopes LV, Cunha RA, Kull B, Fredholm BB, Ribeiro JA. Adenosine A(2A) receptor facilitation of hippocampal synaptic transmission is dependent on tonic A(1) receptor inhibition. Neuroscience. 2002;112:319–29.
111. Rebola N, et al. Enhanced adenosine A2A receptor facilitation of synaptic transmission in the hippocampus of aged rats. J Neurophysiol. 2003;90:1295–303.
112. Tebano MT, et al. Adenosine A(2A) receptors are required for normal BDNF levels and BDNF-induced potentiation of synaptic transmission in the mouse hippocampus. J Neurochem. 2008;104:279–86.
113. Shindou T, et al. Presynaptic adenosine A2A receptors enhance GABAergic synaptic transmission via a cyclic AMP dependent mechanism in the rat globus pallidus. Br J Pharmacol. 2002;136:296–302.
114. Cristóvão-Ferreira S, et al. A1R-A2AR heteromers coupled to Gs and G i/0 proteins modulate GABA transport into astrocytes. Purinergic Signal. 2013;9:433–49.
115. Linden J. Molecular approach to adenosine receptors: receptor-mediated mechanisms of tissue protection. Annu Rev Pharmacol Toxicol. 2001;41:775–87.
116. Reppert SM, Weaver DR, Stehle JH, Rivkees SA. Molecular cloning and characterization of a rat A1-adenosine receptor that is widely expressed in brain and spinal cord. Mol Endocrinol Baltim Md. 1991;5:1037–48.
117. Jarvis MF, Williams M. Direct autoradiographic localization of adenosine A2 receptors in the rat brain using the A2-selective agonist, [3H]CGS 21680. Eur J Pharmacol. 1989;168:243–6.
118. Cunha RA, et al. Evidence for functionally important adenosine A2a receptors in the rat hippocampus. Brain Res. 1994;649:208–16.
119. Kirk IP, Richardson PJ. Further characterization of [3H]-CGS 21680 binding sites in the rat striatum and cortex. Br J Pharmacol. 1995;114:537–43.

120. Rebola N, Canas PM, Oliveira CR, Cunha RA. Different synaptic and subsynaptic localization of adenosine A2A receptors in the hippocampus and striatum of the rat. Neuroscience. 2005;132:893–903.
121. Cunha RA, Ribeiro JA. Purinergic modulation of [(3)H]GABA release from rat hippocampal nerve terminals. Neuropharmacology. 2000;39:1156–67.
122. Rombo DM, et al. Synaptic mechanisms of adenosine A2A receptor-mediated hyperexcitability in the hippocampus. Hippocampus. 2015;25:566–80.
123. Borycz J, et al. Differential glutamate-dependent and glutamate-independent adenosine A1 receptor-mediated modulation of dopamine release in different striatal compartments. J Neurochem. 2007;101:355–63.
124. Garção P, et al. Functional interaction between pre-synaptic α6β2-containing nicotinic and adenosine A2A receptors in the control of dopamine release in the rat striatum. Br J Pharmacol. 2013;169:1600–11.
125. Cunha RA, Johansson B, Fredholm BB, Ribeiro JA, Sebastião AM. Adenosine A2A receptors stimulate acetylcholine release from nerve terminals of the rat hippocampus. Neurosci Lett. 1995;196:41–4.
126. Rodrigues RJ, Canas PM, Lopes LV, Oliveira CR, Cunha RA. Modification of adenosine modulation of acetylcholine release in the hippocampus of aged rats. Neurobiol Aging. 2008;29:1597–601.
127. Barraco RA, Helfman CC, Anderson GF. Augmented release of serotonin by adenosine A2a receptor activation and desensitization by CGS 21680 in the rat nucleus tractus solitarius. Brain Res. 1996;733:155–61.
128. Okada M, et al. Differential effects of adenosine receptor subtypes on release and reuptake of hippocampal serotonin. Eur J Neurosci. 1999;11:1–9.
129. Barraco RA, Clough-Helfman C, Goodwin BP, Anderson GF. Evidence for presynaptic adenosine A2a receptors associated with norepinephrine release and their desensitization in the rat nucleus tractus solitarius. J Neurochem. 1995;65:1604–11.
130. Lopes LV, Cunha RA, Ribeiro JA. Increase in the number, G protein coupling, and efficiency of facilitatory adenosine A2A receptors in the limbic cortex, but not striatum, of aged rats. J Neurochem. 1999;73:1733–8.
131. Canas PM, Duarte JMN, Rodrigues RJ, Köfalvi A, Cunha RA. Modification upon aging of the density of presynaptic modulation systems in the hippocampus. Neurobiol Aging. 2009;30:1877–84.
132. Costenla AR, et al. Enhanced role of adenosine A(2A) receptors in the modulation of LTP in the rat hippocampus upon ageing. Eur J Neurosci. 2011;34:12–21.
133. Cunha RA, Constantino MC, Sebastião AM, Ribeiro JA. Modification of A1 and A2a adenosine receptor binding in aged striatum, hippocampus and cortex of the rat. Neuroreport. 1995;6:1583–8.
134. Pagonopoulou O, Angelatou F. Reduction of A1 adenosine receptors in cortex, hippocampus and cerebellum in ageing mouse brain. Neuroreport. 1992;3:735–7.
135. Meerlo P, et al. Ageing-related decline in adenosine A1 receptor binding in the rat brain: an autoradiographic study. J Neurosci Res. 2004;78:742–8.
136. Von Lubitz DKJE, Paul IA, Bartus RT, Jacobson KA. Effects of chronic administration of adenosine A1 receptor agonist and antagonist on spatial learning and memory. Eur J Pharmacol. 1993;249:271–80.
137. Vollert C, Forkuo GS, Bond RA, Eriksen JL. Chronic treatment with DCPCX, an adenosine A1 antagonist, worsens long-term memory. Neurosci Lett. 2013;548:296–300.
138. Brakeman PR, et al. Homer: a protein that selectively binds metabotropic glutamate receptors. Nature. 1997;386:284–8.
139. Tu JC, et al. Coupling of mGluR/Homer and PSD-95 complexes by the shank family of postsynaptic density proteins. Neuron. 1999;23:583–92.
140. Roche KW, et al. Homer 1b regulates the trafficking of group I metabotropic glutamate receptors. J Biol Chem. 1999;274:25953–7.

141. Jia Z, et al. Selective abolition of the NMDA component of long-term potentiation in mice lacking mGluR5. Learn Mem Cold Spring Harb N. 1998;5:331–43.
142. Ugolini A, Corsi M, Bordi F. Potentiation of NMDA and AMPA responses by the specific mGluR5 agonist CHPG in spinal cord motoneurons. Neuropharmacology. 1999;38:1569–76.
143. Awad H, Hubert GW, Smith Y, Levey AI, Conn PJ. Activation of metabotropic glutamate receptor 5 has direct excitatory effects and potentiates NMDA receptor currents in neurons of the subthalamic nucleus. J Neurosci. 2000;20:7871–9.
144. Mannaioni G, Marino MJ, Valenti O, Traynelis SF, Conn PJ. Metabotropic glutamate receptors 1 and 5 differentially regulate CA1 pyramidal cell function. J Neurosci. 2001;21:5925–34.
145. Ferreira DG, et al. α-synuclein interacts with PrP(C) to induce cognitive impairment through mGluR5 and NMDAR2B. Nat Neurosci. 2017;20:1569–79.
146. Sarantis K, Tsiamaki E, Kouvaros S, Papatheodoropoulos C, Angelatou F. Adenosine $A_2A$ receptors permit mGluR5-evoked tyrosine phosphorylation of NR2B (Tyr1472) in rat hippocampus: a possible key mechanism in NMDA receptor modulation. J Neurochem. 2015;135:714–26.
147. Batalha VL, et al. Adenosine A(2A) receptor blockade reverts hippocampal stress-induced deficits and restores corticosterone circadian oscillation. Mol Psychiatry. 2013;18:320–31.
148. Laurent C, et al. A2A adenosine receptor deletion is protective in a mouse model of Tauopathy. Mol Psychiatry. 2016;21:97–107.
149. Viana da Silva S, et al. Early synaptic deficits in the APP/PS1 mouse model of Alzheimer's disease involve neuronal adenosine A2A receptors. Nat Commun. 2016;7:11915.
150. Orr AG, et al. Astrocytic adenosine receptor A2A and Gs-coupled signaling regulate memory. Nat Neurosci. 2015;18:423–34.
151. Li P, et al. Optogenetic activation of intracellular adenosine A2A receptor signaling in the hippocampus is sufficient to trigger CREB phosphorylation and impair memory. Mol Psychiatry. 2015;20:1339–49.
152. Albasanz JL, Rodríguez A, Ferrer I, Martín M. Adenosine A2A receptors are up-regulated in Pick's disease frontal cortex. Brain Pathol Zurich Switz. 2006;16:249–55.
153. Horgusluoglu-Moloch E, et al. Targeted neurogenesis pathway-based gene analysis identifies ADORA2A associated with hippocampal volume in mild cognitive impairment and Alzheimer's disease. Neurobiol Aging. 2017;60:92–103.
154. van Gelder BM, et al. Coffee consumption is inversely associated with cognitive decline in elderly European men: the FINE study. Eur J Clin Nutr. 2007;61:226–32.
155. Ritchie K, et al. The neuroprotective effects of caffeine: a prospective population study (the three City study). Neurology. 2007;69:536–45.
156. Maia L, de Mendonça A. Does caffeine intake protect from Alzheimer's disease? Eur J Neurol. 2002;9:377–82.
157. Lindsay J, et al. Risk factors for Alzheimer's disease: a prospective analysis from the Canadian study of health and aging. Am J Epidemiol. 2002;156:445–53.
158. Cao C, et al. High blood caffeine levels in MCI linked to lack of progression to dementia. J Alzheimers Dis JAD. 2012;30:559–72.
159. Ascherio A, et al. Prospective study of caffeine consumption and risk of Parkinson's disease in men and women. Ann Neurol. 2001;50:56–63.
160. Ross GW, et al. Association of coffee and caffeine intake with the risk of Parkinson disease. JAMA. 2000;283:2674–9.
161. Fredholm BB. Adenosine actions and adenosine receptors after 1 week treatment with caffeine. Acta Physiol Scand. 1982;115:283–6.
162. Fredholm BB. Astra award lecture. Adenosine, adenosine receptors and the actions of caffeine. Pharmacol Toxicol. 1995;76:93–101.
163. Popat RA, et al. Coffee, ADORA2A, and CYP1A2: the caffeine connection in Parkinson's disease. Eur J Neurol. 2011;18:756–65.
164. Huang Z-L, et al. Adenosine A2A, but not A1, receptors mediate the arousal effect of caffeine. Nat Neurosci. 2005;8:858–9.

165. Ledent C, et al. Aggressiveness, hypoalgesia and high blood pressure in mice lacking the adenosine A2a receptor. Nature. 1997;388:674–8.
166. Alsene K, Deckert J, Sand P, de Wit H. Association between A2a receptor gene polymorphisms and caffeine-induced anxiety. Neuropsychopharmacol Off Publ Am Coll Neuropsychopharmacol. 2003;28:1694–702.
167. Cornelis MC, El-Sohemy A, Campos H. Genetic polymorphism of the adenosine A2A receptor is associated with habitual caffeine consumption. Am J Clin Nutr. 2007;86:240–4.
168. Simons SB, Caruana DA, Zhao M, Dudek SM. Caffeine-induced synaptic potentiation in hippocampal CA2 neurons. Nat Neurosci. 2011;15:23–5.
169. Costa MS, Botton PH, Mioranzza S, Souza DO, Porciúncula LO. Caffeine prevents age-associated recognition memory decline and changes brain-derived neurotrophic factor and tyrosine kinase receptor (TrkB) content in mice. Neuroscience. 2008;153:1071–8.
170. Arendash GW, et al. Caffeine protects Alzheimer's mice against cognitive impairment and reduces brain beta-amyloid production. Neuroscience. 2006;142:941–52.
171. Arendash GW, et al. Caffeine reverses cognitive impairment and decreases brain amyloid-beta levels in aged Alzheimer's disease mice. J Alzheimers Dis JAD. 2009;17:661–80.
172. Chu Y-F, et al. Crude caffeine reduces memory impairment and amyloid β(1-42) levels in an Alzheimer's mouse model. Food Chem. 2012;135:2095–102.
173. Laurent C, et al. Beneficial effects of caffeine in a transgenic model of Alzheimer's disease-like tau pathology. Neurobiol Aging. 2014;35:2079–90.
174. Franceschi C, Garagnani P, Parini P, Giuliani C, Santoro A. Inflammaging: a new immune-metabolic viewpoint for age-related diseases. Nat Rev Endocrinol. 2018;14:576–90.
175. Lucin KM, Wyss-Coray T. Immune activation in brain aging and neurodegeneration: too much or too little? Neuron. 2009;64:110–22.
176. Lee C-K, Weindruch R, Prolla TA. Gene-expression profile of the ageing brain in mice. Nat Genet. 2000;25:294–7.
177. Lu T, et al. Gene regulation and DNA damage in the ageing human brain. Nature. 2004;429:883–91.
178. Perry VH, Matyszak MK, Fearn S. Altered antigen expression of microglia in the aged rodent CNS. Glia. 1993;7:60–7.
179. Ogura K, Ogawa M, Yoshida M. Effects of ageing on microglia in the normal rat brain: immunohistochemical observations. Neuroreport. 1994;5:1224–6.
180. Sheffield LG, Berman NE. Microglial expression of MHC class II increases in normal aging of nonhuman primates. Neurobiol Aging. 1998;19:47–55.
181. Henry CJ, Huang Y, Wynne AM, Godbout JP. Peripheral lipopolysaccharide (LPS) challenge promotes microglial hyperactivity in aged mice that is associated with exaggerated induction of both pro-inflammatory IL-1beta and anti-inflammatory IL-10 cytokines. Brain Behav Immun. 2009;23:309–17.
182. Van Guilder HD, et al. Concurrent hippocampal induction of MHC II pathway components and glial activation with advanced aging is not correlated with cognitive impairment. J Neuroinflammation. 2011;8:138.
183. Wong AM, et al. Macrosialin increases during normal brain aging are attenuated by caloric restriction. Neurosci Lett. 2005;390:76–80.
184. Griffin R, et al. The age-related attenuation in long-term potentiation is associated with microglial activation. J Neurochem. 2006;99:1263–72.
185. Letiembre M, et al. Innate immune receptor expression in normal brain aging. Neuroscience. 2007;146:248–54.
186. Streit WJ, Sammons NW, Kuhns AJ, Sparks DL. Dystrophic microglia in the aging human brain. Glia. 2004;45:208–12.
187. Davies DS, Ma J, Jegathees T, Goldsbury C. Microglia show altered morphology and reduced arborization in human brain during aging and Alzheimer's disease. Brain Pathol Zurich Switz. 2017;27:795–808.
188. Pelvig DP, Pakkenberg H, Stark AK, Pakkenberg B. Neocortical glial cell numbers in human brains. Neurobiol Aging. 2008;29:1754–62.

189. Fabricius K, Jacobsen JS, Pakkenberg B. Effect of age on neocortical brain cells in 90+ year old human females – a cell counting study. Neurobiol Aging. 2013;34:91–9.
190. Grosche A, et al. Versatile and simple approach to determine astrocyte territories in mouse neocortex and hippocampus. PLoS One. 2013;8:e69143.
191. Lalo U, Palygin O, North RA, Verkhratsky A, Pankratov Y. Age-dependent remodelling of ionotropic signalling in cortical astroglia. Aging Cell. 2011;10:392–402.
192. Palygin O, Lalo U, Verkhratsky A, Pankratov Y. Ionotropic NMDA and P2X1/5 receptors mediate synaptically induced Ca2+ signalling in cortical astrocytes. Cell Calcium. 2010;48:225–31.
193. Kress BT, et al. Impairment of paravascular clearance pathways in the aging brain. Ann Neurol. 2014;76:845–61.
194. Zlokovic BV. The blood-brain barrier in health and chronic neurodegenerative disorders. Neuron. 2008;57:178–201.
195. Zlokovic BV. Neurovascular pathways to neurodegeneration in Alzheimer's disease and other disorders. Nat Rev Neurosci. 2011;12:723–38.
196. Kirschen GW, Kéry R, Ge S. The hippocampal neuro-Glio-vascular network: metabolic vulnerability and potential neurogenic regeneration in disease. Brain Plast. 3:129–44.
197. Montagne A, et al. Blood-brain barrier breakdown in the aging human hippocampus. Neuron. 2015;85:296–302.
198. Stranahan AM, Hao S, Dey A, Yu X, Baban B. Blood–brain barrier breakdown promotes macrophage infiltration and cognitive impairment in leptin receptor-deficient mice. J Cereb Blood Flow Metab. 2016;36:2108–21.
199. Floris S, et al. Blood–brain barrier permeability and monocyte infiltration in experimental allergic encephalomyelitis: a quantitative MRI study. Brain. 2004;127:616–27.
200. Cai W, et al. Dysfunction of the neurovascular unit in ischemic stroke and neurodegenerative diseases: an aging effect. Ageing Res Rev. 2017;34:77–87.
201. D'Mello C, Le T, Swain MG. Cerebral microglia recruit monocytes into the brain in response to tumor necrosis factoralpha signaling during peripheral organ inflammation. J Neurosci. 2009;29:2089–102.
202. Kerfoot SM, et al. TNF-alpha-secreting monocytes are recruited into the brain of cholestatic mice. Hepatol Baltim MD. 2006;43:154–62.
203. Town T, Tan J, Flavell RA, Mullan M. T-cells in Alzheimer's disease. NeuroMolecular Med. 2005;7:255–64.
204. Sulzer D, et al. T cells from patients with Parkinson's disease recognize α-synuclein peptides. Nature. 2017;546:656–61.
205. Buckwalter MS, et al. Increased T cell recruitment to the CNS after amyloid beta 1–42 immunization in Alzheimer's mice overproducing transforming growth factor-beta 1. J Neurosci Off J Soc Neurosci. 2006;26:11437–41.
206. Ritzel RM, et al. Age-associated resident memory CD8 T cells in the central nervous system are primed to potentiate inflammation after ischemic brain injury. J Immunol Baltim Md. 2016;1950(196):3318–30.
207. Mrdjen D, et al. High-dimensional single-cell mapping of central nervous system immune cells reveals distinct myeloid subsets in health, aging, and disease. Immunity. 2018;48:380–95.e6.
208. Dulken BW, et al. Single-cell analysis reveals T cell infiltration in old neurogenic niches. Nature. 2019;571:205–10.

# Mitochondrial Function in Aging

# 4

S. L. Morales-Rosales, Nadia Alejandra Rivero-Segura,
and M. Königsberg

## Abbreviations

| | |
|---|---|
| $\Delta\Psi m$ | Mitochondrial membrane potential |
| AD | Alzheimer's disease |
| ATP | Adenosine triphosphate |
| BMI | Body mass index |
| DRP1 | Dynamin-related protein 1 |
| ETC | Electron transport chain |
| FA | Fatty acids |
| FAO | Fatty acid oxidation |
| Fis1 | Mitochondrial fission protein 1 |
| IMM | Inner mitochondrial membrane |
| MFF | Mitochondrial fission factor |
| MiD | Mitochondrial division factors |
| MPTP | Mitochondrial permeability transition pore |
| MRC | Mitochondrial respiratory chain |
| mtDNA | Mitochondrial deoxyribonucleic acid |

S. L. Morales-Rosales
División de Ciencias Biológicas y de la Salud, Departamento de Ciencias de la Salud, Universidad Autónoma Metropolitana-Iztapalapa, Mexico City, Mexico

Posgrado en Biología Experimental, Universidad Autónoma Metropolitana-Iztapalapa, Mexico City, Mexico

N. A. Rivero-Segura
División de Investigación Básica, Instituto Nacional de Geriatría, Mexico City, Mexico
e-mail: nrivero@inger.gob.mx

M. Königsberg (✉)
División de Ciencias Biológicas y de la Salud, Departamento de Ciencias de la Salud, Universidad Autónoma Metropolitana-Iztapalapa, Mexico City, Mexico
e-mail: mkf@xanum.uam.mx





J. C. Gomez-Verjan, N. A. Rivero-Segura (eds.), *Clinical Genetics and Genomics of Aging*, https://doi.org/10.1007/978-3-030-40955-5_4

mtUPR Mitochondrial unfolded protein response
NRF2 Nuclear respiratory factor 2
OMM Outer mitochondrial membrane
OxPhos Oxidative phosphorylation
PARL Presenilin-associated rhomboid-like
PD Parkinson's disease
PGC-1α Peroxisome proliferator-activated receptor γ
Pol-$^{\gamma}$ Polymerase gamma
PUFAs Polyunsaturated fatty acids
RNA Ribonucleic acid
ROS Reactive oxygen species
TCA Tricarboxylic acid cycle
TFAM Mitochondrial transcription factor A

## Introduction

The world is experiencing considerable growth in its older population [1]. This change in population composition has increased emphasis on the treatment of chronic diseases as they have become the primary cause of physical and mental disability. Nowadays, the aging field is devoted not only to increase lifespan but to improve health span; thus, understanding the mechanisms that underlay to the aging process might help to find treatments for age-related diseases and improve the elderlies' quality of life [2].

During aging, the normal physiological functions of an organism gradually decline, and this deficiency has been proposed as the main risk factor to develop multiple diseases that contribute to morbidity and mortality. Recently, López-Otin et al. described nine hallmarks of aging whose alteration might induce the aging process and which are the following: genomic instability, telomere shortening, epigenetic alterations, impaired proteostasis, deregulated nutrient sensing, cellular senescence, altered communication, stem cell exhaustion, and mitochondrial dysfunction [3]. In this chapter, we will review the main implications of mitochondrial dysfunction, mitochondrial dynamics failure (fission and fusion), mitochondrial turnover (mitophagy and biogenesis), and, finally, mitochondrial metabolism. Since mitochondrial decline in quality and activity represents a key feature for the development of aging and age-related diseases, as we will describe in the following paragraphs.

Most studies in this area have been performed in the classical animal models of aging, such as *C. elegans*, yeast, and rodents (mice and rats); however, in this chapter we have attempted to include only representative studies in humans, which were performed in samples of skeletal muscle, heart, and brain obtained from elderly individuals.

## Mitochondrial Physiology

Mitochondria are cellular organelles characterized by a double membrane. The inner mitochondrial membrane (IMM) is invaginated to form folded structures known as cristae that contain the protein complexes of the mitochondrial respiratory chain (MRC) and enclose an inner space, called the mitochondrial matrix, which contains the enzymes of the tricarboxylic acid cycle that provides NADH + $H^+$ and $FADH_2$ as the electron and proton donors. The outer mitochondrial membrane (OMM) surrounds the IMM, creating an intermembrane space that plays a key role in the generation of the mitochondrial membrane potential ($\Delta\Psi m$) necessary for energy generation (meaning ATP). It is known that mitochondria generate reactive oxygen species (ROS) because of the electron transport chain (ETC). Low levels of ROS constitute a physiological signaling mechanism, but high levels, generated under stress, are toxic and might cause damage to mitochondrial components and induce progressive loss of mitochondrial function, like oxidative damage, MRC dysfunction, $\Delta\Psi m$ loss, etc. [4]. Disorders in energy metabolism are a key feature of many human diseases, including metabolic syndromes such as diabetic nephropathy [5], heart failure, neurodegeneration, ischemia-reperfusion injury, and degenerative muscle disorders, among others [6]. With age, mitochondrial membrane potential declines, reducing ATP production and elevating pro-inflammatory molecules and ROS, leading to cell death [7].

Mitochondrial ROS generation has been for a long time related to the molecular damage associated to aging (mitochondrial free radical theory of aging); conversely, recent studies have also shown the involvement of other mitochondrial dysfunctions in the mechanism of aging [8]. Loss of membrane permeability and membrane potential decline have been correlated to reduced ATP synthesis and mitochondrial dysfunction in tissues of old animals [9, 10]. Some studies of the past decades, performed in isolated mitochondria from human liver, skin fibroblasts, brain, and skeletal muscle, have shown that the respiratory activity of the enzymatic complexes of the ETC decreases gradually during the aging process [11–13]. Moreover, mitochondrial morphology is known to change during aging, as well as the accumulation of mitochondrial disorganization in a large number of organs and tissues [14]. In the following sections, we will describe mitochondrial dynamics (fission, fusion, and turnover) and metabolism changes during aging.

## Mitochondrial DNA (mtDNA) Role in Aging

The widely accepted endosymbiotic mitochondria origin theory states that mitochondria derived from endosymbiotic alpha-proteobacteria, so these organelles are unique since they possess their own genome (mtDNA). The mtDNA is maternally inherited and it displays a circular, double-stranded and supercoiled topology that encompasses 16,569 bp, which encodes 13 protein subunits of the ETC, 22 transfer RNAs, and 2 ribosomal RNAs [15]. The mtDNA is arranged in nucleoids, which are dynamic structures with mitochondrial proteins involved in mtDNA replication and transcription processes, along with mtDNA protection [16]. As the nuclear DNA, mtDNA possesses its own machinery for replication, maintenance, and repair. Some examples of those proteins are (1) *replication machinery* (polymerase gamma (Pol-ɣ, nuclear-encoded), Twinkle, mtSSB, topoisomerase, mitochondrial RNA polymerase, RNase H1, and mitochondrial DNA ligase III) and (2) *maintenance machinery* (Pol-ɣ, TFAM, TFB2M, OPA-1, MGME1, FEN1, and DNA2 helicase/nuclease) [17]. For a more explicit review on mtDNA repair and maintenance in health and disease, please refer to Scheibye-Knudsen et al. (2015) and Akhmedov and Marín-García (2015) [18, 19].

Interestingly, the proximity of mtDNA to the ETC, the main source of ROS generation, and the lack of protective histones make this genome very susceptible to oxidative damage. ROS-induced damage results in point mutations, deletions, and depletions, which have been linked to aging and age-related diseases, by the free radical theory of aging, postulated by Denham Harman in 1956 and which was later reformed as the mitochondrial free radical theory of aging [20]. It has been shown that in humans mutations in mtDNA appear starting in the third decade of life, mainly in postmitotic tissues such as skeletal muscle, heart, and brain [21]. Recent studies have shown that stem cells also carry initial mtDNA mutations that increase with clonal expansion over time; the threshold of mutated mtDNA reaches a pathologic level during aging leading to mitochondria dysfuntion, and concomitantly the tissues function [22]. This phenomenon has been called the clonal expansion theory. Along with this theory and independently from the lineage of the cells (stem or postmitotic cells), it has also been shown that as organisms age, there is an increment in mtDNA mutations and a failure to repair them, so the pathways implicated in these processes have become interesting targets to study by the biomedical research. Lastly, changes in mitochondria competence or activity can result in epigenetic changes that alter lifespan [23] and deserve further research. For a complete review on mtDNA mutations in human health and diseases, please refer to MITOMAP (https://www.mitomap.org/MITOMAP).

## Mitochondrial Dynamics

Mitochondria are not only the energy producers of the cell, but they are essential organelles that play critical roles in intracellular processes [24]. Mitochondria can display different morphological states according to their enviroment and cellular physiology, thus promoting the formation of large elongated networks or small single spheroidal organelles. The mitochondrial morphology is highly dynamic and depends on a delicate balance between two opposing processes, fusion and fission, which normally occur in a healthy cell [25]. Maintenance of mitochondrial morphology, in a stable and balanced way, is crucial for the optimal mitochondrial function. Otherwise, physiological consequences and even diverse diseases arise, as seen in aging and age-related diseases, for instance, mammalian cells with senescence phenotype showed abnormalities in either process of fission or fusion [25].

Mitochondrial dynamics involve fission and fusion processes; as mentioned above, both events are in constant activity and must be in an equilibrated state. Mitochondrial dynamics respond to cellular needs to control the mitochondrial shape, size, and number conforming a functional network that is in constant change throughout cell life.

## Mitochondrial Fission

This process refers to the mitochondrial membrane constriction that drives mitochondrial division; this is necessary for many cellular processes like the correct mitochondrial distribution during cell division, mitochondrial quality control, intracellular distribution, interaction with other organelles, and nutrient-rich condition increases [26]. Furthermore, fission is a fundamental process in differentiated cells like neurons and muscle fibers, where fragmentation of damaged mitochondrion is needed to remove them via mitophagy and then renew the mitochondrial pull by biogenesis [27, 28].

The main protein which regulates fission is the cytosolic GTPase dynamin-related protein 1 (Drp1), which translocates to the mitochondria and attaches to the different adaptors anchored to the mitochondrial outer membrane like mitochondrial fission factor (Mff), mitochondrial fission protein 1 (Fis1), and mitochondrial division factors 49 and 51 kDa (MiD49 and MiD51) [26, 27]. Then Drp1 oligomerizes and constricts the mitochondrial membrane. The adaptors that interact with Drp1 can participate in physiological or pathological fission. Increased Fis1 activity has been related to cell stress activation, which augments mitochondrial fission during neurodegenerative diseases. Thus, the inhibition of Drp1-Fis1 interaction has beneficial effects by decreasing pathological mitochondrial fission. However, Drp1-Mff interaction has been related to basal (physiological) fission; therefore, the inhibition of this interaction diminishes ATP synthesis and might cause neurological and motor deficits, suggesting that Mff is essential for efficient mitochondrial activity [29].

## Mitochondrial Fusion

In order to fuse, the outer mitochondrial membrane (OMM) and the inner mitochondrial membrane (IMM) obey the following order: the first membrane that gets fused is the OMM by the action of mitofusins 1 and 2 (Mfn1, Mfn2), followed by the fusion of the IMM controlled by the optic atrophy 1 protein (Opa1). This phenomenon is activated when the cell demands high energy supply and the mitochondria fuse to form a network that optimizes ATP synthesis. In some cases, fusion leads to the combination of two mitochondria with mtDNA mutations in order to rescue them by cross-complementation [26, 30]. Interestingly, Opa1 has additional roles besides its fusion activity; it maintains the mitochondrial cristae shape and participates in the formation of the pore that releases cytochrome c and promotes apoptotic cell death [31, 32].

## Mitochondrial Turnover

The maintenance of the mitochondrial mass is essential for cellular health. So, to fulfill the mitochondrial turnover processes, the mitophagy (mitochondrial elimination) and the mitochondrial biogenesis take place in a coordinated manner. Any alteration in such processes promotes cellular dysfunction, which may lead to cell death or cellular senescence.

Macroautophagy, which is mainly called autophagy, is a process in which the cell eliminates useless or harmful cellular components, like cytoplasmic content, and even complete organelles. The components or organelles are engulfed by a double-membrane system termed autophagosome which fuses with the lysosomes that provides the hydrolytic enzymes necessary for the digestion of the autophagosome content [33]. There are two types of autophagy, a nonselective one that is activated mainly under starvation conditions and whose principal function is to recycle cytoplasmic components to provide simple substrates that will be used to produce energy and for the synthesis of new macromolecules. The second type is a selective one that eliminates specific targets like damaged protein complexes or defective organelles that need to be renewed in order to ensure the adequate cellular function [34]. Selective autophagy is classified regarding their specific target, i.e., reticulophagy eliminates endoplasmic reticulum, xenophagy eliminates pathogens, and mitophagy eliminates mitochondria, among others [35].

Mitophagy is a process that selectively degrades dysfunctional and irreversibly damaged mitochondrion. A depolarized membrane characterizes damaged mitochondria, as well as ATP synthesis decline, increased ROS, or mtDNA alterations. If damaged mitochondria were not eliminated, the mitochondrial network would be impaired, and as a consequence, the cells and the tissue would be affected [36, 37]. Active degradation of dysfunctional mitochondria is vital for cell survival, so mitophagy acts in a coordinated manner with mitochondrial biogenesis to ensure the mitochondrial network equilibrium [38, 39].

Damaged mitochondria are singled out and degraded through the activities of PTEN-induced kinase 1 (PINK1) and the ubiquitin E3 ligase Parkin, which work together to keep cells healthy by removing damaged mitochondria [40]. In normal conditions, PINK1 importation from the cytosol into the mitochondria is carried out by the mitochondrial translocases TIM and TOM and depends on the mitochondrial membrane potential. PINK1 is transported across the IMM, where it is cleaved by the protease presenilin-associated rhomboid-like (PARL) and is returned to the cytosol, where the proteasome system is in charge of its degradation [41–43].

When mitochondrion is damaged, the membrane potential is lost, and consequently PINK1 cannot be imported through the IMM, and it accumulates in the OMM. PINK1 increment in the OMM is recognized by Parkin, who ubiquitinates it, along with other OMM proteins such as Mfn2, which allow the recruitment of the adaptor SQSTM1/p62 that will recruit LC3 to tether the ubiquitinated proteins of the impaired mitochondrion into the autophagosome. PINK1 and Parkin interaction is necessary for the initiation of the mitophagy process, and they act as a marker of the dysfunctional mitochondrion that needs to be removed [44, 45].

### Mitochondrial Biogenesis

Mitochondrial biogenesis is induced as a response to the bioenergetics demands. This response includes an increase in mitochondrial mass. In order to synthesize new mitochondria, it is necessary to start from pre-existing mitochondria, so mitochondrial biogenesis is not a de novo process [46]. It requires the transcription of genes from both nuclear and mtDNA. It also needs the participation of the mitochondrial transcription factor A (TFAM) and the transcriptional family of peroxisome proliferator-activated receptor γ (PPARγ, nuclear-encoded) coactivator-1 alpha (PGC-1α, nuclear-encoded) [47]. PGC-1α regulates the expression of nuclear respiratory factors 1 and 2 (NRF1 and NRF2) that are coregulators that act together with PGC-1α to transcribe the mitochondrial proteins like COX IV, β-ATP synthetase, and mtTFA (TFAM), among others [48]; for this reason, PGC-1α is considered the principal regulator for mitochondrial biogenesis.

After transcription and translation, the mitochondrial proteins must be imported into the mitochondria through the TOM complex and then ensembled there with the aid of different proteins. This process will not be described here because it goes beyond the scope of this chapter.

## Mitochondrial Dynamics in Age-Related Neurodegenerative Diseases

During aging, the fission and fusion activity is altered, leading to cellular dysfunction. Some studies support the hypothesis that during aging mitochondrial fragmentation is increased. However, apparently the most important thing is the alteration in the fusion and fission balance, which may compromise the cell, leading to diverse diseases related to the aging process. The correct homeostasis in mitochondrial dynamics is essential to maintain a healthy network architecture, and the balanced fusion and fission events are needed to prolong lifespan/health span [10]. In particular, the brain and the heart are some examples of the organs that are most severely impacted by the loss of mitochondrial dynamics, since these tissues have a very high energetic demand. Alterations in the mitochondrial dynamics have been related to neurodegenerative diseases and two examples will be described below.

## Mitochondrial Dynamics in Parkinson's Disease (PD)

The loss of dopaminergic neurons in the *substantia nigra* is responsible for the resting tremor, rigidity, and bradykinesia. Very few cases of PD are caused by an autosomal recessive mutation in *PINK1* and *Parkin* genes [49]; PINK1/Parkin dysfunction leads to an increased Drp1-mediated mitochondrial fission that is an essential factor that contributes to neuronal death in PD [50]. Besides neuronal death, mitochondrial fission was observed in skin fibroblasts of PD patients [51], as well as reduced complex I activity in the *substantia nigra*, suggesting a mitochondrial fission-function axis dysregulation as part of the disease onset and progression [52].

## Mitochondrial Dynamics in Alzheimer's Disease (AD)

This disease is characterized by progressive senile or pre-senile dementia with associated biochemical features, such as selective neuronal loss, synaptic alterations leading to loss of connectivity between neurons, neurofibrillary degeneration, and extracellular deposits of αβ plaques [53]. Altered morphology of the mitochondria in AD has been reported, since small abnormal mitochondria with defects in the structures of the cristae have been observed in the patient's neurons. In the brains of postmortem patients, an abnormal expression of proteins that are involved in the mitochondrial dynamics (Drp1 and Fis1) has been reported, as well as a decrease in the expression of Mfn1, Mfn2, and Opa1 [54]. A consequence of AD is the accumulation of β-amyloid protein, which can generate the production of nitric oxide, which can activate Drp1 through S-nitrosylation, increasing the processes of mitochondrial fission, synaptic loss, and neuronal damage [55].

## Mitochondrial Dynamics in Heart and Skeletal Muscle

Mitochondrial morphology and activity changes are associated with normal aging in heart and muscle cells leading to a dysfunction in those tissues. Muscular cells are nondividing specialized cells that require high energy demand; for that reason mitochondrial quality control is very important for the well-functioning of cardiac and skeletal tissues. In Table 4.1 we summarize the impact of aging in the mitochondrial dynamics in skeletal muscle, heart, and brain in healthy elderly individuals.

# Mitochondrial Metabolism in Aging

As many authors state, aging is mainly characterized by the dysfunction at both molecular and organelle levels, which concomitantly leads to organ failure [69]. Mainly, metabolism impairment affects the whole organism lifespan [70]. In this context, beyond other roles exhibited by mitochondria, such as amino acid metabolism, pyridine synthesis, phospholipid modifications, calcium regulation, autophagy, ROS production, and survival [71], mitochondria are the main source

**Table 4.1** Main mitochondrial dynamics proteins that are altered in human tissues during the aging process

| Tissue/ organ | Fission | Fusion | Biogenesis | Mitophagy | Refs |
|---|---|---|---|---|---|
| Skeletal muscle | Increased fragmentation<br>Decreased Drp1 protein | Increased interconnected mitochondrial network<br>Decreased Mfn2 and Opa1 gene expression<br>Opa1 protein decline | PGC-1α, Sirt3 pathway is less activated<br>PGC-1α mRNA is less abundant and less TFAM protein levels | Reduced transcript of LAMP2, increased lipofuscins that affect autophagy flux | [56–61] |
| Heart | Increased Drp1 | Decreased Mfn1, Mfn2<br>Increased Opa1 | Diminished PGC-1α | Deregulated mitophagy, reduction in Pink1 protein levels | [62–66] |
| Brain | Increased Drp1 and Fis1 (mRNA and protein)<br>Increased SON-Drp1, nitrosylation of Drp1 | Decreased Mfn1, Mfn2, and Opa1 (mRNA and protein) | Reduced levels of PGC-1α, TFAM | Lysosomal activity is compromised, and the accumulation of autophagosomes is observed | [54, 55, 67, 68] |

of ATP production, and as a stress response the OxPhos impairment is directly responsible for the mitochondrial dynamics and turnover. Moreover, this mitochondrial activity is severely altered in human age-related diseases such as cancer, type 2 diabetes, liver and kidney disease, osteoporosis, sarcopenia, frailty, and cardiovascular and neurodegenerative diseases [72]. Furthermore, aging is characterized by several damages in cellular and organ metabolism failure, and in other studies, the risk for metabolic disorders is highly associated with age-related diseases that affect lifespan, and interestingly these conditions exhibit mitochondrial dysfunction [73].

Aging is a complex process as a time-dependent progressive loss of physiological integrity, leading to impaired function and increased vulnerability to death [74], and as we described above, aging is highly associated with mtDNA mutations; in fact heteroplasmy incidence increases with age, while lower mtDNA copy number has been reported in aged populations as well as mitochondria morphology, abundance, and oxidative phosphorylation activity [75, 76]. Interestingly, in aging the significant amount of these mutations converges in sites that encode structural subunits of the ETC such as complexes I and III [77], leading to OxPhos uncoupling and mitochondrial dysfunction in aged population. Since there are several limitations to study mitochondrial metabolism in human samples, in this section we briefly described the implications of mitochondrial metabolism for aging in the most studied and high energy demand human tissues, such as skeletal muscle, heart, and brain.

## Mitochondrial Metabolism in Aged Skeletal Muscle

During aging skeletal muscle considerably loses muscle mass and strength, and since it also decreases its regenerative capacity, the result is a poor and restricted physical performance in elderly individuals [78]. Additionally, several authors state that skeletal muscle also exhibits an impaired metabolism that includes both insulin resistance and mitochondrial dysfunction in men and women from the third to the fourth decade of life [65]. This observation suggests that before the skeletal muscle loss appear, there must be cellular and metabolic biomarkers that appear first. Moreover, sarcopenia is defined as the atrophy of skeletal muscle and the decline in muscle strength. It also has a characteristic phenotype that includes a reduction in muscle mass and quality as well as a shift in fiber-type distribution, changes in protein synthesis, reduced cell regeneration, and replacement of muscle with fat and increased fibrosis. This phenotype has been attributed to inflammatory mediators, proteolytic activation, increased apoptosis, and mitochondrial rearrangements (changes in mitochondrial dynamics as mentioned before) [79].

Interestingly, it has been reported a significant ATP reduction and oxygen consumption in elderly individuals; therefore, mitochondrial dysfunction has been proposed as the driving force which underlies both muscle-skeletal aging and sarcopenia, as well as other age-related diseases. However, it is important to consider that due to the differences in the methodologies to evaluate mitochondrial oxygen consumption, such as isolated mitochondria or detergent permeabilized muscle fibers, there are many controversies regarding the differences between mitochondrial dysfunctions in aged populations.

Despite the previous observation, in this section, we summarize the most relevant features described in mitochondrial energy metabolism that were performed in human samples from skeletal muscle. In this sense, in several studies mitochondrial damage measurements, such as the decrease in the mitochondrial content (number, mass and size), loss of mitochondrial dynamics, reduction in the mtDND copy number, the mitochondrial protein expression, the mitochondrial activity (ATP production), the decrease in mitochondrial enzymatic activities, and the increase in mitochondrial ROS production, appear as conventional biomarkers in an age-dependent manner in human samples from the *gastrocnemius*, *vastus lateralis*, and *soleus* muscles. Moreover, these muscles are the most affected in sarcopenia [80]. In agreement with this evidence, a study performed in 146 healthy men and women from 18 to 89 years demonstrated that mtDNA and mRNA abundance, as well as the mitochondrial ATP production, declined with advancing age [81]. Also, this study showed that mitochondrial proteins involved in mitochondrial bioenergetics, such as NADH dehydrogenase, pyruvate dehydrogenase (lipoamide) alpha 1, ubiquitous mitochondrial creatine kinase, citrate synthase, isocitrate dehydrogenase 2 ($NADP^+$), chain A ubiquitous mito-creatine kinase, adenine nucleotide translocator, aspartate aminotransferase 2, aconitase 2, and ubiquinol-cytochrome c reductase core protein I, significantly decreased in older individuals in comparison to the younger, suggesting that age-related functional changes in muscles are accompanied by a continuous decline in mitochondrial capacity for oxidative phosphorylation independent from gender. For instance, the Baltimore Longitudinal Study of Aging measured the link between decrease mitochondrial oxidative capacity and the altered walking performance in male participants from 24 to 97 years; interestingly, the results revealed that the impaired mitochondrial oxidative capacity directly affected the muscle performance and strength [82].

Gueugneau et al. performed an extensive proteomic analysis that unveiled the effect of aging on mitochondrial metabolism; this study was performed in samples from the *vastus lateralis* obtained from post-menopausal ($n = 13$ from 76 to 82 years) and adult women ($n = 11$, 48–61 years). The results showed that 67 proteins were differentially expressed in post-menopausal women in comparison to the adult ones; from these proteins a considerable amount corresponds to mitochondrial energy metabolism at tricarboxylic acid cycle (TCA), ETC, and OxPhos levels (pyruvate dehydrogenase E1 component subunit-β, dihydrolipoyl dehydrogenase, aconitase hydratase, NADH dehydrogenase iron-sulfur protein 2 of complex I, cytochrome b-c1 subunit from complex III and subunit 5A of cytochrome c oxidase of complex IV, ATP synthase subunit-β) [83]. With these data, the authors confirmed mitochondrial participation in muscle decline with aging and offered a new perspective about the role that estrogens might play in muscle decline and highlighted their importance for further studies.

In line with the free radical theory of aging, evidence suggests that mitochondrial ROS production is responsible for the mutations in the mtDNA-encoded genes of complexes I and IV, leading to the decrease in their activity and contributing concomitantly to the mitochondrial metabolism impairment in aged muscle [84]. As seen in several studies performed in human biopsies of skeletal muscle, the content of several mitochondrial proteins as well as the mtDNA decreased with age, whereas the level of oxidative DNA lesions, measured by the oxidation marker 8-oxo-deoxyguanosine, increased.

On the other side, in the literature several intervention studies have demonstrated that the effects of aging muscle decline could be prevented by exercise or by the combination of exercise and the consumption of food supplements, such as omega-3 polyunsaturated fatty acids (n-3-PUFAs), since these interventions demonstrated a significant increase in muscle mass, strength, regenerative capacity, mitochondrial respiratory capacity, and reestablishment of the mitochondrial metabolism [85, 86]. For example, Kent and Fitzgerald highlighted the importance of exercise training to increase the mitochondrial biogenesis and ATP production in muscle from an elderly population by the activation of the master regulator of the mitochondrial biogenesis PGC-1α [87]. Another study performed in 12 older (65–85 years) individuals that consumed 3.9 g of n-3-PUFAs during 16 weeks revealed that this treatment required exercise to improve the mitochondrial respiratory capacity levels [86]. Among other intervention studies, the caloric restriction in humans resulted beneficial at the cardiovascular and muscular levels and decreased the risk of tumorigenesis and atherosclerosis [88]. Additionally, studies performed in human skeletal muscle during caloric restriction showed that under this condition the transcription profile resembled the transcriptional profile of younger individuals. Among the signaling pathways activated under this condition are IGF-1/insulin pathway, inflammation, and mitochondrial biogenesis, which interestingly are also associated with longevity [89].

All the previous studies were performed in healthy elderly individuals, whose body mass index was normal (BMI = 18.5–24.9); however, a recent study performed in overweighted older individuals from the HIPA cohort ($n = 18$ around $85 \pm 6$ years and BMI = $28 \pm 1.7$) demonstrated that overweight induces a metabolic switch from oxidative to lactic acid fermentation metabolism that undermines muscle integrity (*vastus lateralis*) leading to sarcopenia and frailty. The mechanism that underlies this effect has been associated with a significant decrease in the catalytic subunit of the mitochondrial complexes I, III, IV, and ATP synthase subunits [90]. Therefore, it would be interesting to analyze whether intervention therapies, such as exercise and caloric restriction, could help to restore the normal function of mitochondria or revert the metabolic switch in this and other elderly cohorts.

In other studies and to avoid the surgical procedure to obtain human biopsies, Tyrell and collaborators developed a blood-based bioenergetic profiling strategy to measure systemic mitochondrial function that showed a similar OxPhos capacity in monocytes and platelets compared to permeabilized skeletal muscle [91]. Although this strategy results an attractive alternative to assess human mitochondrial metabolism, this test has been only performed in African green monkeys and requires to be studied in human samples. However, it seems promising for the aging bioenergetics field.

## Mitochondrial Metabolism in the Aged Heart

Chaudhary et al. state that despite the advances in medical and therapeutic sciences, age is one of the main risk factors for the development of cardiovascular diseases in the older population [92]. As we age the heart exhibits morphological and cellular changes that impact on its performance, for instance, the number of myocytes decreases and the size of the cardiomyocytes increases; additionally the accumulation of lipid and fibrosis areas also increases, and mitochondrial ROS production augments considerably. Together with these, elderly individuals show decreased ability to tolerate stress and the heart becomes more susceptible to hypertension and failure, due to the increased arterial stiffness in comparison to younger people. Interestingly, this phenomenon has been related to altered mitochondrial metabolism [93, 94].

To understand how aging impairs mitochondrial heart metabolism, it is essential to mention that the heart possesses two mitochondrial subpopulations that differ in both morphology and function. The first ones are the subsarcolemmal mitochondria, located beneath the plasma membrane, and the second ones are the interfibrillar mitochondria, located between the myofibrils [95]. The interfibrillar mitochondria seem responsible for heart disease during aging, since this population has shown alterations in morphology and function; in the subsequent paragraphs, we will focus on studies performed in this subpopulation.

The primary source of ATP in the heart is the fatty acid oxidation (FAO), via mitochondrial β-oxidation (<70%), and just a minor percentage of ATP comes from glucose metabolism. As we age, heart metabolism suffers a shift and turns glucose-dependent [96]. Despite this metabolic shift, the aged heart increases the expression of CD36, a protein that transports fatty acids (FA), and concomitantly increases FA uptake. However, since FAO is decreased, they tend to accumulate [93]. In a study performed in healthy young and old individuals, it was shown that during aging a decline in myocardial FA utilization and oxidation is observed, without altering the rates of glucose consumption [97]. Moreover, the activity from the complexes III and IV decreases significantly and the respirasomes (ETC complexes organization) are altered; this leads to a decrease in mitochondrial respiration and impaired OxPhos [98].

Another study performed on isolated mitochondria from the left atrial appendage tissue from aged patients free of atrial pathologies (≥65 years, $n = 26$) revealed that ETC complex I activity and the protein content of NDUFB (subunit of complex I), UQCRC2 (subunit of complex III), and COX2 (subunit of complex IV) significantly decreased, in comparison to young patients. Moreover, this study also reported that aging altered the expression profile of genes that encode for mitochondrial proteins implicated in mitochondrial bioenergetics in the heart. The main altered pathways were substrate metabolism (30%), OxPhos (13%), and TCA cycle (6%), as well as particular mitochondrial genes such as NDUFA6 (NADH, dehydrogenase ubiquinone 1 alpha subunit 6), ATP5G1, ACO2, IDH2, ME2, and PDHA1, which were downregulated in elderly patients [99]. This study provides valuable information about the association between the downregulation of genes involved in mitochondrial energetics and OxPhos with aging and simultaneously highlights the target that complex I and OxPhos represent in order to improve energy efficiency in the heart. Interestingly no significant differences were observed in sex distribution.

Likewise, some authors have suggest that defects in OxPhos might be associated with the increased propensity to open the mitochondrial permeability transition pore (MPTP) that rises apoptosis during aging and which has been explained due to the decrease in the mitochondrial cardiolipin content [100]. Although the mechanisms that lead to mitochondrial metabolism shifts in human aging are not completely understood, the literature reports that the failure in the mitochondrial metabolism of aged heart might be associated with mutations in the mtDNA. In this sense, the aged heart shows an increase over 15-fold on mtDNA mutations in comparison to hearts from young people [101]. Mutations in genes that encode *Polg-a*, responsible for mtDNA repair machinery, cytochrome b, and several subunits of the OxPhos system, lead to mitochondrial dysfunction and the concomitant protein oxidation that induces apoptosis. Interestingly, the mtDNA copy number from both subpopulations does not change with age, as it occurs in skeletal muscle and liver [93]. Besides, another study reported that cytochrome oxidase (complex IV) content and activity decreased in mitochondria obtained form aged human hearts [102]. Moreover, beyond mtDNA mutations in aging, mitochondrial metabolism might be affected by the regulation of mtDNA transcription factors such as STAT-3 and p53, which regulate the catalytic subunits of ETC complexes [103]. Unfortunately, these data have only been observed in murine models of aging and require further verification in human samples.

## Mitochondrial Metabolism in the Aged Brain

In normal conditions, the brain consumes around 25% of the total body glucose via glycolysis and mitochondrial OxPhos [104]. So besides the mitochondrial dynamics dysfunctions described above, during aging there is also a decline in energy production that directly impacts on neurotransmission, neuronal potential, and in excitotoxicity, leading to metabolic disorders and age-related neurodegenerative conditions (stroke and neurodegenerative disorders) [105]. Therefore, delving into the mitochondrial energy metabolism in the aged brain might bring clues about the potential therapeutic targets to prevent the decline in neuronal function, cognition, learning, and memory.

One of the main characteristics in the aged brain is a 30% decrease in the mitochondrial metabolism from neurons and glia compared to young subjects; this effect correlates with a reduction in neuronal ETC activity and an increase in oxidant production, suggesting that the decline in the mitochondrial metabolism might be responsible for brain dysfunction [106]. Moreover, it has been suggested that the decay in mitochondrial energy metabolism is also related to the decrease in $NAD^+$ availability and abnormal $NAD^+$/NADH ratio. An in vivo, non-invasive study, performed in healthy individuals from 21 to 68 years ($n$ = 17), showed that $NAD^+$/NADH ratio diminished in an age-dependent manner, and this effect was associated with a decrease in the $NAD^+$ levels, thus suggesting that this might be responsible for the shift of glucose-dependent metabolism toward a slower oxygen metabolism and a lower ATP production during aging [107]. These studies, developed in healthy individuals, are relevant since they bring information about metabolic features in healthy aging that could help to distinguish the threshold where mitochondrial energy metabolism failure becomes harmful for the brain, as occurs in PD, AD, and stroke.

It is known that AD patients show a TCA cycle disruption which concomitantly alters the ETC and the OxPhos activity [108]. In this sense, a genome-wide transcriptome study performed in late-onset AD patients aged 73–85 years revealed that several nuclear-encoded genes and mitochondrially encoded subunits of the ETC were under-expressed in specific brain regions, such as the posterior cingulate cortex and the CA1 area of the hippocampus, supporting the hypothesis that defects in the ETC underlie mitochondrial dysfunction and the following reduced energy production in AD [109]. Other factors that might contribute to hypometabolism in the aged brain are the increase in mtDNA mutations; nevertheless, this requires further investigation in human samples. For instance, in a respiratory chain enzymology study performed in neurons from idiopathic PD patients, the ETC complexes I and II were affected, and their mtDNA showed multiple deletions [110]. Besides, mutations in Polg result in mitochondrial defects in complexes I and IV [111] in *substantia nigra* from PD patients [111].

Finally, the literature also reports that several signaling pathways, such as insulin/IGF1 (IIS), JNK, and AMPK, modulate mitochondrial metabolism, and probably the disruption of these pathways also compromised mitochondrial function, as occurs in insulin-resistant patients [112].

## Concluding Remarks

The mitochondrial function has always been of paramount importance when studying aging and age-related diseases. At first view, this seems evident since mitochondria are responsible for providing energy for cellular functions, and they also participate in other relevant cellular processes as mentioned above. However, due to the difficulty of obtaining human samples, the knowledge obtained in elderly people is sparse. Despite this limitation, here we describe a tissue-specific signature of changes in mitochondrial energy metabolism and dynamics. For instance, as we age, the heart turns from a mitochondrial-dependent metabolism to glycolytic metabolism, while the neurons decrease both glycolysis and mitochondrial metabolism. Additionally, we also delve into mitochondrial dynamics in healthy aging and age-related disease that appear, summarized in Fig. 4.1.

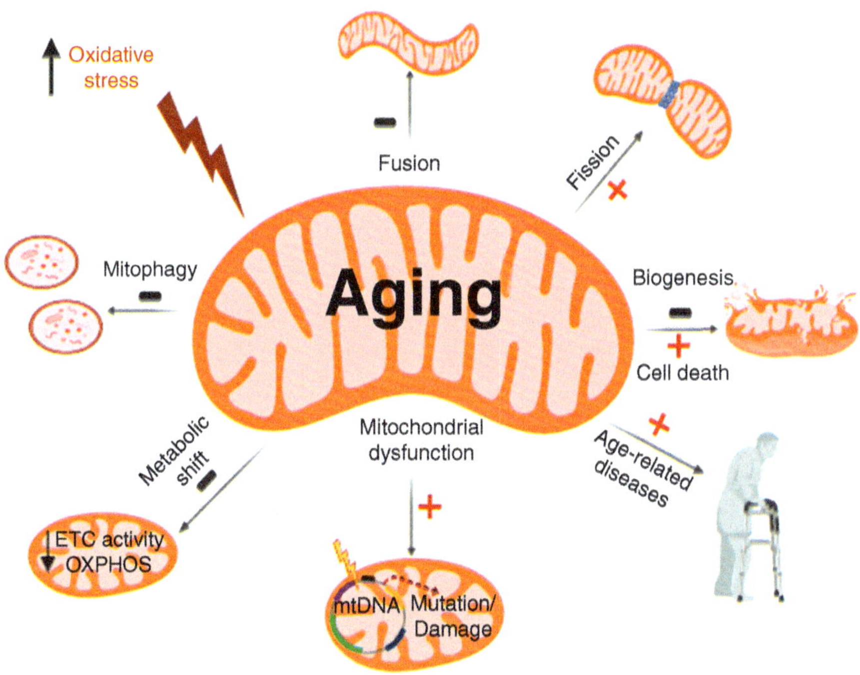


Fig. 4.1 Mitochondrial functions that appear altered in human aging. As we mention in this chapter, mitochondrial functions such as fission, fusion, biogenesis, mitophagy, and metabolism become altered as the organism ages. Therefore, this organelle could be considered as a promising target in aging

On the other hand, some interesting questions that remain to be resolved are how the alterations in mitochondrial dynamics are related to the energy metabolism, the decrease in the synthesis of ATP, and the generation of ROS? Although there are some ideas about it, very little is known. It should also be understood other mitochondrial processes that could be altered during old age, and that were almost not treated in this chapter, such as the transport of proteins into the mitochondria, the mitochondrial unfolded protein response (mtUPR), and the communication between the nuclear and mitochondrial genome.

All the previous suggests that the mitochondrial field still poses interesting crossroads that when studied will bring quite promising targets to improve human healthy aging.

**Acknowledgments** This work was supported by CONACYT grant FOSSIS-272256, as well as the "Red Temática de Investigación en Salud y Desarrollo Social" from CONACYT. Morales-Rosales is a CONACYT scholarship holder (CVU 718720 and scholarship number 702613). Authors thank Ariadna Guerrero-Cruz for the artwork.

## References

1. Suzman R, Beard JR, Boerma T, Chatterji S. Health in an ageing world – what do we know? Lancet. 2015;385:484–6.
2. Shadrach JL, Wagers AJ. Stem cells for skeletal muscle repair. Philos Trans R Soc Lond Ser B Biol Sci. 2011;366:2297–306.
3. López-Otín C, Blasco MA, Partridge L, Serrano M, Kroemer G. The hallmarks of aging. Cell. 2013;153:1194–217.
4. Webb M, Sideris DP, Biddle M. Modulation of mitochondrial dysfunction for treatment of disease. Bioorg Med Chem Lett. 2019;29:1270–7.
5. Salatto CT, Miller RA, Cameron KO, et al. Selective activation of AMPK β 1-containing isoforms improves kidney function in a rat model of diabetic nephropathy. J Pharmacol Exp Ther. 2017;361:303–11.
6. Murphy MP, Hartley RC. Mitochondria as a therapeutic target for common pathologies. Nat Rev Drug Discov. 2018;17:865.
7. Sivapathasuntharam C, Sivaprasad S, Hogg C, Jeffery G. Improving mitochondrial function significantly reduces the rate of age related photoreceptor loss. Exp Eye Res. 2019;185:107691.
8. Payne, B. A., & Chinnery, P. F. Mitochondrial dysfunction in aging: much progress but many unresolved questions. Biochimica et Biophysica Acta (BBA)-Bioenergetics. 2015;1847(11):1347–53.
9. Sastre J, Pallardó FV, Plá R, Pellín A, Juan G, O'Connor JE, Estrela JM, Miquel J, Viña J. Aging of the liver: age-associated mitochondrial damage in intact hepatocytes. Hepatology. 1996;24:1199–205.
10. Hagen TM, Yowe DL, Bartholomew JC, Wehr CM, Do KL, Park J-Y, Ames BN. Mitochondrial decay in hepatocytes from old rats: membrane potential declines, heterogeneity and oxidants increase. Proc Natl Acad Sci U S A. 1997;94:3064–9.
11. Greco M, Villani G, Mazzucchelli F, Bresolin N, Papa S, Attardi G. Marked aging-related decline in efficiency of oxidative phosphorylation in human skin fibroblasts. FASEB J. 2003;17:1706–8.
12. Ojaimi J, Masters CL, Opeskin K, McKelvie P, Byrne E. Mitochondrial respiratory chain activity in the human brain as a function of age. Mech Ageing Dev. 1999;111:39–47.
13. Trounce I, Byrne E, Marzuki S. Decline in skeletal muscle mitochondrial respiratory chain function: possible factor in ageing. Lancet. 1989;1:637–9.

14. Harman D. Aging: a theory based on free radical and radiation chemistry. J Gerontol. 1956;11:298–300.
15. Takamatsu C, Umeda S, Ohsato T, Ohno T, Abe Y, Fukuoh A, Shinagawa H, Hamasaki N, Kang D. Regulation of mitochondrial D-loops by transcription factor a and single-stranded DNA-binding protein. EMBO Rep. 2002;3:451–6.
16. Pinto M, Moraes CT. Mechanisms linking mtDNA damage and aging. Free Radic Biol Med. 2015;85:250–8.
17. DeBalsi KL, Hoff KE, Copeland WC. Role of the mitochondrial DNA replication machinery in mitochondrial DNA mutagenesis, aging and age-related diseases. Ageing Res Rev. 2017;33:89–104.
18. Scheibye-Knudsen M, Fang EF, Croteau DL, Wilson DM 3rd, Bohr VA. Protecting the mitochondrial powerhouse. Trends Cell Biol. 2015;25:158–70.
19. Akhmedov AT, Marín-García J. Mitochondrial DNA maintenance: an appraisal. Mol Cell Biochem. 2015;409:283–305.
20. Harman D. Aging: a theory based on free radical and radiation chemistry. Berkeley: University of California Radiation Laboratory; 1955.
21. Bua E, Johnson J, Herbst A, Delong B, McKenzie D, Salamat S, Aiken JM. Mitochondrial DNA–deletion mutations accumulate intracellularly to detrimental levels in aged human skeletal muscle fibers. Am J Hum Genet. 2006;79:469–80.
22. Taylor RW, Barron MJ, Borthwick GM, et al. Mitochondrial DNA mutations in human colonic crypt stem cells. J Clin Invest. 2003;112:1351–60.
23. Booth LN, Brunet A. The aging epigenome. Mol Cell. 2016;62:728–44.
24. Pustylnikov S, Costabile F, Beghi S, Facciabene A. Targeting mitochondria in cancer: current concepts and immunotherapy approaches. Transl Res. 2018;202:35–51.
25. Westermann B. Mitochondrial fusion and fission in cell life and death. Nat Rev Mol Cell Biol. 2010;11:872–84.
26. Youle RJ, van der Bliek AM. Mitochondrial fission, fusion, and stress. Science. 2012;337:1062–5.
27. Romanello V, Scalabrin M, Albiero M, Blaauw B, Scorrano L, Sandri M. Inhibition of the fission machinery mitigates OPA1 impairment in adult skeletal muscles. Cell. 2019;8:597.
28. Misgeld T, Schwarz TL. Mitostasis in neurons: maintaining mitochondria in an extended cellular architecture. Neuron. 2017;96:651–66.
29. Kornfeld OS, Qvit N, Haileselassie B, Shamloo M, Bernardi P, Mochly-Rosen D. Interaction of mitochondrial fission factor with dynamin related protein 1 governs physiological mitochondrial function in vivo. Sci Rep. 2018;8:14034.
30. Malka F et al. Separate fusion of outer and inner mitochondrial membranes. PubMed – NCBI. https://www.ncbi.nlm.nih.gov/pubmed/16113651. Accessed 5 Jul 2019.
31. Frezza C, Cipolat S, Martins de Brito O, et al. OPA1 controls apoptotic cristae remodeling independently from mitochondrial fusion. Cell. 2006;126:177–89.
32. Olichon A, Baricault L, Gas N, Guillou E, Valette A, Belenguer P, Lenaers G. Loss of OPA1 perturbates the mitochondrial inner membrane structure and integrity, leading to cytochrome c release and apoptosis. J Biol Chem. 2003;278:7743–6.
33. Levine B, Klionsky DJ. Development by self-digestion: molecular mechanisms and biological functions of autophagy. Dev Cell. 2004;6:463–77.
34. Wang Y, Qin Z-H. Coordination of autophagy with other cellular activities. Acta Pharmacol Sin. 2013;34:585–94.
35. Stolz A, Ernst A, Dikic I. Cargo recognition and trafficking in selective autophagy. Nat Cell Biol. 2014;16:495–501.
36. Wallace, D. C. A mitochondrial paradigm of metabolic and degenerative diseases, aging, and cancer: a dawn for evolutionary medicine. Annu. Rev. Genet. 2005;39:359–407.
37. Abdellatif M, Sedej S, Carmona-Gutierrez D, Madeo F, Kroemer G. Autophagy in cardiovascular aging. Circ Res. 2018;123:803–24.
38. Linton PJ et al. This old heart: cardiac aging and autophagy. PubMed – NCBI. https://www.ncbi.nlm.nih.gov/pubmed/25543002. Accessed 5 Jul 2019.

39. Xiao B, Sanders MJ, Carmena D, et al. Structural basis of AMPK regulation by small molecule activators. Nat Commun. 2013;4:3017.
40. Zhuang N, Li L, Chen S, Wang T. PINK1-dependent phosphorylation of PINK1 and Parkin is essential for mitochondrial quality control. Cell Death Dis. 2016;7:e2501.
41. Sekine S, Youle RJ. PINK1 import regulation; a fine system to convey mitochondrial stress to the cytosol. BMC Biol. 2018;16:2.
42. Narendra DP, Jin SM, Tanaka A, Suen D-F, Gautier CA, Shen J, Cookson MR, Youle RJ. PINK1 is selectively stabilized on impaired mitochondria to activate Parkin. PLoS Biol. 2010;8:e1000298.
43. Zhou C, Huang Y, Shao Y, May J, Prou D, Perier C, Dauer W, Schon EA, Przedborski S. The kinase domain of mitochondrial PINK1 faces the cytoplasm. Proc Natl Acad Sci U S A. 2008;105:12022–7.
44. Vives-Bauza C, Zhou C, Huang Y, et al. PINK1-dependent recruitment of Parkin to mitochondria in mitophagy. Proc Natl Acad Sci U S A. 2010;107:378–83.
45. Thai PN, Seidlmayer LK, Miller C, Ferrero M, Dorn GW II, Schaefer S, Bers DM, Dedkova EN. Mitochondrial quality control in aging and heart failure: influence of ketone bodies and Mitofusin-stabilizing peptides. Front Physiol. 2019;10:382.
46. Shiota, T., Traven, A., & Lithgow, T. Mitochondrial biogenesis: cell-cycle-dependent investment in making mitochondria. Current Biology. 2015;25(2):R78–R80.
47. Bouchez C, Devin A. Mitochondrial biogenesis and mitochondrial reactive oxygen species (ROS): a complex relationship regulated by the cAMP/PKA signaling pathway. Cell. 2019. https://doi.org/10.3390/cells8040287.
48. Wu Z, Puigserver P, Andersson U, et al. Mechanisms controlling mitochondrial biogenesis and respiration through the thermogenic coactivator PGC-1. Cell. 1999;98:115–24.
49. Pickrell, A. M., & Youle, R. J. The roles of PINK1, parkin, and mitochondrial fidelity in Parkinson's disease. Neuron. 2015;85(2):257–73.
50. Wang H, Song P, Du L, et al. Parkin ubiquitinates Drp1 for proteasome-dependent degradation: implication of dysregulated mitochondrial dynamics in Parkinson disease. J Biol Chem. 2011;286:11649–58.
51. Exner N, Treske B, Paquet D, et al. Loss-of-function of human PINK1 results in mitochondrial pathology and can be rescued by Parkin. J Neurosci. 2007;27:12413–8.
52. Schapira, A. H. Etiology of Parkinson's disease. Neurology. 2006; 66(10 suppl 4), S10–S23.
53. Baloyannis SJ. Mitochondrial alterations in Alzheimer's disease. J Alzheimers Dis. 2006;9:119–26.
54. Reddy PH, Tripathi R, Troung Q, et al. Abnormal mitochondrial dynamics and synaptic degeneration as early events in Alzheimer's disease: implications to mitochondria-targeted antioxidant therapeutics. Biochim Biophys Acta. 2012;1822:639–49.
55. Cho D-H, Nakamura T, Fang J, Cieplak P, Godzik A, Gu Z, Lipton SA. S-nitrosylation of Drp1 mediates beta-amyloid-related mitochondrial fission and neuronal injury. Science. 2009;324:102–5.
56. Marzetti E, Calvani R, Cesari M, Buford TW, Lorenzi M, Behnke BJ, Leeuwenburgh C. Mitochondrial dysfunction and sarcopenia of aging: from signaling pathways to clinical trials. Int J Biochem Cell Biol. 2013;45:2288–301.
57. Iqbal S, Ostojic O, Singh K, Joseph A-M, Hood DA. Expression of mitochondrial fission and fusion regulatory proteins in skeletal muscle during chronic use and disuse. Muscle Nerve. 2013;48:963–70.
58. Tezze C, Romanello V, Desbats MA, et al. Age-associated loss of OPA1 in muscle impacts muscle mass, metabolic homeostasis, systemic inflammation, and epithelial senescence. Cell Metab. 2017;25:1374–89.e6.
59. Favaro G, Romanello V, Varanita T, et al. DRP1-mediated mitochondrial shape controls calcium homeostasis and muscle mass. Nat Commun. 2019;10:2576.
60. Buso A, Comelli M, Picco R, et al. Mitochondrial adaptations in elderly and young men skeletal muscle following 2 weeks of bed rest and rehabilitation. Front Physiol. 2019;10:474.

61. Ghosh S, Lertwattanarak R, Lefort N, et al. Reduction in reactive oxygen species production by mitochondria from elderly subjects with normal and impaired glucose tolerance. Diabetes. 2011;60:2051–60.
62. Chen L, Gong Q, Stice JP, Knowlton AA. Mitochondrial OPA1, apoptosis, and heart failure. Cardiovasc Res. 2009;84:91–9.
63. Niemann B, Chen Y, Teschner M, Li L, Silber R-E, Rohrbach S. Obesity induces signs of premature cardiac aging in younger patients: the role of mitochondria. J Am Coll Cardiol. 2011;57:577–85.
64. Niemann B, Pan R, Teschner M, Boening A, Silber R-E, Rohrbach S. Age and obesity-associated changes in the expression and activation of components of the AMPK signaling pathway in human right atrial tissue. Exp Gerontol. 2013;48:55–63.
65. Boengler K, Kosiol M, Mayr M, Schulz R, Rohrbach S. Mitochondria and ageing: role in heart, skeletal muscle and adipose tissue. J Cachexia Sarcopenia Muscle. 2017;8:349–69.
66. Billia F, Hauck L, Konecny F, Rao V, Shen J, Mak TW. PTEN-inducible kinase 1 (PINK1)/Park6 is indispensable for normal heart function. Proceedings of the National Academy of Sciences. 2011;108(23):9572–77.
67. Manczak M, Calkins MJ, Reddy PH. Impaired mitochondrial dynamics and abnormal interaction of amyloid beta with mitochondrial protein Drp1 in neurons from patients with Alzheimer's disease: implications for neuronal damage. Hum Mol Genet. 2011;20:2495–509.
68. Kerr JS, Adriaanse BA, Greig NH, Mattson MP, Cader MZ, Bohr VA, Fang EF. Mitophagy and Alzheimer's disease: cellular and molecular mechanisms. Trends Neurosci. 2017;40: 151–66.
69. Srivastava, S. The mitochondrial basis of aging and age-related disorders. Genes. 2017;8(12):398.
70. Kitada M, Ogura Y, Monno I, Koya D. The impact of dietary protein intake on longevity and metabolic health. EBioMedicine. 2019;43:632–40.
71. Herst PM, Rowe MR, Carson GM, Berridge MV. Functional mitochondria in health and disease. Front Endocrinol. 2017;8:296.
72. López-Lluch G, Hernández-Camacho JD, Fernández-Ayala DJM, Navas P. Mitochondrial dysfunction in metabolism and ageing: shared mechanisms and outcomes? Biogerontology. 2018;19:461–80.
73. Long YC, Tan TMC, Takao I, Tang BL. The biochemistry and cell biology of aging: metabolic regulation through mitochondrial signaling. Am J Physiol Endocrinol Metab. 2014;306:E581–91.
74. Zhang R, Wang Y, Ye K, Picard M, Gu Z. Independent impacts of aging on mitochondrial DNA quantity and quality in humans. BMC Genomics. 2017;18:890.
75. Hebert SL, Lanza IR, Nair KS. Mitochondrial DNA alterations and reduced mitochondrial function in aging. Mech Ageing Dev. 2010;131:451–62.
76. Liu D, Li H, Lu J, Bai Y. Tissue-specific implications of mitochondrial alterations in aging. Front Biosci. 2013;5:734–47.
77. Nissanka N, Moraes CT. Mitochondrial DNA damage and reactive oxygen species in neurodegenerative disease. FEBS Lett. 2018;592:728–42.
78. Hughes VA, Frontera WR, Wood M, Evans WJ, Dallal GE, Roubenoff R, Fiatarone Singh MA. Longitudinal muscle strength changes in older adults: influence of muscle mass, physical activity, and health. J Gerontol A Biol Sci Med Sci. 2001;56:B209–17.
79. Lenk K, Schuler G, Adams V. Skeletal muscle wasting in cachexia and sarcopenia: molecular pathophysiology and impact of exercise training. J Cachexia Sarcopenia Muscle. 2010;1:9–21.
80. Carter HN, Chen CCW, Hood DA. Mitochondria, muscle health, and exercise with advancing age. Physiology. 2015;30:208–23.
81. Short KR, Bigelow ML, Kahl J, Singh R, Coenen-Schimke J, Raghavakaimal S, Nair KS. Decline in skeletal muscle mitochondrial function with aging in humans. Proc Natl Acad Sci. 2005;102:5618–23.

82. Zane AC, Reiter DA, Shardell M, Cameron D, Simonsick EM, Fishbein KW, Studenski SA, Spencer RG, Ferrucci L. Muscle strength mediates the relationship between mitochondrial energetics and walking performance. Aging Cell. 2017;16:461–8.
83. Gueugneau M, Coudy-Gandilhon C, Gourbeyre O, et al. Proteomics of muscle chronological ageing in post-menopausal women. BMC Genomics. 2014;15:1165.
84. Peterson CM, Johannsen DL, Ravussin E. Skeletal muscle mitochondria and aging: a review. J Aging Res. 2012;2012:1–20.
85. Distefano G, Goodpaster BH. Effects of exercise and aging on skeletal muscle. Cold Spring Harb Perspect Med. 2018. https://doi.org/10.1101/cshperspect.a029785.
86. Lalia AZ, Dasari S, Robinson MM, Abid H, Morse DM, Klaus KA, Lanza IR. Influence of omega-3 fatty acids on skeletal muscle protein metabolism and mitochondrial bioenergetics in older adults. Aging. 2017;9:1096–129.
87. Kent JA, Fitzgerald LF. In vivo mitochondrial function in aging skeletal muscle: capacity, flux, and patterns of use. J Appl Physiol. 2016;121:996–1003.
88. Fontana L, Meyer TE, Klein S, Holloszy JO. Long-term calorie restriction is highly effective in reducing the risk for atherosclerosis in humans. Proc Natl Acad Sci U S A. 2004;101:6659–63.
89. Mercken EM, Crosby SD, Lamming DW, et al. Calorie restriction in humans inhibits the PI3K/AKT pathway and induces a younger transcription profile. Aging Cell. 2013;12:645–51.
90. Potes Y, Pérez-Martinez Z, Bermejo-Millo JC, et al. Overweight in the elderly induces a switch in energy metabolism that undermines muscle integrity. Aging Dis. 2019;10:217–30.
91. Tyrrell DJ, Bharadwaj MS, Jorgensen MJ, Register TC, Molina AJA. Blood cell respirometry is associated with skeletal and cardiac muscle bioenergetics: implications for a minimally invasive biomarker of mitochondrial health. Redox Biol. 2016;10:65–77.
92. Chaudhary KR, El-Sikhry H, Seubert JM. Mitochondria and the aging heart. J Geriatr Cardiol. 2011;8:159–67.
93. Lesnefsky EJ, Chen Q, Hoppel CL. Mitochondrial metabolism in aging heart. Circ Res. 2016;118:1593–611.
94. Sun Z. Aging, arterial stiffness, and hypertension. Hypertension. 2015;65:252–6.
95. Palmer JW, Tandler B, Hoppel CL. Biochemical properties of subsarcolemmal and interfibrillar mitochondria isolated from rat cardiac muscle. J Biol Chem. 1977;252:8731–9.
96. Wei Y-H, Wu S-B, Ma Y-S, Lee H-C. Respiratory function decline and DNA mutation in mitochondria, oxidative stress and altered gene expression during aging. Chang Gung Med J. 2009;32:113–32.
97. Kates AM, Herrero P, Dence C, Soto P, Srinivasan M, Delano DG, Ehsani A, Gropler RJ. Impact of aging on substrate metabolism by the human heart. J Am Coll Cardiol. 2003;41:293–9.
98. Gómez LA, Monette JS, Chavez JD, Maier CS, Hagen TM. Supercomplexes of the mitochondrial electron transport chain decline in the aging rat heart. Arch Biochem Biophys. 2009;490:30–5.
99. Emelyanova L, Preston C, Gupta A, et al. Effect of aging on mitochondrial energetics in the human atria. J Gerontol A Biol Sci Med Sci. 2018;73:608–16.
100. Paradies G, Paradies V, Ruggiero FM, Petrosillo G. Changes in the mitochondrial permeability transition pore in aging and age-associated diseases. Mech Ageing Dev. 2013;134:1–9.
101. Chistiakov DA, Sobenin IA, Revin VV, Orekhov AN, Bobryshev YV. Mitochondrial aging and age-related dysfunction of mitochondria. Biomed Res Int. 2014;2014:238463.
102. Müller-Höcker J. Cytochrome-c-oxidase deficient cardiomyocytes in the human heart – an age-related phenomenon. A histochemical ultracytochemical study. Am J Pathol. 1989;134:1167–73.
103. Wegrzyn J, Potla R, Chwae J-Y, et al. Function of mitochondrial Stat3 in cellular respiration. Science. 2009;323:793–7.
104. Yin F, Sancheti H, Patil I, Cadenas E. Energy metabolism and inflammation in brain aging and Alzheimer's disease. Free Radic Biol Med. 2016;100:108–22.

105. Selvaraji S, Poh L, Natarajan V, Mallilankaraman K, Arumugam TV. Negative conditioning of mitochondrial dysfunction in age-related neurodegenerative diseases. Cond Med. 2019;2:30–9.
106. Boumezbeur F, Mason GF, de Graaf RA, Behar KL, Cline GW, Shulman GI, Rothman DL, Petersen KF. Altered brain mitochondrial metabolism in healthy aging as assessed by in vivo magnetic resonance spectroscopy. J Cereb Blood Flow Metab. 2010;30:211–21.
107. Zhu X-H, Lu M, Lee B-Y, Ugurbil K, Chen W. In vivo NAD assay reveals the intracellular NAD contents and redox state in healthy human brain and their age dependences. Proc Natl Acad Sci U S A. 2015;112:2876–81.
108. Blass JP, Sheu RK, Gibson GE. Inherent abnormalities in energy metabolism in Alzheimer disease. Interaction with cerebrovascular compromise. Ann N Y Acad Sci. 2000;903:204–21.
109. Liang WS, Reiman EM, Valla J, et al. Alzheimer's disease is associated with reduced expression of energy metabolism genes in posterior cingulate neurons. Proc Natl Acad Sci U S A. 2008;105:4441–6.
110. Grünewald A, Rygiel KA, Hepplewhite PD, Morris CM, Picard M, Turnbull DM. Mitochondrial DNA depletion in respiratory chain-deficient Parkinson disease neurons. Ann Neurol. 2016;79:366–78.
111. Reeve A, Meagher M, Lax N, Simcox E, Hepplewhite P, Jaros E, Turnbull D. The impact of pathogenic mitochondrial DNA mutations on substantia nigra neurons. J Neurosci. 2013;33:10790–801.
112. Lowell BB. Mitochondrial dysfunction and type 2 diabetes. Science. 2005;307:384–7.

# Genomic Tools Used in Molecular Clinical Aging Research

5

Alfredo García-Venzor
and Edna Ayerim Mandujano-Tinoco

## Abbreviations

| | |
|---|---|
| ChIP | Chromatin immunoprecipitation |
| ChIP-seq | ChIP sequencing |
| DMR | Differentially methylated regions |
| DNA | Deoxyribonucleic acid |
| DNAmet | DNA methylation |
| FACS | Fluorescence-activated cell sorting |
| LCM | Laser capture microdissection |
| mtDNA | Mitochondrial DNA |
| NGS | Next-generation sequencing |
| RNA | Ribonucleic acid |
| RNA-seq | RNA sequencing |
| scRNA-seq | Single-cell RNA-seq |
| SCS | Single-cell sequencing |
| SMS | Single-molecule sequencing |
| WES | Whole-exome sequencing |
| WGS | Whole-genome sequencing |

A. García-Venzor
Epigenetics Laboratory, Instituto Nacional de Medicina Genómica, Mexico City, Mexico

E. A. Mandujano-Tinoco (✉)
Laboratory of Connective Tissue, Instituto Nacional de Rehabilitación "Luis Guillermo Ibarra Ibarra", Mexico City, Mexico



J. C. Gomez-Verjan, N. A. Rivero-Segura (eds.), *Clinical Genetics and Genomics of Aging*, https://doi.org/10.1007/978-3-030-40955-5_5

## Introduction

In recent decades, biological and biomedical research has developed different technologies that generate enormous quantities of biological data, which have been grouped under the generic name of high-throughput "-omics" technologies. The "omics" technologies have been used for several applications such as genomic, exomic, transcriptomic, proteomic, metagenomic, microbiome, and metabolomic analysis. The growing use of high-throughput technologies is mainly due to a considerable reduction in sequencing costs and an increase in the data obtained from each analysis [1]. For example, first-generation sequencing (e.g., Sanger sequencing and shotgun sequencing) owed the first human genome assembly in the Human Genome Project (HGP). However, this project spent 3.4 billion dollars, took 13 years to complete, and required the collaboration of hundreds of international research groups. With the advent of next-generation sequencing technologies (NGS technologies) in 2007, the cost of whole-genome sequencing dropped rapidly. Then, the introduction of HiSeq X by Illumina in 2014 allowed the sequencing of the complete human genome by USD 1000, and with this machine 16 complete human genomes can be sequenced at a depth of 30X in only 3 days [2]. Common next-generation applications include DNA-seq, RNA-seq, ChIP-seq, and methyl-seq.

Next-generation sequencing results are millions to billions of short sequence reads that are sequenced simultaneously, allowing a high speed in data production. The biochemistry and the specific methods for template library production, amplification, and fragment sequencing vary from any technology, but all of them use a massive matrix configuration, like microarray technologies, to sequence millions of fragments in parallel. The sequencing is usually done by microscopic observation and recording of optical phenomena during the sequential and iterative cycle of the serial extension of a DNA template by a DNA polymerase or a ligase [3, 4].

All next-generation sequencing platforms use similar workflows. The overall workflow for an NGS experiment is schematized in Fig. 5.1. To begin an NGS sequencing experiment, biological material must be obtained, genomic DNA is used in whole-genome sequencing (WGS) and whole-exome sequencing (WES), and RNA is used for complete transcriptome sequencing (RNA-seq) or the sequencing of specific transcript populations (small RNA or miRNA sequencing). The second stage is the library construction, in which the DNA or RNA molecules are sheared randomly or in a controlled manner to obtain small fragments of DNA or RNA. In the case of RNA being the starting material, it is necessary to synthesize the first and second cDNA strands. The double-stranded DNA fragments (obtained after the second strand synthesis in RNA-seq experiments) are ligated with adaptor sequences in both ends; these adaptor sequences include: (1) an index sequence to identify the sample from which each read comes, (2) sequences allowing fragment immobilization in the matrix, and (3) sequences needed for fragment amplification and sequencing. The mixture of adaptor-bound double-stranded DNA fragments from a sample is known as the library, which is then denatured and immobilized as single-stranded DNA molecules on a solid surface (a planar matrix or beads). Once the library is immobilized in the sequencing surface, different strategies (bridge

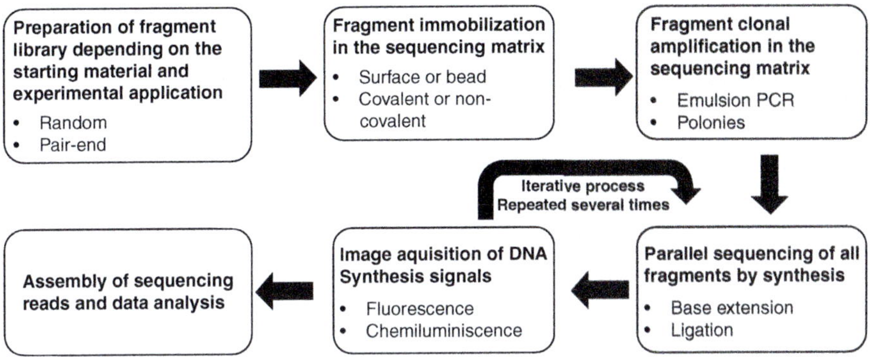


**Fig. 5.1** Next-generation sequencing experiments' general workflow. The general phases requiring an NGS experiment, including the different experimental approaches that could be used in each step, are schematized. The first phase is the construction of a double-stranded cDNA library. After library construction, the cDNA fragments are immobilized in the sequencing matrix (horizontal surface or beads) through covalent or non-covalent binding. Once immobilized, each fragment is amplified by emulsion PCR or polonies (clusters of millions of identical sequences). Then, the fragments are individually sequenced in parallel by base extension (DNA polymerization reaction) or by ligation (ligase reaction). The incorporation of every new base generates a signal that could be fluorescent or chemiluminescent. The data generated by the sequencing of every cDNA fragment is analyzed in terms of quality and biological representativeness

PCR [5], emulsion PCR [6], or in situ polonies [7]) are used to clonally amplify each DNA fragment generating millions of "clusters" consisting of thousands of copies of the same fragment. These individual clusters form a DNA cluster array that is now sequenced by the action of an enzyme: DNA polymerase or DNA ligase. The addition of each new base by the sequencing enzyme produces an optic signal in the form of fluorescence or chemiluminescence that can be recorded as images using a CCD camera. Sequential images of each nucleotide-addition step allow the construction of each fragment sequence; these fragments could be then assembled into larger sequence contigs to assembly the whole-genome sequence or can be used to determine the relative frequency of every transcript in RNA-seq experiments.

In NGS sequencing experiments, planning is generally performed based on the sequencing coverage. Sequencing coverage is defined as the average number of reads that align with known reference bases. Sequencing coverage refers to the number of times that each base in a reference genome was sequenced or the number of reads containing that base. Each sequencing experiment has specific coverage requirements and depends mainly on the read length, genome size, application (if it is for WGS, WES, or RNA-seq or if it is pretended to find low represented mutations in a population or low-expression transcripts), established guidelines in the literature, gene expression level, genome complexity, and error rate of sequencing methodology [8–11]. To achieve desirable results, optimal sequencing coverage should be defined based on these criteria. Three different metrics are used to evaluate NGS coverage: interquartile range (IQR), which measures the variability in coverage values between bases and indicates nonuniform coverage distribution in the data obtained; mean read depth, which measures the average of how many reads are probable to align in a given reference base position; and raw read depth, which is the total number of reads obtained per sample and divided by reference genome size; this parameter does not consider the number of aligned reads and can be larger than the aligned read depth [10].

One of the major drawbacks in NGS technologies is the relatively small reads obtained, which are up to 500pb length in pyrosequencing (Roche 454 genome sequencer) and roughly 50pb for Illumina Gene Analyzer. In order to generate new sequencing technologies that boost the size of sequencing reads, great efforts have been made to develop single-molecule sequencing (SMS) platforms. In SMS sequencing, synthesis is accomplished by single DNA molecule arrays without the amplification step performed in NGS sequencing platforms. This no-amplification procedure allows an increase in the number of DNA molecules tested to improve the throughput, the absence of PCR reduces the price of sequencing, and this technology also increases the length of sequencing reads [12–14].

In the present chapter, we will review different experimental NGS strategies that have been used in the study of human aging. We also include experiments in animal models that have contributed to obtaining relevant experimental data and great advances in the field. Genomics and its derivative techniques are a great promise to transform biogerontology as they serve to better understand the biological mechanisms underlying the complex phenomenon of aging and age-related diseases.

## Exome and Whole-Genome Sequencing

One common and widely used application of NGS in aging studies is DNA-seq, where the molecule to be analyzed is the genomic DNA of one organism or cell population. In DNA-seq experiments, the whole genomic DNA molecule could be sequenced (whole-genome sequencing, WGS), or it can be directed to specific genomic target regions, for example, the coding regions in the genome called exons (whole-exome sequencing, WES) [15]. This application aims to identify novel genomic variations and to correlate genomic variations with a particular phenotypic trait or disease. These genomic variations are studied in the form of single-nucleotide variants (SNVs), like SNPs, small DNA insertions or deletions (indels), copy number variations (CNVs), or other structural variants (SVs) [1]. WGS approach has the advantage of analyzing the complete genomic material, including non-coding regions (typically transcribed into non-coding RNAs), regulatory regions (such as promoters and enhancers), and introns with splicing regulatory elements. But it has two big disadvantages, the complexity of the analysis and the reduced number of samples analyzed per run. The suggested sequencing coverage for WGS ranges from 15X for homozygous SNVs to 60X for indels [8, 16]. In the case of the WES approach, it has the benefit of focusing only on genomic variants of protein-coding regions that have a direct impact on the phenotype of the cell. The coding regions account for less than 2% of the human genome, thus increasing the number of samples and the sequencing coverage per sequencing run. A disadvantage of this approach is that non-coding regions are not evaluated. The recommended sequencing coverage for WES experiments is 100X for homozygous and heterozygous SNVs [9].

Before the advent of NGS technologies, several scientists were interested in the study of allele variants associated with aging, but they were limited by the lack of aging rate biomarkers. Now with NGS technologies, these biomarkers have been emerged such as the epigenetic clock that is described in the DNA methylation sequencing section of this chapter. In this post-genomic era, different strategies have been developed in order to understand the genetic factors involved in aging [17]. One strategy used is the study of aging in extreme longevity groups of people, called centenarians. Centenarians are a group that can reach an age above 100 years and has an incidence of 1 every 10,000 people [18]. In a pioneering study using extreme longevity people (308 individuals belonging to 137 sibships showing extreme longevity), genome-wide scan analysis identified a region on chromosome 4 associated with extreme longevity [19] that corresponds to the microsomal transfer protein (MTP) [20], which is associated with abetalipoproteinemia and hypobeta lipoproteinemia in humans [21, 22]. Another approach to study the genetic factors involved in longevity consists in assessing allele frequencies from people of different ages, looking for those polymorphisms (SNPs) with enhanced allele frequencies in high-longevity individuals. Those alleles with diminished frequencies in aged individuals may be associated with age-related diseases. Using this approximation, an SNP that shifts isoleucine to valine was identified in the PKA-anchoring protein (AKAP2) gene. This polymorphism is associated with reduced longevity and cardiac disease [23]. Genome-wide association studies (GWAS) have confirmed only three loci that affect longevity: FOXO3A, APOE, and an intergenic locus on chromosome 5q33.3 [24–26].

Interestingly, in a recent WGS study of 17 supercentenarians (110 years or older), any allelic variant significantly associated with long longevity was found [27]. Some scientists have also focused on the study of healthy aging based on the hypothesis that this group of people is possibly enriched in allelic variants that confer reduced risk of age-associated diseases [28]. Novel sequencing of genomes from healthy aging individuals found that healthy aging is a divergent phenotype of exceptional longevity with no significant genetic contribution. Interestingly, the authors found that FOXO3A, a longevity allele, may not be related to healthy aging phenotype [29].

Aging is a complex process usually accompanied by the onset of different diseases like neurodegenerative disorders (Alzheimer's disease and Parkinson's disease), cardiovascular illnesses, and cancer. The study of the genetic basis of these aging-related diseases is another approach in the study of the genomic basis of aging. Genome-wide approaches studying rare allelic variants associated with cognitive aging have revealed that allele variants of apolipoprotein E (APOE), catechol-o-methyl transferase (COMT), brain-derived neurotrophic factor (BDNF), and dystrobrevin-binding protein (DRNBP1) could be involved in cognitive aging rates in humans [30]. Following this approach and using WGS, it was observed a new polymorphism in a chemokine gene cluster (including CCL11) in chromosome 17 which is associated with a late onset of familial Alzheimer's disease [31]. Other studies have used WGS technology to associate other allelic variants (RAB10, MYRF, ASRGL1, TECPR2, and CINP) with Alzheimer's disease and cognitive aging [32–34]. As stated, WGS is important because it also gives information about allele variants of non-coding genes, which are important in the regulation of several processes. Using WGS, it was possible to identify a novel non-coding variant, EN1, which is highly associated with BMD (bone mineral density) and the risk of osteoporotic fractures in aging [35].

Researchers have hypothesized that the aging process may be the result of accelerated accumulation of somatic mutations; these mutations may cause changes (more or less severe) in the primary structure, folding, and function of proteins which finally deteriorates the homeostasis of several tissues. In a pioneering study, the whole genome of two pairs of twins (one pair of 40 years old and other of 100 years old) was sequenced. The results showed that 100-year-old twins were genetically identical and had no increase in the accumulation of somatic mutations in blood [36]. However, another study using WES in which postmortem hippocampal of 52 Alzheimer's patients and blood samples of 11 healthy individuals were analyzed discovered that older Alzheimer's patients accumulated SNVs in genes implicated in PI3K-AKT, MAPK, and AMPK pathways [37]. These results suggest that the higher sequencing depth provided by WES serves to find very low represented SNVs in small fractions of cells.

WES has been extensively used in the analysis of genetic contributors to age-related diseases. In a Turkish family with a history of neurological disorders, a WES study identified NOTCH3 as a previously unknown Alzheimer's disease-associated gene [38]. A similar strategy was used to demonstrate that the TREML2 missense variant pS144G protects against Alzheimer's disease [39]. Using also WES technology, a novel INO80 allele missense variant (Ser818Cys) was identified to be responsible for the premature aging phenotype (aortic hypoplasia, calcific atherosclerosis, systolic hypertension, and premature cataract) [40]. Since INO80 is a chromatin remodeling complex, this result suggests that chromatin structure regulation is associated with aging phenotypes. In Parkinson's disease, WGS of large populations has demonstrated several novel allelic variants in genes (GPATCS2L, UHRF1BP1L, PTPRH, ARSB, and VPS13C) associated with disease onset [41].

Whole-exome sequencing has also been used to study novel allele variants associated with the centenarian phenotype. For example, the WES analysis of the complete coding genome of an Iranian supercentenarian found 14 allelic variants associated with exceptional longevity [42], showing the polygenetic nature of longevity and aging. In contrast, a robust study with a cohort of 100 centenarian individuals (between 98 and 108 years old) from the Georgia Centenarian Study (GCS), the WES analysis found only three alleles (LYST, MDN1, RBMXL1) associated with extremely longevity and also identified several allele variants associated with Alzheimer's disease risk (TREM2, EPHA2, ABCA7, PLD3, MAPT, and NOTCH3) [43].

Studying the aging rate of individual tissues is another way to study aging. In a WES study about the genetic factors influencing the youth aspect of skin in South Korean women, several SNPs were associated with wrinkle severity (rs73064632 in

APOBEC1 gene), with lighter skin color (rs12211728 in CLPSL1 gene), and with skin hydration (rs10412066 in ZNF100 gene) [44]. About cognitive aging, a comparative WES analysis of 56 people of more than 80 years with 22 individuals with Alzheimer's disease showed 3 SNPs (rs2363221, rs2230435, and rs736103) in MAP2K3 (mitogen-activated protein kinase 3) gene, suggesting a biological relation of this gene in age-related memory decline [45]. Even these studies have generated valuable information about the deterioration of some organs, it is also important to focus genome-wide studies in those super-aged healthy individuals with genetic alleles that protect against specific age-related decay processes.

Whole-genome and whole-exome sequencing are technologies that generate robust results and confident candidate genes in a cost-effective larger sample cohort. NGS is thus used to improve the study of the biological aging phenomenon and medical surveillance of the aged population with preventive therapy in people with age-related disease risk alleles. It is also useful to introduce genomic medicine in the medical treatment of old individuals in order to advance into personalized medicine.

## Transcriptome Sequencing

Because aging is a complex phenomenon affected by the interaction of environmental factors and the genetic burden of individuals, genomic research of genotypes is not enough to fully understand aging and its biological associated processes. In this regard, the information about the expression levels of certain genes could shed light on their implications in molecular pathways related to aging and age-related diseases. Transcriptomic assays are a new approximation to study qualitative and quantitative changes in gene expression, allowing the simultaneous analysis of thousands of transcripts. Several high-throughput technologies have been used for transcriptomic analysis, such as SAGE, microarray, and more recently RNA-seq technologies. Pioneering studies used SAGE and microarray technologies to study the transcriptome modifications associated with tissue aging [46]. However, with the advent of NGS, RNA-seq technology was incorporated into aging research. RNA-seq is a robust technology that enables a deep transcriptome analysis as it can identify novel transcripts, gene fusion products, rare splice variants, and low-expression RNAs and reveals gene boundaries at a single-base resolution, which microarrays cannot do [47, 48]. In this section, we will focus on aging biology research based on RNA-seq.

For RNA-seq experiments, the total or fractioned (e.g., only poly (A) + RNA or small size RNA populations) RNA sample is converted into double-stranded cDNA fragments in which adaptors are ligated. The cDNA library is high-throughput sequenced from one of its ends (single-end sequencing) or from both ends (paired-end sequencing) generating millions of 30–400pb reads. The reads are mapped to a reference transcriptome or genome, and the resulting transcript counts represent the cellular transcriptome. Differences in gene expression are calculated based on the number of reads that align with that specific transcript between a control and an experimental condition. RNA-seq results are usually normalized according to the gene length, as larger transcripts have more reads per RNA molecule than shorter transcripts [48, 49].

In aging, transcriptome analyses are used to study the changes in gene expression of specific tissues due to age-related processes. For example, impaired bone formation is a hallmark of age-related bone loss and is regulated by estrogens in post-menopausal women. In an attempt to identify the molecular pathways involved in this bone loss during aging, scientists sequenced the transcriptomes of bone biopsies from young, old, and estrogen-treated old woman. The study found that Wnt/β--catenin regulates age-related bone loss, with a significant downregulation of the LEF1 transcription factor. Interestingly, the estrogen treatment reversed the age-related expression of genes such as INHBB (inhibin beta B polypeptide), indicating an important but narrow impact in transcriptome due to estrogen treatment [50]. Following a similar strategy, the aging effect on gene expression and DNA methylation of bone marrow mesenchymal cells (BMMC) from young and old women has been studied. BMMC are the progenitors for osteoblasts which are necessary for bone deposition. In BMMC from old women, transcriptional changes associated with different molecular pathways (protein synthesis and degradation, mTOR, GAP junction, calcium, melatonin, and NFAT signaling pathways) are mediated by differential DNA methylation of its gene promoters [51]. RNA-seq analyses of kidney samples found that transcriptional changes observed in Renin-expressing cells (CoRL, progenitors of glomerular cells) during aging rely greatly on the sex of the individual [52].

Furthermore, RNA-seq has also been used to study the transcriptome of secreted extracellular vesicles (EVs). These EVs are released by the majority of living cells as intercellular communication players due to their target cell specificity. Types of EV's transcriptome sequencing are exosomes, bilayer membrane vesicles (20–200 nm) packaged with microRNAs (miRNAs), messenger RNAs (mRNAs), long non-coding RNAs (lncRNAs), and proteins [53]. Exosomes are important in biological processes as their cargo molecules regulate cellular physiology in a paracrine manner. Because exosomes are present in all biological fluids, RNA sequencing is an easy way to study exosome cargo and its function. With this approach it was found that the expression of RNAs contained in exosomes, released into the cerebrospinal fluid (CSF) of old patients with Alzheimer's and Parkinson's diseases, changes compared to healthy controls. Also, several of the differentially expressed miRNAs in these exosomes are associated with the disease onset and progression [54].

Biological models like the mouse (*Mus musculus*), fruit fly (*Drosophila melanogaster*), and *Caenorhabditis elegans* are commonly used to study conserved age-associated pathways and physiological processes which could be translated into human aging physiology. In the marine mollusk *Aplysia californica*, neurological aging is studied through behavioral deficits in the tail-withdrawal reflex observed in aged animals. Previously, it was observed that aged animals had a reduced excitation in the sensorial neurons that controls this reflex. Studying the transcriptome of these sensorial neurons in sexually mature and old animals, it was found that the expression of ion channels as well as genes involved in memory and learning is downregulated during aging, while several stress response genes are upregulated [55]. In another study, it was found that 13 upregulated and 16 downregulated transcripts are age-regulated in nematodes (*C. elegans*), zebrafish (*D. rerio*), and mice (*M. musculus*). Posterior RNAi studies demonstrated that the *bcat-1* gene (branched-chain amino acid transferase-1) silencing increases the nematode lifespan due to an increase in branched-chain amino acids (BCAAs) reducing a neuroendocrine signal [56].

Interestingly, this data could suggest that many of the changes in the expression of age-related transcriptomes could represent adaptive changes against aging. Another study used RNA-seq and proteomic approaches to study aging in a model of premature aging cell lines from patients with Hutchinson-Gilford progeria syndrome (HGPS). These analyses revealed that ribose-phosphate pyrophosphokinase 1 (PRPS1) and purine levels were downregulated in progerin expressing cell lines. Interestingly, the supplementation with S-adenosyl methionine (SAMe) reduced the senescence phenotype in cells expressing progerin [57].

One important contribution of RNA-seq to genomic studies is its high confidence in the discovery of novel transcripts such as long non-coding RNAs (lncRNAs) and circular RNAs (circRNAs). These transcripts remained largely undiscovered because its analysis using microarrays was very expensive before NGS technology advent. lncRNAs are a heterogeneous class of RNA transcripts that are not transcribed into proteins, are longer than 200 nt, and are highly spatial-temporal regulated. In a study using prefrontal cortex samples from 2 to 60 years old individuals, it was found that during prefrontal cortex aging, certain groups of lncRNAs change their expression in an age-related manner. Some lncRNAs like MALAT1 or Gomafu were associated with specific age-related phenotypes like age-dependent decrease in neurogenesis [58, 59]. Also, the identification of differentially expressed ncRNAs between young adult (4 months) and aged male mouse livers (28 months) showed that several non-coding RNAs participate in the molecular regulation of age-related changes in the liver. For example, Neat1 is a downregulated lncRNA involved in the paraspeckle formation and nuclear retention of mRNAs in aged livers [60, 61]. Also, mtDNA-transcribed lncRNA (ASncmtRNA2) is a mitochondrially encoded lncRNA which overexpression participates in the regulation of age-associated cardiovascular diseases as it is a non-canonical precursor for hsa-miR-4485 and hsa-miR-1973 microRNAs [62]. These studies demonstrate that not only coding genes (which represent only 2% of the genome sequence) are implicated in aging regulation, but also lncRNAs and microRNAs participate in tissue age-related changes.

circRNAs are non-coding covalently closed single-stranded transcripts produced by joining a 5′ splice donor with a 3′ splice acceptor of their parent molecules, which are usually mRNAs [63]. Recent studies have demonstrated that circular isoforms are more numerous than linear isoforms of the same locus, suggesting an important function for circRNA molecules [64]. It has been proposed that circRNAs could regulate gene expression at various levels by functioning as microRNA sponges or interacting with RNA-binding proteins that regulate translation and decay of certain mRNAs [65, 66]. In the brain, it has also been reported an increase in circRNA expression and accumulation [67, 68]. Studying muscle aging-dependent circRNA regulation in Rhesus monkeys (*Macaca mulatta*), it has been shown that 19 circRNAs decrease their expression in an age-dependent manner [69]. However, the function of these circRNAs during aging is still unknown, and more work is needed in order to unravel the biological significance of these molecules during muscle aging. In rats, the study of circRNA expression during aging in different tissues demonstrated that the expression of these molecules is tissue-specific and is regulated in a sexually dimorphic and age-related fashion [70]. Even with the capacity to identify novel RNA molecules like circRNAs, the prediction and the molecular analysis of their function during tissue aging are still in its initial phases of study.

One limitation for classical RNA-seq assays is the analysis of complex samples, where important gene expression changes occur also in small populations of specific cell types in an entire tissue. Different bioinformatic approaches for cell-type-specific gene expression module analysis in RNA-seq datasets from entire tissues have been developed [71]. In a recent study, the authors used the CellMapper algorithm as a method to predict gene modules expressed selectively in microglial cell populations from RNA-seq datasets derived from entire brain tissues. CellMapper method allowed to predict 31 genes co-expressed with the microglial specific mRNA of TMEM119, suggesting a microglial cell-type-specific expression of this gene module. Through this approach, the authors found that this microglial gene module increased its expression during aging and in age-related diseases such as Alzheimer's. Also, the microglial gene module is mainly expressed in regions of healthy brains which are implicated in Alzheimer's pathology [72]. Microglial cells are the resident myeloid cells of the central nervous system, their gene expression patterns alter during aging, and many of the related genes of Alzheimer's are primarily expressed in microglial cells [73]. The results obtained in this work suggest an important implication of microglial cells in neurodegenerative processes and aging of CNS; however, it is still difficult to attribute a microglial origin to Alzheimer's disease.

The analysis of transcriptomes using RNA-seq technologies has greatly improved our understanding of the complex phenomena of gene expression, revealing a more complex landscape where several loci are transcribed in a spatial-temporal manner and their gene products can be proteins, rRNAs, tRNAs, or miRNAs, but also other non-coding transcripts whose molecular function is not as clear as the other RNA families. The subsequent usage of RNA-seq technologies will clarify some molecular events during aging, related not only to protein functions but also to the regulation of cellular processes by other kinds of RNA molecules.

## Single-Cell Whole-Genome Sequencing

Tissues are composed of different cell types, from different lineages or in the different developmental stages of the same lineage. Also, several studies have demonstrated that even cells from the same type are different at its transcriptome, its epigenome, and even its genome due to errors produced by DNA polymerases during replication [74–76]. This implies that the results obtained by the previously described technologies in this chapter (WGS, WES, and RNA-seq) are usually the average genotype or transcriptome of all different cells in the analyzed sample. Single-cell sequencing addresses this gap by developing a technology that analyzes the genome or transcriptome of several unique cells from a sample [77]. This enables the analysis of gene expression in different developmental stages of a particular lineage, constructing a more precise continuum in the differentiation, the detection, and the analysis of rare populations of cells, or the analysis of outlier phenotypes not easily seen in pooled cell methods [78, 79].

In single-cell sequencing (SCS) experiments, unique cells are isolated from the tissue or sample based on specific biomarkers or specific phenotypes. Currently, most used methods to isolate cells for single-cell experiments include micromanipulation, laser capture microdissection (LCM), fluorescence-activated cell sorting (FACS), and microfluidics. Micromanipulation and microdissection are techniques that do not allow the isolation of a large number of cells in a short time. Both techniques rely on the direct visualization of target cells in a microscope and its isolation using a capillary (micromanipulation) or a laser to cut the cell and isolate it from the tissue. Micromanipulation is used mainly to isolate cells from cultures or early embryos, whereas LCM is used mainly to isolate single cells from slides of fixed tissues. FACS and microfluidics rely on cell characteristics such as expression of a biomarker, size, and light scattering; these techniques can be used to isolate large numbers of cells very fast. FACS uses fluorescent antibodies or probes to mark specific cellular populations and isolate them through the electromagnetic system; however, it requires large cell numbers which is a limitation when working with some sample types. In the case of microfluidics, it uses liquid streaming to isolate single cells in a microfluidic ship with micrometer diameter channels. Microfluidics uses small volumes and requires considerably less number of cells and allows their isolation directly into lysis buffer [80]. Isolation technologies are shown in Fig. 5.2.

Once the cells are isolated, they are usually lysed in a hypotonic buffer, and in the case of RNA-seq, the synthesis of cDNA is needed by using poly(A) tailing or template switching mechanism [81, 82]. Unique molecular identifiers (UMIs) or barcodes (random 4–8 bp sequences) are added to the dscDNA molecules in the reverse transcription step, allowing the assignment of each read to its origin cell [83]. After that, the cDNA library is amplified by PCR or by in vitro transcription. For DNA-seq, high-fidelity unbiased whole-genome amplification (WGA) techniques have been developed as a single cell has a very small amount of DNA (6 pg). Due to the great number of technologies, we urge readers to review these techniques in other specialized manuscripts [80]. Single-cell sequencing application is summarized in Fig. 5.2.

Because aging is characterized by the progressive dysfunction of most organs, single-cell sequencing has been recently used to study the accumulation of somatic mutations in unique cell populations of a specific organ. The analysis of the single-cell transcriptome of 2544 unique human pancreas cells of 8 donors (compassing 60 years frame) showed that islet endocrine cells from old people tend to increase its transcriptional noise and to accumulate genetic errors. Transcriptional noise was observed by an increase in non-cell-type-specific gene expression in these cells and is not caused by the mutational load. This suggests that aging is characterized by a gradual accumulation of epigenetic and genetic errors in independent events and in

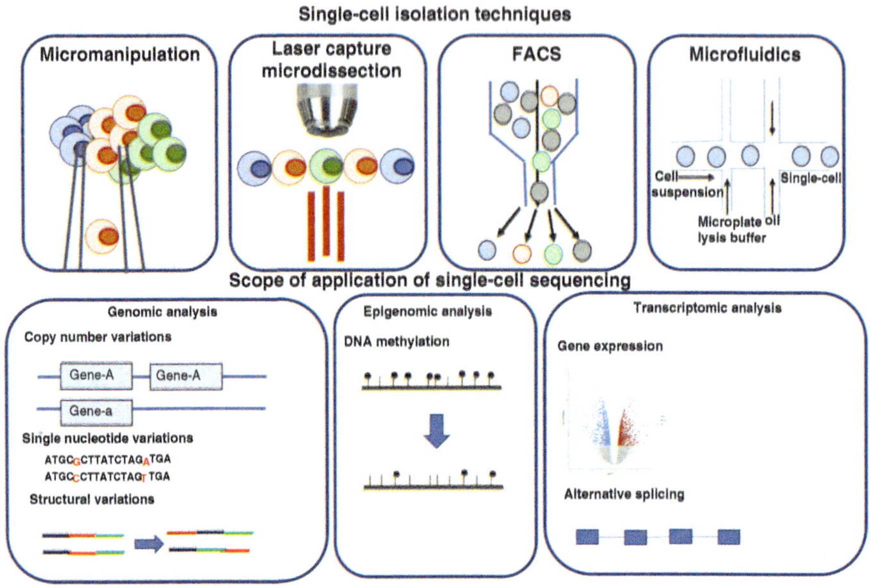


**Fig. 5.2** Single-cell isolation methods and common applications. The upper panels show four common technologies used for single-cell isolation in scNGS experiments: micromanipulation, laser capture microdissection, fluorescence-activated cell sorting (FACS), and microfluidics systems. The lower panels illustrate three common single-cell experimental applications: genomic analysis (scDNA-seq), methylated DNA single-cell sequencing, and transcriptomic analysis (scRNA-seq)

stochastic manner [84]. Interestingly, the transcriptome of single-islet pancreatic cells in young (3 months) and old (26 months) mice showed that only 193 transcripts changed their expression in an age-related way, with no obvious deleterious effect in pancreas physiology [85]. Moreover, the transcriptome of neuronal cell clusters of *D. melanogaster* brains showed that these cells experienced an exponential decrease in RNA content during aging that does not affect the neuronal identity [86].

Single-cell sequencing has also been used to prove if somatic mutations in neurons are associated with neurodegeneration. In this regard, the whole genome of 161 prefrontal and hippocampal individual neurons of healthy individuals and individuals with early-onset neurodegeneration was sequenced, founding that single-nucleotide variants (SNVs) in both groups increased with age and were much more abundant in neurons with neurodegenerative disorders [87].

Single-cell sequencing has helped to support several hypotheses about the cellular and genetic origin of age-related dysfunctions. Since single-cell sequencing allows us to study small populations of cells, it has been possible to find low represented mutations as well as transcriptional events that alter cellular identity. This newly generated data suggests that aging could be the result of mutational accumulation, epigenetic errors, and transcriptional noise that occurs in cells altering the functions of an entire organ.

## Sequencing the Mitochondrial Genome and the Discovery of Age-Related Alterations

The era of the next-generation sequencing technologies has not only offered high-throughput platforms for molecular analysis of the nuclear genome but also provides accurate and sensitive approaches to study the mitochondrial genome.

The human mitochondrial genome (mtDNA) is a double-stranded and circular molecule that codes for 2 rRNAs, 22 tRNAs, and 13 polypeptides that are all components of the oxidative phosphorylation chain [88]. Although mitochondrial functions rely primarily on nuclear-encoded proteins, its genome is essential to regulate the burden of mtDNA mutation and mtDNA copy number to maintain normal cell function [89]. Despite this mitochondrial maintenance, mtDNA is highly subject to mutagenic attacks due to both the limited capability of mitochondrial DNA polymerase to repair DNA damage [90] and the reactive oxygen species released by the oxidative phosphorylation chain [91]. Furthermore, the accumulation of heteroplasmy, a state in which spontaneous mutations occur in different copies of mtDNA, is highly feasible as one mitochondrion contains two to ten copies of mtDNA and each human cell hosts hundreds to thousands of mtDNA copies [92].

Because of the importance of mitochondrial function in regulating cell metabolism, programmed cell death, calcium signaling, and other cellular activities [93], several studies about the link between mtDNA sequence variation and aging have been performed. In this sense, the traditional analysis of the mitochondrial genome consisted only in the detection of the most common mtDNA point mutations and large deletions, which did not allow to find new variations. The Sanger sequencing of the entire mtDNA [94] was then used to find that heteroplasmic variations are probable to arise with growing age [95]; however, these studies are limited due to the elevated point mutation threshold (15%) and the rarely low-to-medium heteroplasmic frequency ratio of this method [96].

Also, mitochondrial gene chip array (MitoChip) has been used to profile the mitoscriptome and to detect heteroplasmic variations in the mitochondrial genomes. This technology enables the sequencing of more than 29 kb of double-stranded DNA with elevated detection and precision rates (99.7–99.9%) and the benefit of shorter testing times and low price [96–98]. Using this kind of genomic approximations, it has been demonstrated that during lifetime, the accumulation of low-level heteroplasmic sequence changes leads to the malfunctioning of the enzymatic complexes of oxidative phosphorylation which is involved in neurodegenerative diseases highly related with aging such as Alzheimer's disease [99].

With the development of NGS based on massively parallel sequencing (MPS) of the entire mitochondrial genome (16,569 bp), thousands of reads are generated for each nucleotide position allowing the detection of all point mutations and deletions guiding the accurate quantification of low-level mtDNA heteroplasmy, deletion breakpoints, multiple deletions, and low-level large deletions [100]. The process for mtDNA-seq does not need to purify mitochondria; it starts from extracted genomic DNA containing both mtDNA and nuclear DNA. mtDNA is enriched through selective amplification with long-range PCR and then subjected to library prep and sequencing. Using these technologies, different studies have realized a comprehensive analysis of the mitochondrial genome of different aged tissues [100]. Li et al. showed, for instance, that dysfunctional mitochondria from old mice's brains have significant accumulation of heteroplasmic mtDNA mutations in the control region, decreasing mtDNA-encoded protein synthesis, and in protein-coding regions leading to important changes in complex I subunit ND5 and complex III subunit CytB, which in turn affects the assembly of respiratory complexes [101]. Also, in platelets isolated from peripheral blood, it was found that a reduced mtDNA copy number is another property implicated in age-dependent mitochondrial dysfunctions [102]. Furthermore, the accumulation of mtDNA mutations results in an inappropriate differentiation of somatic stem cells which is necessary for tissue maintenance during the lifetime of an organism [103].

The translation of the quantity of data acquired with NGS technologies into the research of aging-related mitochondrial processes remains a challenge. Despite the progress that has been made, we still need to reduce the experimental error and detection limitations in order to suggest future clinical applications in the cure of several disorders related to aging.

## DNA Methylation Sequencing

DNA methylation plays a key role in regulating gene expression and is one of the best characterized epigenetic modifications. In mammalian cells, methyl groups are mainly added within a CpG nucleotide at the carbon-5 position of cytosine base [104]. Different techniques have been established over more than two decades to detect CpG methylation; bisulfite conversion, where unmethylated cytosines are converted to uracil, has been the most broadly used and coupled with PCR-based assays, microarrays, and next-generation sequencing [105]. These techniques have different capacities of resolution, quantitation, and throughput, but are generally restricted to short read lengths and have a limited capacity of multiplexing. By contrast, new technologies such as the third-generation single-molecule real-time (SMRT) sequencing and the bisulfite oligonucleotide-capture sequencing (BOCS) allow quantification of multiplexed targeted bisulfite long sequences (near 1.5 kb regions) and absolute quantification of CG and non-CG in specific regions of interest; moreover, whole-genome bisulfite sequencing has provided the capacity of quantitatively profile CpG across an entire genome in a single experiment, although this is an expensive approach that also needs infrastructure and complex computational analyses [106, 107].

The first studies that explore the effects of methylation in aging across multiple tissue types such as fibroblasts, dermis, epidermis, whole blood, and monocytes used human methylation microarrays. These studies reported a general loss of methylation across the genome [108]; however, these array trials examined only a small fraction (27,000–450,000 CpG sites) of the potentially methylated portion of the genome (>28 million CpG sites). With the advancement of the NGS technologies, a study was published in 2012 using whole-genome bisulfite sequencing to explore the relationship between DNA methylation and the aging process by comparing the DNA methylomes of CD4$^+$ T cells of a cohort of 103 newborns and centenaries. The findings indicated that centenarian DNA has lower DNA methylation throughout all genome (promoters, exons, introns, and intergenic regions) than newborn DNA, suggesting dispersed demethylation during lifespan [109]. A more robust methylome-wide study of aging used massively parallel sequencing of whole blood DNA samples from 718 individuals aged between 25 and 92 years to study age-associated differentially methylated regions (DMRs). In this study it was found that although hypomethylated DMRs are more frequently with age, there are also site-specific hypermethylation at several CpG islands and shores, while hypomethylation occurs mainly in regions associated with polycomb/regulatory proteins (EZH2) or histone modifications (e.g., H3K27ac, H3K4m1, m2, and m3) and genes such as protocadherins, homeobox genes, and MAPKs [110].

Other studies have been used NGS technologies to identify age-related methylation changes at single-base resolution in specific tissues, for example, it was reported that global methylation patterns of human epidermis samples from young (18–24) and old (70–75) individuals were very similar, found only a small fraction of genes with highly localized methylation changes that were associated with skin homeostasis such as ERRFI1 (ERBB receptor feedback inhibitor 1) and LDLR (low-density lipoprotein receptor) [111, 112]. These results showed that the global hypomethylation associated with age found in blood or T cells is not conserved in particular tissues as the epidermis.

In addition, bisulfite sequencing has also been used to study whether modifications in DNA methylation are correlated with age-related diseases. In this context, a mouse model of Alzheimer's disease was used to study the methylation profiles of brain samples where a total of 63 DMRs were found. Between those DMRs, hypomethylated sites were the more represented, and gene ontology analyses disclosed that genes associated with DMRs such as Dlgap1, TMEM51, and Eif2ak2 are involved in the development of Alzheimer's disease [112].

Recently, the analysis of a great amount of DNAmet sequencing data has provided one of the most reliable aging biomarkers. An epigenetic clock is a group of CpG sites with particular methylation patterns that are highly related to the chronological age of an individual. This correlation is very robust ($r = 0.9$) for individuals between 20 and 100 years. The epigenetic clock is a breakthrough discovery that will allow novel experimental approaches to understand the biological basis of aging [113]. For example, by using the epigenetic clock as a measure of cellular aging, it was possible to establish that cellular senescence and aging are independent and different phenomena [114].

In summary, changes in DNA methylation associated with aging can be divided into global hypomethylation and local hypermethylation patterns. These patterns cannot be generalized in all tissues because certain DNA methylation modifications are tissue-specific. Next-generation sequencing technologies have significantly improved the age-related DNA methylation research as they have contributed to accurate and sensitive methods to identify the most important genes for which altered methylation contributes to age-related functional decline. Those advances are new promising approaches in the development of therapeutic strategies to the treatment of disorders linked with the inevitable effects of aging.

## Analysis of Protein-DNA Interaction Genome Wide, Chip-Seq

Gene expression changes are the result of differential activity of transcription factors and differential epigenetic marks in the histones of nucleosomes. The study about the interaction of proteins with DNA and its transcriptomic output is very important to understand the changes in regulatory pathways that result in age-related organ decay and to discover regulatory nodes that can be pharmacologically targeted in order to achieve healthy aging. Chromatin immunoprecipitation (ChIP) is a technique for studying protein interactions (transcription factors and post-translationally modified histones) with DNA target sequences in vivo. In ChIP experiments, the cells are cross-linking with formaldehyde or glutaraldehyde to covalently link proteins to its target DNA regions, after that cells are lysed, and chromatin is fragmented into small pieces using sonication. Transcription factors (TF) bounded to DNA regions are recovered using a specific antibody and isolated with magnetic beads coated with streptavidin or protein A. DNA is isolated by cross-linking reverse and purification of DNA molecules. Isolated DNA fragments are sequenced using NGS as described before for DNA sequencing [115]. The principal methodological steps during ChIP-seq experiments are schematized in Fig. 5.3.

ChIP-seq is a powerful tool to study the activity of key transcription factors during aging processes. For example, the analysis of ChIP-seq datasets from kidney cells during human aging showed that the activity of inflammatory associated transcription factors such as NFkB, STAT1, and STAT3 drastically increases during the aging process. Interestingly, the stimulation of renal tubular cells with inflammatory cytokines (IL-6, IFN$\gamma$, and TNF$\alpha$) simulates the age-associated transcriptomic pattern [116].

Post-translational modification of histones, like methylation or acetylation, is also a key player in epigenetic regulation of aging processes. One of the most used approaches to study genome localization of these marks in chromatin is ChIP-seq experiments. This strategy has been used to test the hypothesis about the accumulation of epigenetic marks (H3K4me3, H3K36me3, and H3k27me3) in quiescent-muscle stem cells (qSCs) from aged muscles, founding that an increase in the repressive mark H3K27 impacts the function of old qSCs while young qSCs have several regions of euchromatin marked with H3K4me3 and H3K36me3 and without H3K27me3 [117]. Furthermore, it has been found that the histone variant H2A.Z accumulates during aging and is probably related to cognitive decline. The study of the genomic localization of H2A.Z in neurons of young and old mice reveals that H2A.Z accumulates in the chromatin of aged neurons in comparison with young neurons and is located between different genes [118]. In these studies, the use of ChIP-seq technology has served to complete the picture of the epigenetic landscapes and its deterioration during the aging process.

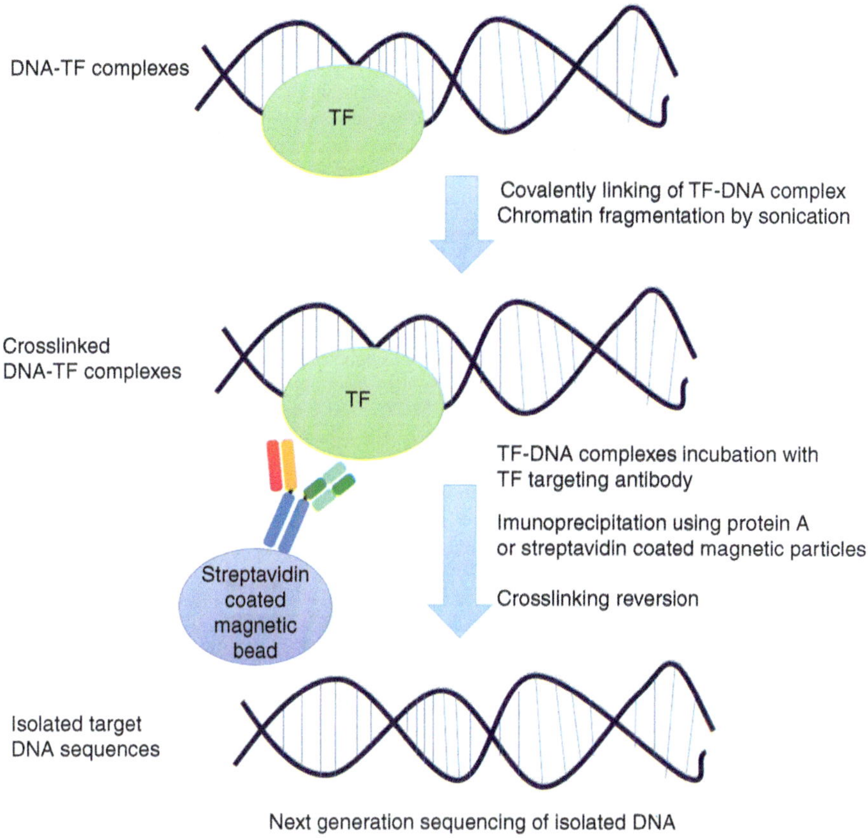


**Fig. 5.3** ChIP-seq experiments' general workflow. The general phases of a ChIP-seq experiment are schematized. The first phase consists on the covalent cross-linking of the DNA-protein interactions; after this, cells are lysed and DNA is fragmented by sonication. The second phase is the isolation of specific protein-DNA complexes using a monoclonal antibody which targets the protein of interest. After DNA-protein isolation, the cross-linking is reversed and DNA is isolated and sequenced

## References


1. Bao R, et al. Review of current methods, applications, and data management for the bioinformatics analysis of whole exome sequencing. Cancer Inform. 2014;13:67–82. https://doi.org/10.4137/CIN.S13779.
2. Hayden E, Technology C. The $1,000 genome. Nature. 2014;507:294–5. https://doi.org/10.1038/507294a.
3. Mitra RD, Shendure J, Olejnik J, Edyta Krzymanska O, Church GM. Fluorescent in situ sequencing on polymerase colonies. Anal Biochem. 2003;320:55–65. https://doi.org/10.1016/s0003-2697(03)00291-4.
4. Shendure J, et al. Accurate multiplex polony sequencing of an evolved bacterial genome. Science. 2005;309:1728–32. https://doi.org/10.1126/science.1117389.

5. Adessi C, et al. Solid phase DNA amplification: characterisation of primer attachment and amplification mechanisms. Nucleic Acids Res. 2000;28:E87. https://doi.org/10.1093/nar/28.20.e87.
6. Dressman D, Yan H, Traverso G, Kinzler KW, Vogelstein B. Transforming single DNA molecules into fluorescent magnetic particles for detection and enumeration of genetic variations. Proc Natl Acad Sci U S A. 2003;100:8817–22. https://doi.org/10.1073/pnas.1133470100.
7. Mitra RD, Church GM. In situ localized amplification and contact replication of many individual DNA molecules. Nucleic Acids Res. 1999;27:e34. https://doi.org/10.1093/nar/27.24.e34.
8. Bentley DR, et al. Accurate whole human genome sequencing using reversible terminator chemistry. Nature. 2008;456:53–9. https://doi.org/10.1038/nature07517.
9. Clark MJ, et al. Performance comparison of exome DNA sequencing technologies. Nat Biotechnol. 2011;29:908–14. https://doi.org/10.1038/nbt.1975.
10. Liu Y, Zhou J, White KP. RNA-seq differential expression studies: more sequence or more replication? Bioinformatics. 2014;30:301–4. https://doi.org/10.1093/bioinformatics/btt688.
11. Ziller MJ, Hansen KD, Meissner A, Aryee MJ. Coverage recommendations for methylation analysis by whole-genome bisulfite sequencing. Nat Methods. 2015;12:230–2., 231 p following 232. https://doi.org/10.1038/nmeth.3152.
12. Ozsolak F, Milos PM. Transcriptome profiling using single-molecule direct RNA sequencing. Methods Mol Biol. 2011;733:51–61. https://doi.org/10.1007/978-1-61779-089-8_4.
13. Ozsolak F, Milos PM. RNA sequencing: advances, challenges and opportunities. Nat Rev Genet. 2011;12:87–98. https://doi.org/10.1038/nrg2934.
14. Zhou X, et al. The next-generation sequencing technology and application. Protein Cell. 2010;1:520–36. https://doi.org/10.1007/s13238-010-0065-3.
15. Choi M, et al. Genetic diagnosis by whole exome capture and massively parallel DNA sequencing. Proc Natl Acad Sci U S A. 2009;106:19096–101. https://doi.org/10.1073/pnas.0910672106.
16. Fang H, et al. Reducing INDEL calling errors in whole genome and exome sequencing data. Genome Med. 2014;6:89. https://doi.org/10.1186/s13073-014-0089-z.
17. Kaeberlein M. Genome-wide approaches to understanding human ageing. Hum Genomics. 2006;2:422–8.
18. Perls TT, Bochen K, Freeman M, Alpert L, Silver MH. Validity of reported age and centenarian prevalence in New England. Age Ageing. 1999;28:193–7. https://doi.org/10.1093/ageing/28.2.193.
19. Puca AA, et al. A genome-wide scan for linkage to human exceptional longevity identifies a locus on chromosome 4. Proc Natl Acad Sci U S A. 2001;98:10505–8. https://doi.org/10.1073/pnas.181337598.
20. Geesaman BJ, et al. Haplotype-based identification of a microsomal transfer protein marker associated with the human lifespan. Proc Natl Acad Sci U S A. 2003;100:14115–20. https://doi.org/10.1073/pnas.1936249100.
21. Di Leo E, et al. Mutations in MTP gene in abeta- and hypobeta-lipoproteinemia. Atherosclerosis. 2005;180:311–8. https://doi.org/10.1016/j.atherosclerosis.2004.12.004.
22. Gregg RE, Wetterau JR. The molecular basis of abetalipoproteinemia. Curr Opin Lipidol. 1994;5:81–6.
23. Kammerer S, et al. Amino acid variant in the kinase binding domain of dual-specific A kinase-anchoring protein 2: a disease susceptibility polymorphism. Proc Natl Acad Sci U S A. 2003;100:4066–71. https://doi.org/10.1073/pnas.2628028100.
24. van den Akker EB, Deelen J, Slagboom PE, Beekman M. Exome and whole genome sequencing in aging and longevity. Adv Exp Med Biol. 2015;847:127–39. https://doi.org/10.1007/978-1-4939-2404-2_6.
25. Flachsbart F, et al. Association of FOXO3A variation with human longevity confirmed in German centenarians. Proc Natl Acad Sci U S A. 2009;106:2700–5. https://doi.org/10.1073/pnas.0809594106.

26. Willcox BJ, et al. FOXO3A genotype is strongly associated with human longevity. Proc Natl Acad Sci U S A. 2008;105:13987–92. https://doi.org/10.1073/pnas.0801030105.
27. Gierman HJ, et al. Whole-genome sequencing of the world's oldest people. PLoS One. 2014;9:e112430. https://doi.org/10.1371/journal.pone.0112430.
28. Lacaze P, et al. The Medical Genome Reference Bank: a whole-genome data resource of 4000 healthy elderly individuals. Rationale and cohort design. Eur J Hum Genet. 2019;27:308–16. https://doi.org/10.1038/s41431-018-0279-z.
29. Erikson GA, et al. Whole-genome sequencing of a healthy aging cohort. Cell. 2016;165:1002–11. https://doi.org/10.1016/j.cell.2016.03.022.
30. Harris SE, Deary IJ. The genetics of cognitive ability and cognitive ageing in healthy older people. Trends Cogn Sci. 2011;15:388–94. https://doi.org/10.1016/j.tics.2011.07.004.
31. Lalli MA, et al. Whole-genome sequencing suggests a chemokine gene cluster that modifies age at onset in familial Alzheimer's disease. Mol Psychiatry. 2015;20:1294–300. https://doi.org/10.1038/mp.2015.131.
32. Ridge PG, et al. Linkage, whole genome sequence, and biological data implicate variants in RAB10 in Alzheimer's disease resilience. Genome Med. 2017;9:100. https://doi.org/10.1186/s13073-017-0486-1.
33. Vardarajan BN, et al. Whole genome sequencing of Caribbean Hispanic families with late-onset Alzheimer's disease. Ann Clin Transl Neurol. 2018;5:406–17. https://doi.org/10.1002/acn3.537.
34. Alexander J, et al. Neuropathology-driven whole-genome sequencing study points to novel candidate genes for healthy brain aging. Alzheimer Dis Assoc Disord. 2019;33:7–14. https://doi.org/10.1097/WAD.0000000000000294.
35. Zheng HF, et al. Whole-genome sequencing identifies EN1 as a determinant of bone density and fracture. Nature. 2015;526:112–7. https://doi.org/10.1038/nature14878.
36. Ye K, et al. Aging as accelerated accumulation of somatic variants: whole-genome sequencing of centenarian and middle-aged monozygotic twin pairs. Twin Res Hum Genet. 2013;16:1026–32. https://doi.org/10.1017/thg.2013.73.
37. Park JS, et al. Brain somatic mutations observed in Alzheimer's disease associated with aging and dysregulation of tau phosphorylation. Nat Commun. 2019;10:3090. https://doi.org/10.1038/s41467-019-11000-7.
38. Guerreiro RJ, et al. Exome sequencing reveals an unexpected genetic cause of disease: NOTCH3 mutation in a Turkish family with Alzheimer's disease. Neurobiol Aging. 2012;33:1008 e1017–23. https://doi.org/10.1016/j.neurobiolaging.2011.10.009.
39. Benitez BA, et al. Missense variant in TREML2 protects against Alzheimer's disease. Neurobiol Aging. 2014;35:1510 e1519–26. https://doi.org/10.1016/j.neurobiolaging.2013.12.010.
40. Shameer K, Klee EW, Dalenberg AK, Kullo IJ. Whole exome sequencing implicates an INO80D mutation in a syndrome of aortic hypoplasia, premature atherosclerosis, and arterial stiffness. Circ Cardiovasc Genet. 2014;7:607–14. https://doi.org/10.1161/CIRCGENETICS.113.000233.
41. Jansen IE, et al. Discovery and functional prioritization of Parkinson's disease candidate genes from large-scale whole exome sequencing. Genome Biol. 2017;18:22. https://doi.org/10.1186/s13059-017-1147-9.
42. Akhtarkhavari T, et al. Genetic investigation of an Iranian supercentenarian by whole exome sequencing. Arch Iran Med. 2015;18:688–97, 0151/810/AIM.009.
43. Nygaard HB, et al. Whole exome sequencing of an exceptional longevity cohort. J Gerontol A Biol Sci Med Sci. 2018; https://doi.org/10.1093/gerona/gly098.
44. Chang YH, et al. Use of whole-exome sequencing to determine the genetic basis of signs of skin youthfulness in Korean women. J Eur Acad Dermatol Venereol. 2017;31:e138–41. https://doi.org/10.1111/jdv.13904.
45. Huentelman MJ, et al. Associations of MAP 2K3 gene variants with superior memory in superagers. Front Aging Neurosci. 2018;10:155. https://doi.org/10.3389/fnagi.2018.00155.
46. Anisimov SV, Boheler KR. Aging-associated changes in cardiac gene expression: large scale transcriptome analysis. Adv Gerontol. 2003;11:67–75.

47. Xing W, et al. Long non-coding RNAs in aging organs and tissues. Clin Exp Pharmacol Physiol. 2017;44(Suppl 1):30–7. https://doi.org/10.1111/1440-1681.12795.
48. Wang Z, Gerstein M, Snyder M. RNA-Seq: a revolutionary tool for transcriptomics. Nat Rev Genet. 2009;10:57–63. https://doi.org/10.1038/nrg2484.
49. Stark R, Grzelak M, Hadfield J. RNA sequencing: the teenage years Nat Rev Gen. 2019. https://doi.org/10.1038/s41576-019-0150-2.
50. Farr JN, et al. Effects of age and estrogen on skeletal gene expression in humans as assessed by RNA sequencing. PLoS One. 2015;10:e0138347. https://doi.org/10.1371/journal.pone.0138347.
51. Roforth MM, et al. Global transcriptional profiling using RNA sequencing and DNA methylation patterns in highly enriched mesenchymal cells from young versus elderly women. Bone. 2015;76:49–57. https://doi.org/10.1016/j.bone.2015.03.017.
52. Wang Y, et al. Sex differences in transcriptomic profiles in aged kidney cells of renin lineage. Aging (Albany NY). 2018;10:606–21. https://doi.org/10.18632/aging.101416.
53. de la Torre Gomez C, Goreham RV, Bech Serra JJ, Nann T, Kussmann M. "Exosomics"-a review of biophysics, biology and biochemistry of exosomes with a focus on human breast milk. Front Genet. 2018;9:92. https://doi.org/10.3389/fgene.2018.00092.
54. Saugstad JA, et al. Analysis of extracellular RNA in cerebrospinal fluid. J Extracell Vesicles. 2017;6:1317577. https://doi.org/10.1080/20013078.2017.1317577.
55. Greer JB, Schmale MC, Fieber LA. Whole-transcriptome changes in gene expression accompany aging of sensory neurons in Aplysia californica. BMC Genomics. 2018;19:529. https://doi.org/10.1186/s12864-018-4909-1.
56. Mansfeld J, et al. Branched-chain amino acid catabolism is a conserved regulator of physiological ageing. Nat Commun. 2015;6:10043. https://doi.org/10.1038/ncomms10043.
57. Mateos J, et al. Next-generation sequencing and quantitative proteomics of Hutchinson-Gilford progeria syndrome-derived cells point to a role of nucleotide metabolism in premature aging. PLoS One. 2018;13:e0205878. https://doi.org/10.1371/journal.pone.0205878.
58. Barry G, Guennewig B, Fung S, Kaczorowski D, Weickert CS. Long non-coding RNA expression during aging in the human subependymal zone. Front Neurol. 2015;6:45. https://doi.org/10.3389/fneur.2015.00045.
59. He Z, Bammann H, Han D, Xie G, Khaitovich P. Conserved expression of lincRNA during human and macaque prefrontal cortex development and maturation. RNA. 2014;20:1103–11. https://doi.org/10.1261/rna.043075.113.
60. White RR, et al. Comprehensive transcriptional landscape of aging mouse liver. BMC Genomics. 2015;16:899. https://doi.org/10.1186/s12864-015-2061-8.
61. Chen LL, Carmichael GG. Altered nuclear retention of mRNAs containing inverted repeats in human embryonic stem cells: functional role of a nuclear noncoding RNA. Mol Cell. 2009;35:467–78. https://doi.org/10.1016/j.molcel.2009.06.027.
62. Bianchessi V, et al. The mitochondrial lncRNA ASncmtRNA-2 is induced in aging and replicative senescence in endothelial cells. J Mol Cell Cardiol. 2015;81:62–70. https://doi.org/10.1016/j.yjmcc.2015.01.012.
63. Yang D, Yang K, Yang M. Circular RNA in aging and age-related diseases. Adv Exp Med Biol. 2018;1086:17–35. https://doi.org/10.1007/978-981-13-1117-8_2.
64. Guo JU, Agarwal V, Guo H, Bartel DP. Expanded identification and characterization of mammalian circular RNAs. Genome Biol. 2014;15:409. https://doi.org/10.1186/s13059-014-0409-z.
65. Hansen TB, et al. Natural RNA circles function as efficient microRNA sponges. Nature. 2013;495:384–8. https://doi.org/10.1038/nature11993.
66. Ashwal-Fluss R, et al. circRNA biogenesis competes with pre-mRNA splicing. Mol Cell. 2014;56:55–66. https://doi.org/10.1016/j.molcel.2014.08.019.
67. Calarco JA, et al. Regulation of vertebrate nervous system alternative splicing and development by an SR-related protein. Cell. 2009;138:898–910. https://doi.org/10.1016/j.cell.2009.06.012.

68. Brown JB, et al. Diversity and dynamics of the Drosophila transcriptome. Nature. 2014;512:393–9. https://doi.org/10.1038/nature12962.
69. Abdelmohsen K, et al. Circular RNAs in monkey muscle: age-dependent changes. Aging (Albany NY). 2015;7:903–10. https://doi.org/10.18632/aging.100834.
70. Mahmoudi E, Cairns MJ. Circular RNAs are temporospatially regulated throughout development and ageing in the rat. Sci Rep. 2019;9:2564. https://doi.org/10.1038/s41598-019-38860-9.
71. Nelms BD, et al. CellMapper: rapid and accurate inference of gene expression in difficult-to-isolate cell types. Genome Biol. 2016;17:201. https://doi.org/10.1186/s13059-016-1062-5.
72. Bonham LW, Sirkis DW, Yokoyama JS. The transcriptional landscape of microglial genes in aging and neurodegenerative disease. Front Immunol. 2019;10:1170. https://doi.org/10.3389/fimmu.2019.01170.
73. Plaza-Zabala A, Sierra-Torre V, Sierra A. Autophagy and microglia: novel partners in neurodegeneration and aging. Int J Mol Sci. 2017;18:598. https://doi.org/10.3390/ijms18030598.
74. Huang S. Non-genetic heterogeneity of cells in development: more than just noise. Development. 2009;136:3853–62. https://doi.org/10.1242/dev.035139.
75. Li L, Clevers H. Coexistence of quiescent and active adult stem cells in mammals. Science. 2010;327:542–5. https://doi.org/10.1126/science.1180794.
76. Shalek AK, et al. Single-cell RNA-seq reveals dynamic paracrine control of cellular variation. Nature. 2014;510:363–9. https://doi.org/10.1038/nature13437.
77. Hwang B, Lee JH, Bang D. Single-cell RNA sequencing technologies and bioinformatics pipelines. Exp Mol Med. 2018;50:96. https://doi.org/10.1038/s12276-018-0071-8.
78. Trapnell C, et al. The dynamics and regulators of cell fate decisions are revealed by pseudotemporal ordering of single cells. Nat Biotechnol. 2014;32:381–6. https://doi.org/10.1038/nbt.2859.
79. Stubbington MJT, et al. T cell fate and clonality inference from single-cell transcriptomes. Nat Methods. 2016;13:329–32. https://doi.org/10.1038/nmeth.3800.
80. Liang J, Cai W, Sun Z. Single-cell sequencing technologies: current and future. J Genet Genomics. 2014;41:513–28. https://doi.org/10.1016/j.jgg.2014.09.005.
81. Tang F, et al. mRNA-Seq whole-transcriptome analysis of a single cell. Nat Methods. 2009;6:377–82. https://doi.org/10.1038/nmeth.1315.
82. Ramskold D, et al. Full-length mRNA-Seq from single-cell levels of RNA and individual circulating tumor cells. Nat Biotechnol. 2012;30:777–82. https://doi.org/10.1038/nbt.2282.
83. Macosko EZ, et al. Highly parallel genome-wide expression profiling of individual cells using nanoliter droplets. Cell. 2015;161:1202–14. https://doi.org/10.1016/j.cell.2015.05.002.
84. Enge M, et al. Single-cell analysis of human pancreas reveals transcriptional signatures of aging and somatic mutation patterns. Cell. 2017;171:321–30.e314. https://doi.org/10.1016/j.cell.2017.09.004.
85. Xin Y, et al. Single-cell RNAseq reveals that pancreatic beta-cells from very old male mice have a young gene signature. Endocrinology. 2016;157:3431–8. https://doi.org/10.1210/en.2016–1235.
86. Davie K, et al. A single-cell transcriptome atlas of the aging drosophila brain. Cell. 2018;174:982–98. e920. https://doi.org/10.1016/j.cell.2018.05.057.
87. Lodato MA, et al. Aging and neurodegeneration are associated with increased mutations in single human neurons. Science. 2018;359:555–9. https://doi.org/10.1126/science.aao4426.
88. Taanman JW. The mitochondrial genome: structure, transcription, translation and replication. Biochim Biophys Acta. 1999;1410:103–23. https://doi.org/10.1016/s0005-2728(98)00161-3.
89. Alston CL, Rocha MC, Lax NZ, Turnbull DM, Taylor RW. The genetics and pathology of mitochondrial disease. J Pathol. 2017;241:236–50. https://doi.org/10.1002/path.4809.
90. DeBalsi KL, Hoff KE, Copeland WC. Role of the mitochondrial DNA replication machinery in mitochondrial DNA mutagenesis, aging and age-related diseases. Ageing Res Rev. 2017;33:89–104. https://doi.org/10.1016/j.arr.2016.04.006.
91. Islam MT. Oxidative stress and mitochondrial dysfunction-linked neurodegenerative disorders. Neurol Res. 2017;39:73–82. https://doi.org/10.1080/01616412.2016.1251711.

92. Stewart JB, Chinnery PF. The dynamics of mitochondrial DNA heteroplasmy: implications for human health and disease. Nat Rev Genet. 2015;16:530–42. https://doi.org/10.1038/nrg3966.
93. Koch RE, Josefson CC, Hill GE. Mitochondrial function, ornamentation, and immunocompetence. Biol Rev Camb Philos Soc. 2017;92:1459–74. https://doi.org/10.1111/brv.12291.
94. Tang S, et al. Transition to next generation analysis of the whole mitochondrial genome: a summary of molecular defects. Hum Mutat. 2013;34:882–93. https://doi.org/10.1002/humu.22307.
95. Sondheimer N, et al. Neutral mitochondrial heteroplasmy and the influence of aging. Hum Mol Genet. 2011;20:1653–9. https://doi.org/10.1093/hmg/ddr043.
96. Duan M, Tu J, Lu Z. Recent advances in detecting mitochondrial DNA heteroplasmic variations. Molecules. 2018;23:E323. https://doi.org/10.3390/molecules23020323.
97. Maitra A, et al. The human MitoChip: a high-throughput sequencing microarray for mitochondrial mutation detection. Genome Res. 2004;14:812–9. https://doi.org/10.1101/gr.2228504.
98. Raju R, Jian B, Hubbard W, Chaudry I. The mitoscriptome in aging and disease. Aging Dis. 2011;2:174–80.
99. Casoli T, Spazzafumo L, Di Stefano G, Conti F. Role of diffuse low-level heteroplasmy of mitochondrial DNA in Alzheimer's disease neurodegeneration. Front Aging Neurosci. 2015;7:142. https://doi.org/10.3389/fnagi.2015.00142.
100. Palculict ME, Zhang VW, Wong LJ, Wang J. Comprehensive mitochondrial genome analysis by massively parallel sequencing. Methods Mol Biol. 2016;1351:3–17. https://doi.org/10.1007/978-1-4939-3040-1_1.
101. Li H, et al. Aging-associated mitochondrial DNA mutations alter oxidative phosphorylation machinery and cause mitochondrial dysfunctions. Biochim Biophys Acta Mol basis Dis. 2017;1863:2266–73. https://doi.org/10.1016/j.bbadis.2017.05.022.
102. Zhang R, Wang Y, Ye K, Picard M, Gu Z. Independent impacts of aging on mitochondrial DNA quantity and quality in humans. BMC Genomics. 2017;18:890. https://doi.org/10.1186/s12864-017-4287-0.
103. Norddahl GL, et al. Accumulating mitochondrial DNA mutations drive premature hematopoietic aging phenotypes distinct from physiological stem cell aging. Cell Stem Cell. 2011;8:499–510. https://doi.org/10.1016/j.stem.2011.03.009.
104. Li E, Zhang Y. DNA methylation in mammals. Cold Spring Harb Perspect Biol. 2014;6:a019133. https://doi.org/10.1101/cshperspect.a019133.
105. Frommer M, et al. A genomic sequencing protocol that yields a positive display of 5-methylcytosine residues in individual DNA strands. Proc Natl Acad Sci U S A. 1992;89:1827–31. https://doi.org/10.1073/pnas.89.5.1827.
106. Yang Y, et al. Quantitative and multiplexed DNA methylation analysis using long-read single-molecule real-time bisulfite sequencing (SMRT-BS). BMC Genomics. 2015;16:350. https://doi.org/10.1186/s12864-015-1572-7.
107. Masser DR, et al. Analysis of DNA modifications in aging research. Geroscience. 2018;40:11–29. https://doi.org/10.1007/s11357-018-0005-3.
108. Koch CM, Wagner W. Epigenetic-aging-signature to determine age in different tissues. Aging (Albany NY). 2011;3:1018–27. https://doi.org/10.18632/aging.100395.
109. Heyn H, et al. Distinct DNA methylomes of newborns and centenarians. Proc Natl Acad Sci U S A. 2012;109:10522–7. https://doi.org/10.1073/pnas.1120658109.
110. McClay JL, et al. A methylome-wide study of aging using massively parallel sequencing of the methyl-CpG-enriched genomic fraction from blood in over 700 subjects. Hum Mol Genet. 2014;23:1175–85. https://doi.org/10.1093/hmg/ddt511.
111. Raddatz G, et al. Aging is associated with highly defined epigenetic changes in the human epidermis. Epigenetics Chromatin. 2013;6:36. https://doi.org/10.1186/1756-8935-6-36.
112. Zhang S, et al. Genome-wide analysis of DNA methylation profiles in a senescence-accelerated mouse prone 8 brain using whole-genome bisulfite sequencing. Bioinformatics. 2017;33:1591–5. https://doi.org/10.1093/bioinformatics/btx040.

113. Horvath S, Raj K. DNA methylation-based biomarkers and the epigenetic clock theory of ageing. Nat Rev Genet. 2018;19:371–84. https://doi.org/10.1038/s41576-018-0004-3.
114. Lowe D, Horvath S, Raj K. Epigenetic clock analyses of cellular senescence and ageing. Oncotarget. 2016;7:8524–31. https://doi.org/10.18632/oncotarget.7383.
115. Furey TS. ChIP-seq and beyond: new and improved methodologies to detect and characterize protein-DNA interactions. Nat Rev Genet. 2012;13:840–52. https://doi.org/10.1038/nrg3306.
116. O'Brown ZK, Van Nostrand EL, Higgins JP, Kim SK. The inflammatory transcription factors NFkappaB, STAT1 and STAT3 drive age-associated transcriptional changes in the human kidney. PLoS Genet. 2015;11:e1005734. https://doi.org/10.1371/journal.pgen.1005734.
117. Liu L, et al. Chromatin modifications as determinants of muscle stem cell quiescence and chronological aging. Cell Rep. 2013;4:189–204. https://doi.org/10.1016/j.celrep.2013.05.043.
118. Stefanelli G, et al. Learning and age-related changes in genome-wide H2A.Z binding in the mouse hippocampus. Cell Rep. 2018;22:1124–31. https://doi.org/10.1016/j.celrep.2018.01.020.

# Molecular Biomarkers of Aging Studies in Humans

# 6

G. Pedraza-Vázquez, A. Alarcón-Aguilar, and A. Luna-López

## Abbreviations

| | |
|---|---|
| AMPK | AMP-activated protein kinase |
| BMI | Body mass index |
| CAT | Catalase |
| CHO | Chinese hamster ovary cells |
| COPD | Chronic obstructive pulmonary disease |
| CRP | C-reactive protein |
| DHEA | Dehydroepiandrosterone |
| DNA | Deoxyribonucleic acid |
| GDF-8 | Growth differentiation factor 8 |
| GH | Growth hormone |
| GM-CSF | Granulocyte-macrophage colony-stimulating factor |
| GPx | Glutathione peroxidase |
| GR | Glutathione reductase |
| GSH | Reduced glutathione |
| GSSG | Oxidized glutathione |
| GST | Glutathione S-transferase |

G. Pedraza-Vázquez
Posgrado en Biología Experimental, Universidad Autónoma Metropolitana-Iztapalapa, Mexico City, Mexico
e-mail: gpv@xanum.uam.mx

A. Alarcón-Aguilar
Departamento de Ciencias de la Salud, Universidad Autónoma Metropolitana-Iztapalapa, Mexico City, Mexico
e-mail: adyalagui@xanum.uam.mx

A. Luna-López (✉)
Departamento de Investigación Básica, Instituto Nacional de Geriatría, Mexico City, Mexico
e-mail: aluna@inger.gob.mx



J. C. Gomez-Verjan, N. A. Rivero-Segura (eds.), *Clinical Genetics and Genomics of Aging*, https://doi.org/10.1007/978-3-030-40955-5_6

| | |
|---|---|
| HIV | Human immunodeficiency virus |
| IFN-γ | Interferon γ |
| IGF-1 | Insulin-like growth factor 1 |
| IL-10 | Interleukin 10 |
| IL-12 | Interleukin 12 |
| IL-1Ra | Interleukin-1 receptor antagonist |
| IL-1ß | Interleukin 1ß |
| IL-2 | Interleukin 2 |
| IL-4 | Interleukin 4 |
| IL-6 | Interleukin 6 |
| NF-κB | Nuclear factor κB |
| OS | Oxidative stress |
| ROS | Reactive oxygen species |
| SASP | Senescence-associated secretory phenotype |
| SOD | Superoxide dismutase |
| T3 | Triiodothyronine |
| T4 | Thyroxine |
| TGF-ß | Transforming growth factor ß |
| TNF-α | Tumor necrosis factor α |
| TRH | Thyrotropin-releasing hormone |

## Introduction

Aging is a natural and irreversible process characterized by a progressive decay in physiological, biochemical, and structural functions of individuals. Aging is a multifactorial process that can be affected by two main factors: environmental and genetic. Environmental factors are nutrition, pathologies, pollution exposure, physical activity, and microbiota, while genetic factors are issues that have been associated with antioxidant and DNA damage responses, the fidelity of genetic information transfer, the efficiency of protein degradation, the extent of cellular responsiveness to stress, the mechanisms of epigenetic regulation, and the ability to elongate telomeres. All of them can determine how fast we age. Traditionally, aging studies had used several model organisms, from yeast to mammals, especially rodents (rats and mice). Most of the studies are made under controlled conditions, where only a few variables are observed, and the subjects are members of the same strain with the same genetic backgrounds or the same mutations. The information that so far has been obtained about aging has helped us to describe different factors that influence this process and that are the fundamental concepts of the various theories of aging. However, these theories do not fully explain the aging process in the different models of aging study. This is the case of the study of aging in humans, where it is very difficult to control the environmental and genetic variables. That is why issues haven't been solved such as the following: How does time influence aging? When do we start to age? How do we know we are old? Is it possible to delay aging? Those and more questions are the cornerstones for aging studies. Biological aging has been associated with the decrease in the repair and regeneration capacity of tissues and organs; it is a time-dependent process. This reduction can be observed by an increase in the acquisition of diseases and functional and reproductive disability, which eventually lead to death. On the other hand, it has been observed that in humans, people with the same chronological age exhibit different trajectories in the decrease of physiological functions associated with biological aging and what complicates the understanding of the molecular and physiological phenomena that drive the complex and multifactorial processes that underlie biological aging in humans.

To try to answer those questions in humans, many epidemiologic, demographic, nutritional, cellular, and molecular studies have been done in order to allow us to understand the aging process. It is important to consider that some of the biomarkers that have been proposed for the study of aging in humans, such as epigenetic biomarkers, telomere length and telomerase activity, stem cell exhaustion, cellular proteostasis, senescence, and the stress response capacity of organisms, among the most important, are very complex for evaluation in humans. This is mainly due to the difficulty of obtaining human samples, since these processes turn out to be highly invasive and dangerous. In addition, the results obtained in a tissue are not necessarily replicable in other tissues, so we should consider that the biomarkers of aging often turn out to be tissue-specific. One of the most interesting examples in this regard is the length of telomeres, since this parameter could hardly be determined in tissues composed mostly of post-mitotic cells, such as muscle (myofibrils), heart (cardiomyocyte), and central nervous system (neurons). Therefore, in this chapter we will discuss the diverse molecular biomarkers that have been proposed for aging studies in humans.

## Molecular Biomarkers for Inflammation in Aging

Inflammation is the physiological process associated with tissue repair against damage generated by several endogenous and external factors. Chronic age-related diseases such as type II diabetes, cardiovascular diseases, arthritis, sarcopenia, frailty, and neurodegenerative diseases have been associated with a dysregulation of the inflammatory response [1, 2]. Such dysregulation of the inflammatory response is a chronic process and it is known as inflammaging [3]. To evaluate this condition, there have been proposed several molecular biomarkers like the systemic balance between pro-inflammatory and anti-inflammatory cytokines, which is a very useful and easy tool, because it can be performed with a single blood sample from the patient.

The main pro-inflammatory biomarkers associated with aging are TNF-α, IL-6, IL-1ß, and C-reactive protein (CRP). Elevated levels of these molecules have been associated with metabolic failures, chronic inflammation, sarcopenia, and neurodegenerative diseases [4–6]. On the other hand, the most important anti-inflammatory biomarkers are IL-10 and IL-4 that are commonly decreased in age-related diseases compared to healthy adults [7–10]. Nevertheless, care must be taken with these determinations because sometimes an elevation in IL-10 and IL-4 could be attributed to a compensatory response against inflammaging [11–14]. Therefore, in order to have a better understanding of the inflammatory status observed during aging, it has been proposed to determine the balance between pro-inflammatory and anti-inflammatory cytokines through the implementation of the IL-6/IL-10, TNF-α/IL-4, and TNF-α/IL-10 ratios [15, 16].

Comparative evaluations of the inflammatory profile in elderly patients against young and adult patients have shown that the levels of pro-inflammatory cytokines are slightly elevated in inflammaging (IL-2, IL-6, IL-8, and GM-CSF), meanwhile levels of anti-inflammatory cytokines (IL-4 and IL-10) are slightly lower in inflammaging. IFN-γ and TNF-α did not show significative differences among studied populations [17].

Sarcopenia is an age-related syndrome where it is observed a strength decay in skeletal muscle mass composition and functionality. This syndrome can be exacerbated by obesity, another physiological phenomenon that has increased in the past few years. This factor increases the muscle dysfunction, along with the comorbidity and mortality in elderly patients. It has been reported that both local inflammation (adipose tissue and muscular tissue) and systemic inflammation (inflammaging) strongly influence sarcopenia development. In fact, adipose tissue secretes molecules known as adipokines, which regulate functions like appetite, energetic management, glucose and lipid metabolism, insulin secretion, fat distribution, and immune regulation [18, 19]. One of the most interesting adipokines of the age-related sarcopenic obesity is adiponectin, which is associated with the AMPK activation and NF-κB signaling inhibition that leads to a decay of TNF-α and IFN-γ levels and also an increment of IL-10 and IL-1Ra [20]. Leptin is another important adipokine associated with obesity and insulin resistance. Leptin has been reported to have pro-inflammatory properties. High levels of this adipokine increase IL-6, IL-12, and TNF-α, also involving monocytes [21]. It is important to mention that the inflammatory biomarkers that have been described are the most representative inflammatory molecules in aging; however, there are other specific inflammatory biomarkers for age-related diseases that require further analysis due to their relation with other diseases.

## Molecular Biomarkers for Oxidative Stress

There are many theories that try to explain the nature of aging; however, none of them can explain every aspect of the biology of aging. One of the most accepted and studied is the one proposed by Denham Harman in 1956. This theory proposed that during lifespan organisms accumulate oxidative damage in their biomolecules. Oxidative damage is generated by reactive oxygen species (ROS), which are the product of aerobic metabolism. The main metabolic processes associated with ROS production are electron transport chain, purine metabolism, and immune response [22–24]. In order to prevent oxidative damage in the biomolecules, organisms have developed several strategies against the deleterious effects generated by ROS. Those mechanisms are known as antioxidant responses, and they involve enzymatic antioxidants and non-enzymatic antioxidants.

The unbalance between ROS production and antioxidant defense is known as oxidative stress (OS). In other words, OS is a state where the level of ROS is higher than the antioxidant capacity. OS is a physiological phenomenon that increases with aging, and it has been associated with a reduction of the mechanisms for cellular damage repair. Nonetheless, high levels of ROS can also be generated by exogenous factors such as radiation and pollution and human factors like nutrition, sedentarism, drugs, and microbe interaction during life [25]. In order to establish the main OS biomarkers of aging, we divided them into three categories: ROS production, oxidized biomolecules, and antioxidant response.

The main ROS generated in cells are superoxide radical ($O_2$•-), hydrogen peroxide ($H_2O_2$), and hydroxyl radical (OH•-). The first two are produced in the aerobic metabolism: $O_2$•- is produced in complexes I and III of the electron transport chain [22], as well as a product of xanthine oxidase in purine metabolism, and by the NADPH oxidase in the immune response [23]. Superoxide radical is transformed into $H_2O_2$ by the superoxide dismutase (SOD), which has three different isoforms: mitochondrial, cytosolic, and extracellular [26]. Finally, when these two ROS react with free iron, they produce the hydroxyl radical in two different mechanisms: Weiss reaction and Fenton reaction [27]. Unfortunately, ROS are highly reactive, and their half-life is too short, so their quantification represents a technical challenge in in vivo models, so that is why this determination is mainly performed in vitro.

An indirect way to measure OS is to evaluate the damage generated by ROS, in other words, determining the concentration of oxidized biomolecules. The main biomolecules that can be evaluated to this end are lipids, proteins, and nucleic acids. Therefore, the main biomarkers for lipid peroxidation are malondialdehyde (MDA) and 4-hydroxynonenal (4-HNE), which are generated from the peroxidation of polyunsaturated fatty acids. The formation of these lipid peroxides can be described as a process where ROS react with lipids containing a carbon-carbon double bond in their structure. This process implies the extraction of a carbon atom and an oxygen insertion; the product of the reaction is peroxyl radical or lipidic hyperoxide. Finally, due to the reactive nature of this radicals, MDA and 4-HNE are formed in order to achieve a more stable structure [28].

The principal biomarkers for oxidized proteins are protein carbonyls and 3-nitrotyrosine (3-NT). Protein carbonyls are generated due to the oxidation of the α-carbon of proline, arginine, lysine, threonine, and other amino acid residues, having as a final product a carbonyl group and the fragmentation of the protein, resulting in a decay of function. 3-NT formation involves the addition of the -$NO_2$ group in carbon three of the tyrosine residue in a polypeptide; this also causes the protein to lose its function [29, 30].

One of the most important biomarkers for genomic and mitochondrial DNA oxidative damage is 8-hydroxydeoxyguanosine (8-OHdG). This DNA adduct is formed as a result of the reaction of hydroxyl radical with carbon eight of guanosine. The importance of this product lies on the fact of its abundance over the DNA and is considered as a mutagenic damage. The evidence suggests that 8-OHdG lesions in DNA during replication result in somatic mutations. These mutations have been associated with a decay in the physiological functionality of the individuals, like in aging. 8-OHdG determination and analysis can be performed in several human samples like urine, as well as tissue and blood biopsies. Due to its relative stability compared to other DNA adducts, 8-OHdG is considered one of the most reliable OS biomarkers in aging [30, 31].

To evaluate the capacity of the antioxidant response of the organisms during aging, it has been proposed to determine the activity of the main enzymes of the antioxidant response: superoxide dismutase (SOD) metabolizes superoxide radical, while catalase (CAT) and glutathione peroxidase (GPx) metabolize hydrogen peroxide. It is important to say that GPx enzyme uses γ-glutamyl-cysteinyl-glycine, also known as reduced glutathione (GSH), as a cofactor. Other enzymes used as biomarkers of aging are glutathione reductase (GR), an enzyme that transforms oxidized glutathione (GSSG) into GSH using NADPH as a substrate, and glutathione S-transferase (GST), an enzyme that inactivates lipid and protein radicals using the thiol of the GSH cysteine. Glutathione is a very important part of the antioxidant response against OS, because of its direct and indirect involvement in ROS elimination, due to its capacity to neutralize the free radicals and by being a substrate for the antioxidant enzymes.

Studies in different elderly patients' populations have shown that high levels of the OS biomarkers like MDA, 4-HNE, 3-NT, protein carbonyls, and 8-OHdG associate with age-related diseases (sarcopenia, frailty, neurodegenerative diseases, osteoporosis, and osteopenia). Also, it has been observed a decay in the activity of the antioxidant enzymes SOD, CAT, GPx, and GR, and the GSSG/GSH ratio is elevated [28, 32–35].

Interestingly, longitudinal studies of distinct populations where OS biomarkers have been evaluated show contradictory results. Some of them show elevated levels of MDA in elderly patients until 80 years of age, but after 90 years of age there is a significant decay of MDA levels. Moreover, the antioxidant response in both populations showed similar levels of GSH, GSSG, GSSG/GSH ratio, and CAT, GPx, and GR enzymatic activity. This study was performed strictly on a healthy population, so the variations in OS biomarkers between octogenarian and nonagenarian groups might be related to genetic or adaptive factors that might allow them to have a better response to overcome OS [36]. Another study, performed on normal populations, showed lower levels of MDA in octogenarian compared to nonagenarian populations. There, a progressive decay of CAT, SOD, GR, and GPx enzymatic activity during aging was observed. This study was conducted in patients with certain lipidic profile, BMI, and age. However, it presents some limitations like the lack of evidence of age-related diseases and GSSG/GSH ratio, which could have helped to understand better the effect of OS over aging [37].

## Molecular Biomarkers for Hormones in Aging

In the postulates that have been used to define aging, we can find the decay of the physiological functions of the individuals, which can be interpreted as the incapacity of old organisms to maintain homeostasis against environmental and metabolic stress in their daily life. The endocrine system has a relevant function in homeostasis control and, therefore, hormones are key regulators during a lifespan. During the individual lifespan, there are hormonal changes in order to regulate homeostasis in many situations, which include nutrition, energetic metabolism, reproduction, growth, and tissue repair. During aging, it is common to have a reduced amount of secreted hormones, which translates to loss of reproductive functions and growth, including the loss of muscle mass, strength, bone, skin, insulin-related problems, fat gain, and effects over the immune function [38]. The most important hormonal biomarkers in aging are growth hormone (GH), testosterone, dehydroepiandrosterone (DHEA), insulin-like growth factor 1 (IGF-1), estradiol, thyroid-stimulating hormone (TSH), vitamin D, ghrelin, adiponectin, and leptin.

#### Growth Hormone

GH levels drastically decrease during lifespan, which means that elderly patients may have very low levels of this hormone compared to young ones. There is a great number of reports that discuss the role of GH in aging. In some age-related diseases, it has been observed that low levels of GH are associated with extended lifespan in humans. The phenotype of humans with a deficiency either of GH secretion or GH receptors displays a short height and a low incidence of age-related diseases like cancer and diabetes mellitus [39]. In recent years, it has been demonstrated that these individuals have high levels of adiponectin with great sensitivity to insulin despite the higher percentage of body fat [40]. Moreover, high levels of GH in patients with acromegalia show reduced longevity [41]. In syndromes like gigantism, it has been observed an excessive secretion of GH in the early stages of life; the high levels of GH can be associated then with a risk of mortality. The patients with gigantism are also more likely to suffer from diabetes, cardiovascular diseases, and cancer. The symptomatology observed in acromegalia resembles the effects of chronological age, where the incidence of age-related diseases is higher, and it could be interpreted as accelerated aging [42]. Other studies show that in healthy elderly patients that are descendants of long-lived individuals, the levels of GH are lower than the healthy elderly patients that are descendants of non-long-lived individuals [43]. Generally, the results obtained in different studies show that organisms that have lower concentrations of GH have greater longevity.

### Insulin-Like Growth Factor 1

Insulin-like growth factor 1 (IGF-1) regulates several cellular processes like senescence, apoptosis, growth, metabolism, mitochondrial impairment, inflammation, and autophagy. Like the GH, IGF-1 has been associated with longevity and aging, because it has been reported that the levels of this hormone tend to decrease over the years [44]. It has been shown that IGF-1 displays higher levels in patients with age-related diseases, like diabetes, cardiovascular diseases, neurodegenerative diseases, and obesity, compared to healthy elderly patients [44–46]. In a study with nonagenarians, low concentrations of IGF-1 were detected; therefore, this hormone has been associated with greater functionality and longevity [43]. Similar results were observed in a study with a population of long-lived Japanese women with low concentrations of IGF-1 [47].

## Testosterone

Testosterone is one of the main sexual hormones that participates in embryogenesis, sexual activity, and men reproduction. Also, many studies revealed that testosterone participates in male general health. It has been reported that low concentrations of testosterone are associated with age-related diseases like diabetes, Alzheimer's disease, arteriosclerosis, cardiovascular diseases, osteoporosis, and cancer [48–50]. Some studies report testosterone concentration reduction with age [51–53].

### Dehydroepiandrosterone

Protective steroid hormones tend to decrease over the years, like dehydroepiandrosterone with its active metabolite dehydroepiandrosterone sulfate (DHEA-S). These two endogenous steroid hormones are synthesized from cholesterol and are secreted by the suprarenal cortex and are the most abundant steroid hormones in the bloodstream [54, 55]. DHEA is a precursor useful in steroidogenesis, where it is metabolized to androstenedione, which can be metabolized to estrone and estradiol in female and to testosterone in male. Production of DHEA reaches its higher point in adult life, and then it starts to decay over time. In the past few years, new evidence suggests an important association between the levels of DHEA-S and aging [56]. DHEA is considered a pleiotropic hormone because it has been associated with cardiovascular diseases, chronic obstructive pulmonary disease (COPD), osteoporosis, neurodegenerative diseases, metabolic diseases, muscle function decay, and other age-related diseases [57–59].

## Thyroid-Stimulating Hormone

Thyroid hormones are involved in the basal metabolism regulation and actively participate in several physiological processes such as growth, embryogenesis, and energetic metabolism. It has been demonstrated that the dysregulation of the thyroid axis results in strong alterations within the energetic balance. The thyroid gland is regulated by thyrotropin-releasing hormone (TRH), which regulates the secretion of TSH from the pituitary gland. Activation of thyroxine (T4) to triiodothyronine (T3) by the enzyme type 2 5-deiodinase is a key mechanism that regulates the metabolism in peripheral tissues. Signals of this hormone are peripheral mainly in the liver, white and brown adipose tissue, and hypothalamus. Thyroid hormones directly stimulate the energetic metabolism by changing the functionality and favoring the expression of genes related to thermogenesis [60]. The relation between thyroid hormones and aging has been reported in some studies. Low expression of thyroid hormones has been associated with greater longevity. During the investigation carried out in project Leiden 85-plus, a prospective study that took place in the city of Leiden in the Netherlands, high levels of TSH were associated with lower mortality in participants between 85 and 90 years old. Also, in the Leiden Longevity Study, the case of a family with extraordinary longevity showed slightly higher levels of circulating TSH and lower levels of T4 and T3 were associated with greater longevity [61]. In general, TSH increases during the lifespan and lower levels could be associated with age-related diseases [62, 63].

## Vitamin D

Vitamin D is a micronutrient metabolized in a multifunctional hormone that is essential for human health. Most vitamin D requirements can be synthesized by the organism itself due to sunlight exposure; however, diet plays an important role when it comes to vitamin D supplementation in cases when synthesis is limited or defective [64].

One of the main functions of vitamin D is to preserve calcium homeostasis; when there is a deficiency of vitamin D, the bone mineralization process induces osteomalacia and osteoporosis in adults. There are some reports of risk factors associated with the deficiency of this vitamin like age, malnutrition, obesity, and insufficient solar exposure, among others. Besides bone metabolism, vitamin D participates in several physiological mechanisms and that is why its deficiency is also associated with sarcopenia, physical function, cognitive function, and cardiovascular risk [65, 66].

## Myostatin

During the inevitable process of aging, a gradual loss in muscular mass and strength is inevitable. This starts approximately at the age of 30, and it ends up being determinant to develop a certain grade of incapacity for elderly people. This gradual loss of muscle mass and strength is called sarcopenia. One of the factors that triggers this process is myostatin, also known as GDF-8, which is a protein member of the activin subclass of the transforming growth factor beta (TGF-ß) superfamily. Myostatin is liberated mainly in the skeletal muscle, where it negatively regulates muscle mass through anti-anabolic and pro-catabolic mechanisms, acting directly over the myocytes. Myostatin can be found in three different forms in the plasma: free, bound to its own pro-peptide, and bound to any of its inhibitors. When it is bound to its pro-peptide, myostatin is inactive; this prevents its atrophic functions. The same case occurs when this protein is bound to any of its inhibitors like follistatin. The role of myostatin as a hormone was suggested for the first time in humans when a negative correlation between muscle mass and the concentration of this protein was observed in the serum of patients with HIV and cachexia [67]. This role was reinforced by Zimmers et al. in 2002, when they conducted an experiment introducing CHO (Chinese hamster ovary) cells, which overexpressed myostatin, in healthy mice resulting in high levels of this protein in serum and a massive loss of skeletal muscle [68]. Myostatin has also been negatively associated with muscular function in elderly women [69]. In other studies, it has been reported that high levels of myostatin are linked with the adipose tissue infiltration in the muscle, which affects the muscular function and physical performance [70]. It has also been observed that the levels of myostatin are higher in patients with age-related diseases than in healthy elderly patients [71].

## Concluding Remarks

The study of the human aging process is complex and multifactorial, where genetic and environmental variables are key players in its development. That is why we suggest a series of different biomarkers which include hormonal, inflammatory, and oxidative stress biomarkers. However, it is possible that other biomarkers such as DNA damage, telomere length determination, DNA repair mechanisms and p53 activation, can be considered as biomarkers of aging. Also, another interesting proposal could be to include transcriptomic, proteomic, and epigenetic profiles of the affected organs as molecular biomarkers. Likewise, it is important to consider another age-related biomarker, such as cellular senescence and its senescence-associated secretory phenotype (SASP), also including cell cycle-related proteins and the activity of the ß-galactosidase enzyme. These last biomarkers are vital to understand the aging process; however, the only way to obtain them, in order to get a proper analysis, is to collect biopsies from patients, and sometimes it is not possible because it is harmful. Thus, the whole set of biomarkers that we suggest in this chapter require low-invasive procedures, since they determine the aging process of the patients by collecting peripheral blood.

## References

1. Franceschi C, et al. Inflammaging and 'Garb-aging'. Trends Endocrinol Metab. 2017;28(3):199–212.
2. Strickland M, et al. Relationships between ion channels, mitochondrial functions and inflammation in human aging. Front Physiol. 2019;10:158.
3. Franceschi C, et al. Inflamm-aging. An evolutionary perspective on immunosenescence. Ann N Y Acad Sci. 2000;908:244–54.
4. Fan J, et al. MicroRNA-regulated proinflammatory cytokines in sarcopenia. Mediators Inflamm. 2016;2016:1438686.
5. Pinti M, et al. Circulating mitochondrial DNA increases with age and is a familiar trait: implications for "inflamm-aging". Eur J Immunol. 2014;44(5):1552–62.
6. Michaud M, et al. Proinflammatory cytokines, aging, and age-related diseases. J Am Med Dir Assoc. 2013;14(12):877–82.
7. Li X, et al. The prognostic value of serum cytokines in patients with acute ischemic stroke. Aging Dis. 2019;10(3):544–56.
8. Vettoretti S, et al. Sarcopenia is associated with malnutrition but not with systemic inflammation in older persons with advanced CKD. Nutrients. 2019;11(6):E1378.

9. Forsey RJ, et al. Plasma cytokine profiles in elderly humans. Mech Ageing Dev. 2003;124(4):487–93.
10. Wang T, et al. The efficacy of plasma biomarkers in early diagnosis of Alzheimer's disease. Int J Geriatr Psychiatry. 2014;29(7):713–9.
11. Taipa R, et al. Proinflammatory and anti-inflammatory cytokines in the CSF of patients with Alzheimer's disease and their correlation with cognitive decline. Neurobiol Aging. 2019;76:125–32.
12. Alvarez-Rodriguez L, et al. Aging is associated with circulating cytokine dysregulation. Cell Immunol. 2012;273(2):124–32.
13. D'Anna L, et al. Serum interleukin-10 levels correlate with cerebrospinal fluid amyloid beta deposition in Alzheimer disease patients. Neurodegener Dis. 2017;17(4–5):227–34.
14. Cruz-Almeida Y, et al. Age differences in cytokine expression under conditions of health using experimental pain models. Exp Gerontol. 2015;72:150–6.
15. Wennberg AMV, et al. The cross-sectional and longitudinal associations between IL-6, IL-10, and TNFalpha and cognitive outcomes in the Mayo Clinic study of aging. J Gerontol A Biol Sci Med Sci. 2018;74:1289.
16. Hou R, et al. Peripheral inflammatory cytokines and immune balance in generalised anxiety disorder: case-controlled study. Brain Behav Immun. 2017;62:212–8.
17. Barajas-Gomez BA, et al. Relationship of inflammatory profile of elderly patients serum and senescence-associated secretory phenotype with human breast cancer cells proliferation: role of IL6/IL8 ratio. Cytokine. 2017;91:13–29.
18. Bluher M, Mantzoros CS. From leptin to other adipokines in health and disease: facts and expectations at the beginning of the 21st century. Metabolism. 2015;64(1):131–45.
19. Sakuma K, Yamaguchi A. Sarcopenic obesity and endocrinal adaptation with age. Int J Endocrinol. 2013;2013:204164.
20. Tilg H, Moschen AR. Adipocytokines: mediators linking adipose tissue, inflammation and immunity. Nat Rev Immunol. 2006;6(10):772–83.
21. Procaccini C, Jirillo E, Matarese G. Leptin as an immunomodulator. Mol Asp Med. 2012;33(1):35–45.
22. Wong HS, et al. Production of superoxide and hydrogen peroxide from specific mitochondrial sites under different bioenergetic conditions. J Biol Chem. 2017;292(41):16804–9.
23. Zanotto-Filho A, Schroder R, Moreira JC. Xanthine oxidase-dependent ROS production mediates vitamin a pro-oxidant effects in cultured Sertoli cells. Free Radic Res. 2008;42(6):593–601.
24. Liang X, et al. Cyclic stretch induced oxidative stress by mitochondrial and NADPH oxidase in retinal pigment epithelial cells. BMC Ophthalmol. 2019;19(1):79.
25. Guillaumet-Adkins A, et al. Epigenetics and oxidative stress in aging. Oxid Med Cell Longev. 2017;2017:9175806.
26. Case AJ. On the origin of superoxide dismutase: an evolutionary perspective of superoxide-mediated redox signaling. Antioxidants (Basel). 2017;6(4):E82.
27. Tatsumi H, Tsuchiya Y, Sakamoto K. Sensitive electrochemical measurement of hydroxyl radical generation induced by the xanthine-xanthine oxidase system. Anal Biochem. 2014;467:22–7.
28. Barrera G, et al. Lipid peroxidation-derived aldehydes, 4-Hydroxynonenal and malondialdehyde in aging-related disorders. Antioxidants (Basel). 2018;7(8):E102.
29. Topkaya SN, et al. Nitration of tyrosine and its effect on DNA hybridization. Biosens Bioelectron. 2018;102:464–9.
30. Kolgiri V, Patil VW. Protein carbonyl content: a novel biomarker for aging in HIV/AIDS patients. Braz J Infect Dis. 2017;21(1):35–41.
31. Kolgiri V, Nagar V, Patil V. Association of serum total bilirubin and plasma 8-OHdG in HIV/AIDS patients. Interv Med Appl Sci. 2018;10(2):76–82.
32. Bellanti F, et al. Oxidative stress is increased in sarcopenia and associated with cardiovascular disease risk in sarcopenic obesity. Maturitas. 2018;109:6–12.
33. Serviddio G, et al. Frailty syndrome is associated with altered circulating redox balance and increased markers of oxidative stress. Int J Immunopathol Pharmacol. 2009;22(3):819–27.

34. Di Domenico F, Tramutola A, Butterfield DA. Role of 4-hydroxy-2-nonenal (HNE) in the pathogenesis of alzheimer disease and other selected age-related neurodegenerative disorders. Free Radic Biol Med. 2017;111:253–61.
35. Jacob KD, et al. Markers of oxidant stress that are clinically relevant in aging and age-related disease. Mech Ageing Dev. 2013;134(3–4):139–57.
36. Martinez de Toda I, et al. Function, oxidative, and inflammatory stress parameters in immune cells as predictive markers of lifespan throughout aging. Oxid Med Cell Longev. 2019;2019:4574276.
37. Kozakiewicz M, et al. Changes in the blood antioxidant defense of advanced age people. Clin Interv Aging. 2019;14:763–71.
38. Jones DP. Redox theory of aging. Redox Biol. 2015;5:71–9.
39. Guevara-Aguirre J, et al. Growth hormone receptor deficiency is associated with a major reduction in pro-aging signaling, cancer, and diabetes in humans. Sci Transl Med. 2011;3(70):70ra13.
40. Guevara-Aguirre J, et al. GH receptor Deficiency in Ecuadorian adults is associated with obesity and enhanced insulin sensitivity. J Clin Endocrinol Metab. 2015;100(7):2589–96.
41. Bartke A. Growth hormone and aging: updated review. World J Mens Health. 2019;37(1):19–30.
42. Bartke A. Can growth hormone (GH) accelerate aging? Evidence from GH-transgenic mice. Neuroendocrinology. 2003;78(4):210–6.
43. van der Spoel E, et al. Growth hormone secretion is diminished and tightly controlled in humans enriched for familial longevity. Aging Cell. 2016;15(6):1126–31.
44. Lee WS, Kim J. Insulin-like growth factor-1 signaling in cardiac aging. Biochim Biophys Acta Mol basis Dis. 2018;1864(5 Pt B):1931–8.
45. Balasubramanian P, Longo VD. Growth factors, aging and age-related diseases. Growth Hormon IGF Res. 2016;28:66–8.
46. Suzuki K, et al. Serum insulin-like growth factor-1 levels in neurodegenerative diseases. Acta Neurol Scand. 2019;139(6):563–7.
47. Tanisawa K, et al. Inverse association between height-increasing alleles and extreme longevity in Japanese women. J Gerontol A Biol Sci Med Sci. 2018;73(5):588–95.
48. Asih PR, et al. Multiple mechanisms linking type 2 diabetes and Alzheimer's disease: testosterone as a modifier. J Alzheimers Dis. 2017;59(2):445–66.
49. Kloner RA, et al. Testosterone and cardiovascular disease. J Am Coll Cardiol. 2016;67(5):545–57.
50. Mohamad NV, Soelaiman IN, Chin KY. A concise review of testosterone and bone health. Clin Interv Aging. 2016;11:1317–24.
51. Huang G, et al. Long-term testosterone administration on insulin sensitivity in older men with low or low-Normal testosterone levels. J Clin Endocrinol Metab. 2018;103(4):1678–85.
52. Buvat J, et al. Testosterone deficiency in men: systematic review and standard operating procedures for diagnosis and treatment. J Sex Med. 2013;10(1):245–84.
53. Harman SM, et al. Longitudinal effects of aging on serum total and free testosterone levels in healthy men. Baltimore longitudinal study of aging. J Clin Endocrinol Metab. 2001;86(2):724–31.
54. Adams JB. Control of secretion and the function of C19-delta 5-steroids of the human adrenal gland. Mol Cell Endocrinol. 1985;41(1):1–17.
55. Morales AJ, et al. Effects of replacement dose of dehydroepiandrosterone in men and women of advancing age. J Clin Endocrinol Metab. 1994;78(6):1360–7.
56. Ferrari E, et al. Age-related changes of the hypothalamic-pituitary-adrenal axis: pathophysiological correlates. Eur J Endocrinol. 2001;144(4):319–29.
57. Pitt B, et al. Eplerenone, a selective aldosterone blocker, in patients with left ventricular dysfunction after myocardial infarction. N Engl J Med. 2003;348(14):1309–21.
58. Zhou S, Glowacki J. Dehydroepiandrosterone and Bone. Vitam Horm. 2018;108:251–71.
59. Karametos I, et al. Chronic obstructive pulmonary disease as a main factor of premature aging. Int J Environ Res Public Health. 2019;16(4):E540.
60. Anon-Hidalgo J, et al. Circulating concentrations of GDF11 are positively associated with TSH levels in humans. J Clin Med. 2019;8(6):E878.

61. van Vliet NA, et al. Thyroid status and mortality in nonagenarians from long-lived families and the general population. Aging (Albany NY). 2017;9(10):2223–34.
62. Chen J, et al. Age-related change in thyroid-stimulating hormone: a cross-sectional study in healthy euthyroid population. Endocr J. 2018;65(11):1075–82.
63. Barbesino G. Thyroid function changes in the elderly and their relationship to cardiovascular health: a mini-review. Gerontology. 2019;65(1):1–8.
64. Wimalawansa SJ. Vitamin D deficiency: effects on oxidative stress, epigenetics, gene regulation, and aging. Biology (Basel). 2019;8(2):E30.
65. Chen CH, et al. Associations between vitamin D deficiency, musculoskeletal health, and cardiometabolic risk among community-living people in Taiwan: age and sex-specific relationship. Medicine (Baltimore). 2018;97(52):e13886.
66. Mathieu SV, et al. Association between 25-hydroxyvitamin D status and components of body composition and glucose metabolism in older men and women. Nutrients. 2018;10(12):E1826.
67. Barrios-Silva LV, et al. Activin subfamily peptides predict chronological age in humans. Physiol Rep. 2018;6(17):e13823.
68. Zimmers TA, et al. Induction of cachexia in mice by systemically administered myostatin. Science. 2002;296(5572):1486–8.
69. Fife E, et al. Relationship of muscle function to circulating myostatin, follistatin and GDF11 in older women and men. BMC Geriatr. 2018;18(1):200.
70. Konopka AR, et al. Relationship between intermuscular adipose tissue infiltration and myostatin before and after aerobic exercise training. Am J Physiol Regul Integr Comp Physiol. 2018;315(3):R461–8.
71. Schafer MJ, et al. Quantification of GDF11 and myostatin in human aging and cardiovascular disease. Cell Metab. 2016;23(6):1207–15.

# Alternative Splicing and Aging 7

J. C. Yustis-Rubio and Juan Carlos Gomez-Verjan

## Abbreviations

| | |
|---|---|
| AD | Alzheimer's disease |
| ALS | Amyotrophic lateral sclerosis |
| AS | Alternative splicing |
| BPS | Branch point site |
| BS | Bloom syndrome |
| CTD | C-terminal domain (CTD) |
| DMD | Duchenne muscular dystrophy |
| ESE | Exonic splicing enhancer |
| ESS | Exonic splicing silencer |
| HAT | Histone acetylase |
| HDAC | Histone deacetylase |
| HGS | Hutchinson-Gilford syndrome |
| hnRNP | Heterogeneous nuclear ribonucleoprotein |
| ISE | Intronic splicing enhancer |
| ISS | Intronic splicing silencer |
| NMD | Nonsense-mediated mRNA decay |
| PD | Parkinson's disease |
| pre-mRNA | Precursor messenger mRNA |
| PTC | Premature termination codons |
| RNAPII | RNA polymerase II |

J. C. Yustis-Rubio
Departamento de Ecología Funcional, Instituto de Ecología, UNAM, Mexico City, Mexico
e-mail: jcyustis@ciencias.unam.mx

J. C. Gomez-Verjan (✉)
División de Ciencias Básicas, Instituto Nacional de Geriatría (INGER), Mexico City, Mexico
e-mail: jverjan@inger.gob.mx



J. C. Gomez-Verjan, N. A. Rivero-Segura (eds.), *Clinical Genetics and Genomics of Aging*, https://doi.org/10.1007/978-3-030-40955-5_7

| | |
|---|---|
| snRNA | Small nuclear RNA |
| snRNP | Small nuclear ribonucleoprotein |
| SR | Serine-arginine-rich proteins |
| SS | Splice sites |
| WS | Werner syndrome |

## Introduction

One of the most striking characteristics of eukaryotic genomes is the discontinuous arrangement of genes, in which protein-coding segments, known as exons, are interrupted by non-coding sequences, known as introns. Through a highly regulated process known as *splicing*, the introns present in the precursor messenger RNA (pre-mRNA) are removed, and exons are joined together, forming the mature form of mRNA. While some genes are constitutively spliced, meaning that they will produce the same mature mRNA from a given pre-mRNA, some can generate different mRNA isoforms from a single pre-mRNA through a process known as alternative splicing (AS). AS is a process by which a single gene can give rise to different transcripts through the differential assembly and organization of the sequences present within the exons/introns of a gene. This process can give rise to a wide variety of transcript isoforms from a small number of genes, increasing both transcriptome and proteome [1, 2].

With the recent development of faster and accurate sequencing technologies and the ever-decreasing costs of sequencing whole transcriptomes, it has become apparent that AS has a significant role in organism development. It is estimated that around 95% of all human protein-coding genes undergo a process of AS [3, 4]. After the sequencing of the human genome and that of other model organisms, it became clear that although humans are significantly more complex both morphologically and behaviorally than mice, fruit flies (*Drosophila melanogaster*), or tapeworms (*Caenorhabditis elegans*), the difference in the number of genes between these organisms was not the reason behind these differences. This meant that something else besides the number of protein-coding genes was responsible for the increasing level of complexity among different organisms. Evidence from the characterization of expressed cDNA clone sequence tags [5, 6], as well as bioinformatic analysis, indicates that AS events seem to increase with organism complexity. These findings suggest that AS has been used throughout evolutionary history as a mechanism through which higher level of molecular complexity can be achieved. In that regard, humans (*Homo sapiens*), compared to other organisms, are the ones that have the highest percentage of AS events for multiexon protein-coding genes (around 88%) with at least 2+ mRNA isoforms per gene (comparatively mouse sits at around 63%, fruit fly 45%, and tapeworm 25%). This information is based upon current genome annotations that do not consider recent RNA-seq data. Recent studies based on RNA-seq of the human transcriptome indicate that >95–100% of human genes generate at least two alternative pre-mRNA isoforms (with an average of seven mRNA isoforms per gene) [3, 4]. These observations support that an increase in the occurrence of AS events is directly correlated with the increase in organism complexity [7].

## Mechanisms of Pre-mRNA Splicing

The underlying molecular mechanisms by which introns are removed from the pre-mRNA seem to be very well conserved among all eukaryotic groups [8]. Intron excision from the pre-mRNA and subsequent exon ligation is mediated by a complex and highly regulated molecular machinery known as the spliceosome. The spliceosome is a ribonucleoprotein (RNA-protein complex) which acts in a dynamic cycle of stepwise reactions that is assembled and disassembled for every single splicing reaction [9]. Several efforts have been made to characterize and determine the structure and function of the different components of the spliceosome throughout the different steps of the cycle. Biochemical and structural analyses have demonstrated that the catalytic center of the spliceosome is composed of RNA [10]. The actual biochemical reactions that take place during a splicing event are two consecutive $S_N2$-type transesterification reactions involving functional groups from three reactive regions present in the pre-mRNA. Two of these regions are present at the 5′ and 3′ end of introns and are known as either 5′ or 3′ splice sites (SS). The other region involved is known as the branch point site (BPS) located near the 3′ end of the intron, around 15–50 nucleotides upstream of the 3′ SS [11]. The sequences that define the 5′ and 3′ SS, as well as the BPS, are very small consensus elements [9].

The primary assembly process of the spliceosome requires the recruitment of several small nuclear ribonucleoprotein (snRNP) subunits, namely, snRNPs U1, U2, U4, U5, and U6, as well as other non-snRNP splicing factors. Each of these snRNP subunits is composed of a specific small nuclear RNA (snRNA), as well as other proteins. These snRNAs are the ones that through a base pairing-based mechanism recognize the specific sequences within the DNA (5′ and 3′ SS, BPS) to differentiate exons from introns. Firstly, the U1 snRNP recognizes the 5′ SS of the mRNA forming the early complex (complex E), meanwhile, the 3′ SS is recognized by the U2 snRNP as well as other associated factors, such as splicing factor 1 (SF1) and U2 auxiliary factors (U2AFs), which are also components of complex E. U2 then recognizes sequences at the BPS and interacts with U1 to form the pre-spliceosome complex (complex A). After the assembly of the complex A, the U4, U5, and U6 snRNPs are recruited as a pre-formed tri-snRNP, forming complex B. This resulting complex B is still catalytically inactive and goes through several changes to form the catalytically active complex B∗. The activation of complex B results in the release of U1 and U4. Complex B∗ can complete the first catalytic step of splicing, generating complex C, which contains exon 1 and the intron-exon 2 lariat intermediate. Complex C undergoes a series of rearrangements to carry out the second catalytic step that results in a post-spliceosomal complex that contains the lariat intron and the spliced exons. In the last step of the cycle, the U2, U5, and U6 snRNPs are released alongside the lariat intron and recycled for additional rounds of splicing. As mentioned before, the splicing process is largely RNA-based, mainly through the U2-U5-U6 snRNP complex [12], which seems to be the active structure that catalyzes both steps of the splicing reaction, but it seems that some proteins are also necessary for the formation of the catalytic site [13].

## Mechanisms and Regulation of Alternative Splicing

The occurrence of different types of AS events is influenced by a wide variety of factors, including splicing regulatory sequences present in the pre-mRNA, differential activities of splicing factors that either activate or repress AS, chromatin density and structure, as well as transcription elongation rates [14]. The different types of AS events include exon skipping, in which an exon is spliced out of the mature mRNA, along with its flanking introns. Intron retention occurs when an intron is included in the mature transcript; alternative 3′ SS and 5′ SS selection events occur when multiple SS are recognized at the same time at either end of an exon. A mutually exclusive AS event can occur when two exons are included in the mature transcript in a mutually exclusive way (either one of the two exons is included); another type of AS event is known as alternative polyadenylation in which the region where the poly(A) tract is localized can vary. In vertebrates, and specifically in humans, the most prevalent AS event is exon skipping [6, 15]. All these events can be combined into even more complex types of AS, giving rise to a wide variety of isoforms from a single transcript.

The SS selection that eventually gives rise to different transcript isoforms from a single gene is determined by a wide variety of elements which can be both cis- and trans-acting. As mentioned earlier, because most SS consensus sequences are poorly conserved, SS by themselves cannot efficiently direct the spliceosome assembly process. For instance, the cis-acting elements include regulatory sequences which can be found both within exons and introns and act as splicing enhancers or silencers, depending on their position as well as their effect on the usage of a SS [14], meaning that within a specific region of the genome, both intronic splicing enhancers (ISE) and silencers (ISS) can be found, as well as exonic splicing enhancers (ESE) and silencers (ESS). These regulatory sequences function mainly as binding sites for trans-acting factors that in turn recruit the snRNP subunits of the spliceosome to a specific site.

The trans-acting elements function through the binding to splicing enhancer or silencer sequences and include both serine-arginine (SR)-rich and heterogeneous nuclear ribonucleoprotein (hnRNP) families of proteins. It is generally considered that SR proteins act as splicing promoters while hnRNP as repressors, although there is evidence indicating that the activities of some of these splicing regulators are determined by the region of the pre-mRNA in which they bind. A recent study has shown that SR proteins can act both as enhancers and silencers of splicing [16]. Interestingly, these proteins can recognize short RNA sequence motifs and can function as splicing enhancers when bound to exons and as repressors of splicing when bound to introns [17]. hnRNPs can also recognize specific binding sequences in RNA, and depending on its binding position, they can also act as both enhancers and silencers of splicing [18].

Alterations of pre-mRNA splicing can give rise to several physiological abnormalities that often lead to disease [19]. Even though the process of splicing itself consists of relatively simple steps, the recognition of correct SS is a daunting task for the splicing machinery given the highly complex organization of the genome. Mutations of these (and other) regulatory regions of splicing can sometimes generate faulty transcripts harboring premature termination codons (PTC) that if translated could lead to defective proteins. The nonsense-mediated mRNA decay (NMD) pathway was first described solely as a post-transcriptional surveillance and quality control mechanism responsible for the degradation of transcripts harboring a PTC that if translated could lead to the production of truncated proteins with deleterious effects for the organism. Evidence has also shown the importance of the NMD pathway as a regulatory mechanism that controls the expression of several naturally occurring transcripts [20]. Recently, it has been shown that not all PTC-containing transcripts trigger the activation of the NMD pathway. Moreover, other transcripts that do not contain a PTC are also targets of NMD [20], which indicates that further studies are needed to understand all the factors involved in the activation of the NMD pathway.

AS can generate transcripts harboring PTCs, and canonically these transcripts should be subject to degradation by NMD; however, the NMD pathway does not degrade these transcripts. Instead, it seems that some of these transcripts were able to "hijack" the NMD pathway to serve as a regulatory mechanism for their transcription [21]. This phenomenon, known as AS-NMD regulation, was first reported as a widely spread mechanism of regulation of a variety of transcripts, both naturally occurring and disease-related [22]. More recent evidence seems to suggest that AS-NMD regulation is not as widespread as initially thought [23], but there is evidence supporting an important role of AS-NMD regulation on specific gene families, including well-known regulators of splicing and AS [24–26]. It would seem that AS-NMD acts mainly as a repressive regulatory mechanism, but there is evidence that it can also be used as a developmental switch [27].

## Coupling of Splicing with Transcription

There has been accumulating evidence showing the coupling of transcription and splicing [14]. The fact that splicing occurs in a cotranscriptional manner is the basis for inferring that transcription elongation rate, chromatin structure, and modifications are coupled with splicing.

One of the key elements that link transcription and splicing is the RNA polymerase II (RNAPII). Transcription elongation rate can affect SS selection and thus the products of AS. A faster elongation rate of transcription encourages skipping of exons with "weak" 3′ SS, while slower elongation rates encourage the inclusion of exons with weak 3′ SS sites [28]. One possible mechanism is that the occupancy of nucleosomes can alter the elongation rate of the RNAPII to facilitate inclusion of weak SS [29]. Nucleosomes can act as barriers for elongating RNAPII altering its elongation rate, as exons flanked by weak SS are more enriched with nucleosomes compared with those containing strong SS [30].

One of the main characteristics of RNAPII is the presence of a C-terminal domain (CTD). Post-translational modifications of this CTD have been shown to play a crucial role in the regulation of its transcriptional activity, particularly phosphorylation. The CTD of RNAPII serves as a scaffold for the recruitment of a wide variety of splicing factors [31], as mutations of the CTD lead to splicing alterations [32]. These post-transcriptional modifications may regulate the physical interactions between the CTD and splicing components creating a binding platform for splicing factors. Apart from nucleosome occupancy, there is evidence that chromatin modifications also have a role in coupling transcription and splicing [33]. Transcriptional elongation rate is regulated by a dynamic cycle of histone acetylation/deacetylation, which is very important for nucleosome dynamics during transcription and is coordinated by the CTD of RNAPII [34]. A wide variety of histone acetyltransferase (HAT) and deacetylase (HDAC) proteins mediate the addition and removal of acetyl groups that modify the interactions between nucleosomes and DNA. During the transcription process, it is necessary that HATs acetylate the nucleosome downstream of the elongation complex in order to destabilize the interactions between histones and DNA. RNAPII elongation causes a displacement of histones, which are subsequently placed onto the DNA behind RNAPII. These deposited nucleosomes are hyperacetylated momentarily. HDAC complexes remove acetylation marks from the chromatin to maintain a stable configuration. This acetylation/deacetylation dynamic can influence the selection of SS in many genes [33].

Chromatin-modifying proteins that recognize and bind specific histone marks can also affect splicing patterns by recruiting several splicing factors to sites of active transcription to modulate the inclusion or exclusion of alternative exons. Specific patterns of histone marks can correlate with particular splicing patterns in many genes [35]. Another evidence is the fact that modulation of histone marks by inhibitors, overexpression of histone modifiers, or knockdown experiment induces changes in the splicing patterns [36].

## Connections Between Alternative Splicing and Human Disease

Recently, a vast amount of evidence supporting pre-mRNA splicing, both constitutive and alternative, as an important regulatory mechanism of organismic complexity in humans gave rise to further research the relevance that pre-mRNA splicing alterations could have on disease [37, 38].

The complex genomic arrangement of eukaryotic genomes comes with the implication that every intron-containing gene requires to undergo the process of splicing, meaning that the proper processing of pre-mRNA into mature transcripts needs to be tightly regulated, and the fact that splicing occurs in a cotranscriptional manner adds another layer of complexity to this process. The downside of the functional versatility that comes with pre-mRNA splicing is that this process can be disrupted through a wide variety of ways and these alterations can end up being the cause of several pathological conditions [37].

According to data from the Human Gene Mutation Database (HGMD), of all the single-nucleotide polymorphisms (SNPs) that are the cause of a disease, around 15% are located within SS sequences and 22% of disease alleles are located within splicing elements, meaning that more than one third of all disease-causing SNPs can alter splicing [39, 40]. Also, evidence from the HGMD suggests that around 10% of human inherited diseases are due to single base-pair substitution mutations located in SS [41]. However, these data only take into account mutations located at the relatively well-conserved SS sequences, but not at other *cis*-acting splicing elements nor mutations located at loci of *trans*-acting splicing elements. Alterations in pre-mRNA splicing can come from a wide variety of alterations, but they are grouped into these categories: mutations of canonical 5′ and 3′ SS, mutations of the BPS, mutations of *cis*-acting regulatory elements, mutations of *trans*-acting splicing elements, and mutations of the splicing machinery.

## Mutations in Splice Sites and Regulatory Sequences

The most common types of splicing-related mutations that occur are those of *cis*-acting elements, such as the core consensus sequences (both 5′ and 3′ SS, as well as the BPS) as well as other splicing regulatory sequences [19]. Among these, familial dysautonomia is a rare recessive disorder in the Ashkenazi Jewish population that affects both the autonomous nervous system and the somatic sensory neurons [42]. Caused by a point mutation in intron 20 (T→C) in the *IKBKAP* gene, that results in the alteration of a 5′ SS weakening the binding of the spliceosome subunit U1, leading to the skipping of exon 20 which results in the introduction of a PTC in exon 21, making the mRNA susceptible to degradation by the NMD pathway [43].

One of the best studied cases of splicing alterations of *cis*-acting elements that end up being the cause of a pathological condition is spinal muscular atrophy (SMA). SMA is a prevalent recessive disorder associated with infant mortality; more than 90% of all cases of SMA are the result of mutations of the *Survival Motor Neuron 1* (*SMN1*) gene. Humans carry two copies of the *SMN* gene: *SMN1* and *SMN2*. SMN is required for proper snRNP synthesis, and its absence leads to degeneration of motor neurons, particularly those of the spinal cord. The main difference between the two copies is the fact that in SMN2 exon 7 is predominantly skipped in most tissues. *SMN2* codes for SMNΔ 7, a partially functional and unstable protein. Loss of *SMN1* leads to a deficit of the SMN protein and the consequent death of motor neurons. SMN2 presents a C→T change at position 6 of exon 7. This single mutation causes two different outcomes: first, the deletion of an ESE, and second, it creates an ESS, which in turn promotes the skipping of exon 7 [44].

Another well-documented case is Duchenne muscular dystrophy (DMD). While genomic deletions of the *dystrophin* gene cause the most severe forms of DMD, some mild forms of DMD are caused by point mutations that affect the splicing patterns [37]. Particularly, a T→A substitution in exon 31 simultaneously generates an

ESS resulting in exon skipping and introduces a PTC [45]. These splicing alterations produce a partially functioning form of the protein, which explains the mild phenotype of the disease.

## Mutations of Splicing Trans-acting and Core Spliceosome Factors

Mutations in *trans*-acting splicing factors, as well as core spliceosome components, can simultaneously affect a significant number of genes. Unlike mutations in *cis*-acting elements, there are relatively few examples of genetic disorders caused by alterations of *trans*-acting factors, including spliceosomal factors, maybe because many of these mutations result in lethality during embryonic development [46].

Amyotrophic lateral sclerosis (ALS) is an adult-onset neurodegenerative disease characterized by the degeneration of upper and lower motor neurons. It is a fatal disorder that ultimately causes death within 2–5 years following diagnosis. Around 10% of cases seem to follow a pattern of Mendelian inheritance and high penetrance [47]. Studies demonstrated that RNA processing plays an essential role in the onset of the disease. Specifically, one of the most important genes for ALS, *TDP-43* (*TARDBP*), an RNA-binding protein, seems to be a major component of cytoplasmic inclusions in motor neurons of ALS patients [48]. TDP-43 is normally localized in the nucleus and it is involved in RNA processing as well as AS and neurons with cytoplasmic aggregations show a depletion of nuclear TDP-43. Recent studies have demonstrated that TDP-43 seems to be a direct regulator of several AS events in the brain [49, 50]. This evidence suggests that the loss of function of TDP-43 seems to be a major determinant factor in ALS.

Retinitis pigmentosa is a disorder characterized by the progressive degeneration of the retina. Mutations in the core spliceosomal factors PRPF3, PRPF8, PRPF31, and SNRNP200 are associated with the onset of the disease [51]. These factors are important for the assembly of the tri-snRNP complex of U4/U6/U5 from the spliceosome [11]. Even though the specific pathological defects seem to indicate a functional role in the retina, the specific splicing abnormalities responsible for the disease remain to be discovered.

## Alternative Splicing and Aging

Aging is characterized by a general decline of the homeostatic capacity of the organism to reach the normal state, leading to a general decline in the physiological and social functions highly associated with mortality. In this context, aging has been associated with several diseases such as cardiovascular and metabolic disorders, many types of cancer, and neurodegenerative diseases as Alzheimer's and Parkinson's diseases, among others [52]. Such age-related decline is associated with tissue damage and several inflammatory processes (inflammaging [53] and immunosenescence [54]); in this context aging seems to be tissue-specific and highly related to genetic expression more than genotype itself. Therefore, AS becomes highly essential since 90% of human protein-coding genes produce multiple transcripts through this process [3], and as previously stated, aberrant splicing events are correlated with age-associated diseases, since most of them lead to aberrant protein formation and, therefore, to misfolded protein accumulation, a process highly related to the molecular pillars of aging [55].

## Alternative Splicing, Progeroid, and Age-Related Diseases

**Werner syndrome (WS)** It is a well-characterized autosomal recessive progeroid syndrome, in which patients developed normally until they reach puberty and then started to experiment wrong physiological development, the suffering of skin and gonadal atrophy, cataracts, type 2 diabetes, osteoporosis, and loss and graying of hair [56]. Most of WS patients reach 54 years old and die of myocardial infarction; mutations on WRN gene (located at chromosome 8p12 that codified for 34 exons encoding a DNA helicase protein) are responsible for such disease [57]. AS is quite essential in WS since due to exon skipping associated with stop codons, indels, or mutations, most of the pathogenic variants on the WRN gene result in helicase protein truncation; additionally pathogenic variants have also been reported in intronic regions [56].

**Hutchinson-Gilford syndrome (HGS)** It is a genetic disease characterized by a dramatic aging phenotype early in childhood [58]. Most of HGS patients die from heart attacks and stroke early in their teens [59]. Interestingly, most cases are characterized by a silent mutation within a single codon of the *LMNA* gene which enhances the use of an internal 5′ SS in exon 11 and leads to the production of a truncated protein (progerin). Its accumulation could lead to abnormally shaped nuclei, loss of heterochromatin distribution, changes in methylation patterns, and misregulation of nuclear proteins, among other changes [60]. Although it is not clear the relationship between HGS and normal aging, evidence suggests that progerin may be involved in the aging process since the number of (+) progerin protein cells increases with age in samples from healthy individuals [61–63].

**Bloom syndrome (BS)** It is an autosomal recessive progeroid disease mainly characterized by early growth deficiency, photosensitive skin changes, immune deficiency, insulin resistance, and a substantially increased risk for the development of multiple cancers [64]. Mutations on the *BLM* gene cause BS; such gene encodes RecQ helicase. Interestingly, such mutations have been found to induce aberrant splicing in which the extra exon 3 s are skipped, and a site mutation on p53 splice acceptor has been found in skin fibroblasts derived from BS patient [65].

**Diabetes** It is a chronic disease characterized by hyperglycemia as a result of pancreas not making enough insulin or due to insulin resistance. In this context, insulin sensitivity is associated with insulin receptor isoform, and studies have demonstrated that insulin receptor type B mRNA variant increases in response to bariatric surgery [66] and weight loss for low caloric diet [67] as well as the genetic expression of several splicing factors involved in the insulin receptor [68]. Particularly in the pathogenesis of diabetes type 1, splicing process in T cells and node stromal cells seems to be involved in the modulation of the immunological response against β cells; interestingly, β cells exposed to cytokines activate AS networks that modulate its viability and susceptibility to immune-induced stress [69, 70].

**Cancer** It is a broad term to refer to several diseases characterized by abnormal cells that possess a very particular genetic expression related with cell survival, accelerated growth and spreading across the body. Since the incidence of most cancers increases as a person ages, it is considered an age-related disease. Several genome-wide association studies suggest a strong relation between AS and cancer due to the plasticity offered by this process [71]. Splicing aberration related with cancer could be divided in four main categories: those related with alteration on tumor suppressor genes and oncogenes, those related with aberration on spliceosomal components, mutations over splicing factors, and changes in the signaling pathways that regulate splicing process; some of these changes are highly significant to cancer hallmarks [72].

**Alzheimer's disease (AD)** It is characterized by a progressive decline in normal cognitive functions, diminishing the performance of memory, attention, language, and visuospatial skills and in executing tasks [73]. Neuropathology of AD includes the accumulation of β-amyloid deposition and accumulation of *Tau*-hyperphosphorylated proteins [74]. Mutations occurring in the intronic regions of presenilin 1 and 2 cause missplicing and lead to abnormal expression of β-amyloid [75]. A variant including exon 7 is the dominant splice form of the amyloid precursor protein gene in AD patients and contributes to β-amyloid accumulation; interestingly, RBFox is a trans-acting regulator that leads to the inclusion or exclusion of exon 7 [76]. ApoE4 a major cholesterol transporter in the brain and cholesterol-rich membrane domains increase β-amyloid production affecting β- and γ-secretase complexes; the proteolysis of apoE4 may lead to a loss of function in its ability to remove β-amyloid. Interestingly, E4 isoform is more prone to proteolysis than other APOE [77]. The inclusion of the exon 10 in *Tau* gene generates an isoform susceptible to microtubule binding involved in the formation of *Tau* into paired helical filaments [74].

**Parkinson's disease (PD)** It is the second most common neurodegenerative disease, characterized by resting tremor, bradykinesia, stiffness of movement, and postural instability; among its physiopathology is caused by protein aggregation in Lewy bodies and loss of dopamine-containing neurons in the substantia nigra of the midbrain [78]. Six genes, including *PARK2*, *SNCAIP*, *LRRK2*, *SNCA*, *SRRM2*, and *MAPT*, are involved in aberrant AS events in PD patients [79]. For instance, several point mutations in *PARK2* splice acceptor or donor sites have been identified in PD patients [80]. On the other side, mutations in *LRRK2* are the most common genetic cause of familial late-onset parkinsonism; most of them are on intronic regions highly susceptible to splicing [81]. Interestingly, oxidant generated AS of *SNCA* plays a central role in dopamine neuron cell death [79]. The *MAPT* gene which encodes Tau is also susceptible to several mutations present within coding regions and reduces its binding activity and decreases the ability of Tau to promote MT assembly [79].

## Conclusions

AS constitutes one of the most important mechanisms for the plasticity of the transcriptome and proteome, since it is not only a spatiotemporal process but it helps to identify critical processes. Growing evidence demonstrates that dysregulation of the AS events is highly implicated in several diseases including those age-related diseases. In this context, it can function to develop biomarkers for such diseases or to develop therapeutic agents. Further research must be performed to improve our understanding of this complicated process.

## References

1. Nilsen TW, Graveley BR. Expansion of the eukaryotic proteome by alternative splicing. Nature. 2010;463(7280):457–63.
2. Blencowe BJ. Alternative splicing: new insights from global analyses. Cell. 2006;126(1):37–47.
3. Wang ET, Sandberg R, Luo S, Khrebtukova I, Zhang L, Mayr C, et al. Alternative isoform regulation in human tissue transcriptomes. Nature. 2008;456(7221):470–6.
4. Pan Q, Shai O, Lee LJ, Frey BJ, Blencowe BJ. Deep surveying of alternative splicing complexity in the human transcriptome by high-throughput sequencing. Nat Genet. 2008;40(12):1413–5.
5. Kim H, Klein R, Majewski J, Ott J, Harrington ED, Boue S, et al. Estimating rates of alternative splicing in mammals and invertebrates (multiple letters). Nat Genet. 2004;36(9):915–7.
6. Kim E, Magen A, Ast G. Different levels of alternative splicing among eukaryotes. Nucleic Acids Res. 2007;35(1):125–31.
7. Chen L, Bush SJ, Tovar-Corona JM, Castillo-Morales A, Urrutia AO. Correcting for differential transcript coverage reveals a strong relationship between alternative splicing and organism complexity. Mol Biol Evol. 2014;31(6):1402–13.
8. Keren H, Lev-Maor G, Ast G. Alternative splicing and evolution: diversification, exon definition and function. Nat Rev Genet. 2010;11(5):345–55.
9. Wahl MC, Will CL, Lührmann R. The spliceosome: design principles of a dynamic RNP machine. Cell. 2009;136(4):701–18.
10. Lee Y, Rio DC. Mechanisms and regulation of alternative Pre-mRNA splicing. Annu Rev Biochem. 2015;84:291–323.
11. Matera AG, Wang Z. A day in the life of the spliceosome. Nat Rev Mol Cell Biol. 2014;15(2):108–21.
12. Fica SM, Tuttle N, Novak T, Li NS, Lu J, Koodathingal P, et al. RNA catalyses nuclear pre-mRNA splicing. Nature. 2013;503(7475):229–34.
13. Galej WP, Oubridge C, Newman AJ, Nagai K. Crystal structure of Prp8 reveals active site cavity of the spliceosome. Nature. 2013;493(7434):638–43.
14. Naftelberg S, Schor IE, Ast G, Kornblihtt AR. Regulation of alternative splicing through coupling with transcription and chromatin structure. Annu Rev Biochem. 2015;84(1):165–98.
15. Sultan M, Schulz MH, Richard H, Magen A, Klingenhoff A, Scherf M, et al. A global view of gene activity and alternative splicing by deep sequencing of the human transcriptome. Science. 2008;321(5891):956–60.

16. Pandit S, Zhou Y, Shiue L, Coutinho-Mansfield G, Li H, Qiu J, et al. Genome-wide analysis reveals SR protein cooperation and competition in regulated splicing. Mol Cell. 2013;50(2):223–35.
17. Änkö ML. Regulation of gene expression programmes by serine-arginine rich splicing factors. Semin Cell Dev Biol. 2014;32:11–21.
18. Motta-Mena LB, Heyd F, Lynch KW. Context-dependent regulatory mechanism of the splicing factor hnRNP L. Mol Cell. 2010;37(2):223–34.
19. Scotti MM, Swanson MS. RNA mis-splicing in disease. Nat Rev Genet. 2016;17(1):19–32.
20. Hug N, Longman D, Cáceres JF. Mechanism and regulation of the nonsense-mediated decay pathway. Nucleic Acids Res. 2015;44(4):1483–95.
21. Hillman RT, Green RE, Brenner SE. An unappreciated role for RNA surveillance. Genome Biol. 2004;5(2):R8.
22. Green RE, Lewis BP, Hillman RT, Blanchette M, Lareau LF, Garnett AT, et al. Widespread predicted nonsense-mediated mRNA decay of alternatively-spliced transcripts of human normal and disease genes. Bioinformatics. 2003;19(Suppl. 1):i118–21.
23. Pan Q, Saltzman AL, Yoon KK, Misquitta C, Shai O, Maquat LE, et al. Quantitative microarray profiling provides evidence against widespread coupling of alternative splicing with nonsense-mediated mRNA decay to control gene expression. Genes Dev. 2006;20(2):153–8.
24. Lareau LF, Inada M, Green RE, Wengrod JC, Brenner SE. Unproductive splicing of SR genes associated with highly conserved and ultraconserved DNA elements. Nature. 2007;446(7138):926–9.
25. Ni JZ, Grate L, Donohue JP, Preston C, Nobida N, O'Brien G, et al. Ultraconserved elements are associated with homeostatic control of splicing regulators by alternative splicing and nonsense-mediated decay. Genes Dev. 2007;21(6):708–18.
26. Saltzman AL, Kim YK, Pan Q, Fagnani MM, Maquat LE, Blencowe BJ. Regulation of multiple core spliceosomal proteins by alternative splicing-coupled nonsense-mediated mRNA decay. Mol Cell Biol. 2008;28(13):4320–30.
27. Boutz PL, Stoilov P, Li Q, Lin CH, Chawla G, Ostrow K, et al. A post-transcriptional regulatory switch in polypyrimidine tract-binding proteins reprograms alternative splicing in developing neurons. Genes Dev. 2007;21(13):1636–52.
28. De La Mata M, Alonso CR, Kadener S, Fededa JP, Blaustein M, Pelisch F, et al. A slow RNA polymerase II affects alternative splicing in vivo. Mol Cell. 2003;12(2):525–32.
29. Hodges C, Bintu L, Lubkowska L, Kashlev M, Bustamante C. Nucleosomal fluctuations govern the transcription dynamics of RNA polymerase II. Science. 2009;325(5940):626–8.
30. Schwartz S, Meshorer E, Ast G. Chromatin organization marks exon-intron structure. Nat Struct Mol Biol. 2009;16(9):990–5.
31. de Almeida SF, Carmo-Fonseca M. The CTD role in cotranscriptional RNA processing and surveillance. FEBS Lett. 2008;582(14):1971–6.
32. McCracken S, Fong N, Yankulov K, Ballantyne S, Pan G, Greenblatt J, et al. The C-terminal domain of RNA polymerase II couples mRNA processing to transcription. Nature. 1997;385(6614):357–60.
33. Zhou HL, Luo G, Wise JA, Lou H. Regulation of alternative splicing by local histone modifications: potential roles for RNA-guided mechanisms. Nucleic Acids Res. 2014;42(2):701–13.
34. Hsin JP, Manley JL. The RNA polymerase II CTD coordinates transcription and RNA processing. Genes Dev. 2012;26(19):2119–37.
35. Luco RF, Misteli T. More than a splicing code: integrating the role of RNA, chromatin and non-coding RNA in alternative splicing regulation. Curr Opin Genet Dev. 2011;21(4):366–72.
36. Luco R, Pan Q, Tominaga K, Blencowe B, Pereira-Smith O, Misteli T. Regulation of alternative splicing by histone modifications. Science. 2010;327(5968):996–1000.
37. Cooper TA, Wan L, Dreyfuss G. RNA and disease. Cell. 2009;136(4):777–93.
38. Padgett RA. New connections between splicing and human disease. Trends Genet. 2012;28(4):147–54.
39. Krawczak M, Thomas NST, Hundrieser B, Mort M, Wittig M, Hampe J, et al. Single base-pair substitutions in exon-intron junctions of human genes: nature, distribution, and consequences for mRNA splicing. Hum Mutat. 2007;28(2):150–8.

40. Lim KH, Ferraris L, Filloux ME, Raphael BJ, Fairbrother WG. Using positional distribution to identify splicing elements and predict pre-mRNA processing defects in human genes. Proc Natl Acad Sci. 2011;108(27):11093–8.
41. Stenson PD, Ball EV, Howells K, Phillips AD, Mort M, Cooper DN. The human gene mutation database: providing a comprehensive central mutation database for molecular diagnostics and personalized genomics. Hum Genomics. 2009;4(2):69–72.
42. Slaugenhaupt SA, Gusella JF. Familial dysautonomia. Curr Opin Genet Dev. 2002;12(3):307–11.
43. Sinha R, Kim YJ, Nomakuchi T, Sahashi K, Hua Y, Rigo F, et al. Antisense oligonucleotides correct the familial dysautonomia splicing defect in IKBKAP transgenic mice. Nucleic Acids Res. 2018;46(10):4833–44.
44. Singh RN, Singh NN. Mechanism of splicing regulation of spinal muscular atrophy genes. Adv Neurobiol. 2018;20:31–61.
45. Disset A, Bourgeois CF, Benmalek N, Claustres M, Stevenin J, Tuffery-Giraud S. An exon skipping-associated nonsense mutation in the dystrophin gene uncovers a complex interplay between multiple antagonistic splicing elements. Hum Mol Genet. 2006;15(6):999–1013.
46. Kalsotra A, Cooper TA. Functional consequences of developmentally regulated alternative splicing. Nat Rev Genet. 2011;12(10):715–29.
47. Pasinelli P, Brown RH. Molecular biology of amyotrophic lateral sclerosis: insights from genetics. Nat Rev Neurosci. 2006;7(9):710–23.
48. Winton MJ, Igaz LM, Wong MM, Kwong LK, Trojanowski JQ, Lee VMY. Disturbance of nuclear and cytoplasmic TAR DNA-binding protein (TDP-43) induces disease-like redistribution, sequestration, and aggregate formation. J Biol Chem. 2008;283(19):13302–9.
49. Polymenidou M, Lagier-Tourenne C, Hutt KR, Huelga SC, Moran J, Liang TY, et al. Long pre-mRNA depletion and RNA missplicing contribute to neuronal vulnerability from loss of TDP-43. Nat Neurosci. 2011;14(4):459–68.
50. Tollervey JR, Curk T, Rogelj B, Briese M, Cereda M, Kayikci M, et al. Characterizing the RNA targets and position-dependent splicing regulation by TDP-43. Nat Neurosci. 2011;14(4):452–8.
51. Mordes D, Luo X, Kar A, Kuo D, Xu L, Fushimi K, et al. Pre-mRNA splicing and retinitis pigmentosa. Mol Vis. 2006;12:1259–71.
52. Laboratories PFG. Epigenetic regulation of ageing. Nat Publ Gr [Internet]. 2015;16(10):593–610. Available from: https://doi.org/10.1038/nrm4048.
53. Franceschi C, Garagnani P, Vitale G, Capri M, Salvioli S. Inflammaging and Garb-aging. Trends Endocrinol Metab. 2017;28(3):199–212.
54. Aw D, Silva AB, Palmer DB. Immunosenescence: emerging challenges for an ageing population. Immunology [Internet]. 2007;120(4):435–46. Available from: https://www.ncbi.nlm.nih.gov/pubmed/17313487.
55. Kennedy BK, Berger SL, Brunet A, Campisi J, Cuervo AM, Epel ES, et al. Geroscience: linking aging to chronic disease. Cell [Internet]. 2014;159(4):709–13. Available from: https://www.ncbi.nlm.nih.gov/pubmed/25417146.
56. Friedrich K, Lee L, Leistritz DF, Nürnberg G, Saha B, Hisama FM, et al. WRN mutations in Werner syndrome patients: genomic rearrangements, unusual intronic mutations and ethnic-specific alterations. Hum Genet [Internet]. 2010;128(1):103–11. Available from: https://doi.org/10.1007/s00439-010-0832-5.
57. Rincón A, Mora L, Rojas JA. Case report Werner's syndrome: understanding the phenotype of premature aging – first case described in Colombia. Case Rep Genet. 2019;2019(8538325):4.
58. Pollex RL, Hegele RA. Hutchinson–Gilford progeria syndrome. Clin Genet [Internet]. 2004;66(5):375–81. Available from: https://doi.org/10.1111/j.1399-0004.2004.00315.x.
59. Lopez-Mejia IC, Vautrot V, De Toledo M, Behm-Ansmant I, Bourgeois CF, Navarro CL, et al. A conserved splicing mechanism of the LMNA gene controls premature aging. Hum Mol Genet [Internet]. 2011;20(23):4540–55. Available from: https://doi.org/10.1093/hmg/ddr385.
60. Rodriguez S, Coppedè F, Sagelius H, Eriksson M. Increased expression of the Hutchinson-Gilford progeria syndrome truncated lamin A transcript during cell aging. Eur J Hum Genet [Internet]. 2009;17(7):928–37. Available from: https://www.ncbi.nlm.nih.gov/pubmed/19172989.

61. McClintock D, Ratner D, Lokuge M, Owens DM, Gordon LB, Collins FS, et al. The mutant form of lamin A that causes Hutchinson-Gilford progeria is a biomarker of cellular aging in human skin. PLoS One [Internet]. 2007;2(12):e1269–e9. Available from: https://www.ncbi.nlm.nih.gov/pubmed/18060063.
62. Cao K, Capell BC, Erdos MR, Djabali K, Collins FS. A lamin A protein isoform overexpressed in Hutchinson-Gilford progeria syndrome interferes with mitosis in progeria and normal cells. Proc Natl Acad Sci U S A [Internet]. 2007;104(12):4949–54. Available from: https://www.ncbi.nlm.nih.gov/pubmed/17360355.
63. Skoczyńska A, Budzisz E, Dana A, Rotsztejn H. New look at the role of progerin in skin aging. Prz Menopauzalny Menopause Rev [Internet]. 2015;14(1):53–8. Available from: https://www.ncbi.nlm.nih.gov/pubmed/26327889.
64. Cunniff C, Bassetti JA, Ellis NA. Bloom's syndrome: clinical spectrum, molecular pathogenesis, and cancer predisposition. Mol Syndromol [Internet]. 2017;8(1):4–23. Available from: https://www.ncbi.nlm.nih.gov/pubmed/28232778.
65. Magnusson KP, Sandström M, Ståhlberg M, Larsson M, Flygare J, Hellgren D, et al. p53 splice acceptor site mutation and increased HsRAD51 protein expression in Bloom's syndrome GM1492 fibroblasts. Gene [Internet]. 2000;246(1):247–54. Available from: http://www.sciencedirect.com/science/article/pii/S0378111900000688.
66. Besic V, Shi H, Stubbs RS, Hayes MT. Aberrant liver insulin receptor isoform a expression normalises with remission of type 2 diabetes after gastric bypass surgery. PLoS One [Internet]. 2015;10(3):e0119270. Available from: https://doi.org/10.1371/journal.pone.0119270.
67. Kaminska D, Hämäläinen M, Cederberg H, Käkelä P, Venesmaa S, Miettinen P, et al. Adipose tissue INSR splicing in humans associates with fasting insulin level and is regulated by weight loss. Diabetologia [Internet]. 2014;57(2):347–51. Available from: https://doi.org/10.1007/s00125-013-3097-4.
68. Juan-Mateu J, Villate O, Eizirik DL. Mechanisms in endocrinology: alternative splicing: the new frontier in diabetes research. Eur J Endocrinol [Internet]. 2016;174(5):R225–38. Available from: https://www.ncbi.nlm.nih.gov/pubmed/26628584.
69. Wong C-M, Xu L, MY-C Y. Alternative mRNA splicing in the pathogenesis of obesity. Int J Mol Sci [Internet]. 2018;19(2):632. Available from: https://www.ncbi.nlm.nih.gov/pubmed/29473878.
70. Dlamini Z, Mokoena F, Hull R. Abnormalities in alternative splicing in diabetes: therapeutic targets. J Mol Endocrinol [Internet]. 2017;59(2):R93–107. Available from: https://jme.bioscientifica.com/view/journals/jme/59/2/JME-17-0049.xml.
71. David CJ, Manley JL. Alternative pre-mRNA splicing regulation in cancer: pathways and programs unhinged. Genes Dev. 2010;24:2343–64.
72. El Marabti E, Younis I. The cancer spliceome: reprograming of alternative splicing in cancer. Front Mol Biosci [Internet]. 2018;5:80. Available from: https://www.ncbi.nlm.nih.gov/pubmed/30246013.
73. Cummings JL. Alzheimer's disease. N Engl J Med [Internet]. 2004;351(1):56–67. Available from: https://doi.org/10.1056/NEJMra040223.
74. Love JE, Hayden EJ, Rohn TT. Alternative splicing in Alzheimer's disease. J Park Dis Alzheimer's Dis [Internet]. 2015;2(2):6. Available from: https://www.ncbi.nlm.nih.gov/pubmed/26942228.
75. Cruts M, Van Broeckhoven C. Presenilin mutations in Alzheimer's disease. Hum Mutat [Internet]. 1998;11(3):183–90. Available from: https://doi.org/10.1002/(SICI)1098-1004(1998)11:3%3C183::AID-HUMU1%3E3.0.CO.
76. Alam S, Suzuki H, Tsukahara T. Alternative splicing regulation of APP exon 7 by RBFox proteins. Neurochem Int [Internet]. 2014;78:7–17. Available from: http://www.sciencedirect.com/science/article/pii/S0197018614001843.
77. Rohn TT. Proteolytic cleavage of apolipoprotein E4 as the keystone for the heightened risk associated with Alzheimer's disease. Int J Mol Sci [Internet]. 2013;14(7):14908–22. Available from: https://www.ncbi.nlm.nih.gov/pubmed/23867607.

78. Dawson TM, Dawson VL. Molecular pathways of neurodegeneration in Parkinson's disease. Science [Internet]. 2003;302(5646):819 LP–822. Available from: http://science.sciencemag.org/content/302/5646/819.abstract.
79. Fu R-H, Liu S-P, Huang S-J, Chen H-J, Chen P-R, Lin Y-H, et al. Aberrant alternative splicing events in Parkinson's disease. Cell Transplant [Internet]. 2013;22(4):653–61. Available from: https://doi.org/10.3727/096368912X655154.
80. Xu L, Lin D, Yin D, Koeffler HP. An emerging role of PARK2 in cancer. J Mol Med [Internet]. 2014;92(1):31–42. Available from: https://doi.org/10.1007/s00109-013-1107-0.
81. Rideout HJ, Stefanis L. The neurobiology of LRRK2 and its role in the pathogenesis of Parkinson's disease. Neurochem Res [Internet]. 2014;39(3):576–92. Available from: https://doi.org/10.1007/s11064-013-1073-5.

# Epigenetics and Ageing

# 8

Nancy Monroy-Jaramillo
and Edgar Ricardo Vázquez-Martínez

## Abbreviations

| | |
|---|---|
| AD | Alzheimer's disease |
| AMPK | AMP-activated protein kinase |
| circRNA | Circular RNA |
| CTCF | CCCTC-binding factor |
| DNMT | DNA methyltransferase |
| ES | Estrogen receptor |
| EWAS | Epigenome-wide association study |
| EZH2 | Enhancer of zeste 2 polycomb repressive complex 2 subunit |
| H2BK20 | Lysine 20 of histone 2B |
| H3K18Ac | Histone 3 acetylated at lysine 18 |
| H3K27me | Histone 3 methylated at lysine 27 |
| H3K4me | Histone 3 methylated at lysine 4 |
| H3K9Ac | Histone 3 acetylated at lysine 9 |
| H3K9me | Histone 3 methylated at lysine 9 |
| H4K12 | Lysine 12 of histone 4 |
| H4K16 | Lysine 16 of histone 4 |
| H4K20me | Histone 4 methylated at lysine 20 |

Nancy Monroy-Jaramillo and Edgar Ricardo Vázquez-Martínez contributed equally to this work.

N. Monroy-Jaramillo (✉)
Departamento de Genética, Instituto Nacional de Neurología y Neurocirugía, Manuel Velasco Suárez, Mexico City, Mexico
e-mail: nancy97@unam.mx

E. R. Vázquez-Martínez (✉)
Unidad de Investigación en Reproducción Humana, Instituto Nacional de Perinatología-Facultad de Química, Universidad Nacional Autónoma de México, Mexico City, Mexico
e-mail: vamer@comunidad.unam.mx



J. C. Gomez-Verjan, N. A. Rivero-Segura (eds.), *Clinical Genetics and Genomics of Aging*, https://doi.org/10.1007/978-3-030-40955-5_8

| | |
|---|---|
| HAT | Histone acetyl transferases |
| HDAC | Histone deacetylases |
| HGS | Hutchinson-Gilford syndrome |
| HOTAIR | HOX antisense intergenic RNA |
| HP1 | Heterochromatin protein 1 |
| KMT1/Suv39 | Histone lysine methyltransferase family encoded by the *EHM1* gene |
| LADs | Lamina-associated domains |
| lncRNA | Long non-coding RNA |
| miRNA | MicroRNAs |
| ncRNA | Non-coding RNA |
| NL | Nuclear lamina |
| NOS2 | Nitric oxide synthase |
| PD | Parkinson's disease |
| PRC2 | Polycomb repressive complex 2 |
| PTGS2 | Cyclooxygenase 2 |
| PTM | Post-translational modification |
| RA | Rheumatoid arthritis |
| RBBP4 | RB Binding Protein 4 |
| RISC | RNA-induced silencing complex |
| ROS | Reactive oxygen species |
| SAHF | Senescence-associated heterochromatic foci |
| SALNR | Senescence-associated lncRNA |
| SMCs | Smooth muscle cells |
| T2D | Type 2 diabetes |
| TADs | Topologically associated domains |
| TERF2 | Telomeric repeat binding factor 2 |
| TOR | Target of rapamycin |
| WHO | World Health Organization |
| XIST | X-inactive-specific transcript |

## Introduction

According to the World Health Organization (WHO), populations around the world are rapidly ageing. For instance, by 2050, one in five people will be 60 years or older, amounting to two billion people worldwide. Increasing life expectancy is accompanied by a higher prevalence of age-related diseases, thus generating a growing demand for primary health care and long-term care [1]. Ageing is an inescapable physiological process involving a physical ability decline [2], but also the cognitive function becomes less effective as a person ages [3]. In this context, it is urgent to assure healthy ageing for all people and to find biomarkers to reduce chronic illnesses or to find strategies to slow its progression.

The molecular bases of ageing are multi factorial, but there are nine distinctive features related to this process, which include genomic instability, telomere shortening, de-regulated nutrient sensing, mitochondrial dysfunction, cellular senescence, stem cell exhaustion, altered cellular senescence, loss of proteostasis and a change in the patterns of epigenetic modifications [4, 5].

## Epigenetics and Ageing

Epigenetics is considered as a dynamic interface between the genome and the environment [6] and refers to the modulation of gene expression without any change in the genomic sequence. Epigenetic changes include DNA methylation, histone modifications, histone variants, and non-coding RNA (ncRNA) interference.

The research of epigenetic modifications is very attractive since these changes are reversible and might be preventable; thus, this makes them potential therapeutic targets to assure a healthy-ageing process and of relevance in cancer and age-related disorders such as neurodegenerative and cardiovascular diseases and inflammation [7, 8]. In addition, epigenetic modifications are regulatory events that may impact other hallmarks of ageing, for instance, silencing DNA repair gene or anti-inflammatory genes [9]. Therefore, in the present chapter, we aim to provide an overview of the current research focused on the participation of epigenetic mechanisms in ageing health and disease, as well as to discuss the perspectives regarding this topic.

## DNA Methylation and Ageing

DNA methylation is the best-characterized and most-stable epigenetic modification, which consists of the covalent addition of a methyl group to a cytosine of a CpG dinucleotide (when a cytosine is followed by a guanine from 5′ to 3′ direction and separated by a phosphate group) in vertebrates and is mediated by the action of three DNA methyltransferases (DNMT1, DNMT3A, and DNMT3B). This modification is involved in the development, differentiation and maintenance of cellular identity as a mechanism responsible for gene expression regulation and maintenance of genomic stability [10]. Therefore, some of the heritable DNA methylation patterns may be retained as an epigenetic mark of cellular memory [11].

DNA methylation can be quantitatively measured by distinct methods and, for this reason, has been evaluated in healthy subjects and in different age-related diseases [12]. There is an established correlation between methylation, CpG frequency, chromatin states, and gene expression; however, the mechanisms and specificity of this process are not fully understood. A high density of clustered CpGs into a certain region of genomic DNA is referred to as CpG islands, and nearly 50% of them are located in the gene-regulatory regions. Overall, DNA methylation in promoter regions is negatively correlated with gene expression, while gene body methylation is positively correlated with expression.

There are numerous studies examining associations between DNA methylation in age across the lifespan and across tissues [13, 14]. In an 8-year longitudinal study was shown a gradual DNA hypomethylation through ageing in repetitive elements, particularly in *Alu* sequences [15]. Thus, evidence demonstrates that gradual change in DNA methylation occurs with age, across the genome and specifically at repetitive DNA elements [16, 17]. Moreover, studies of senescence specifically using human cultured fibroblasts also showed that there is age-dependent compaction of the chromatin (heterochromatinization) [18, 19].

The DNA methylation gradual loss and increase in variability over the lifespan constitutes the epigenetic drift, which is different even in monozygotic tweens. In addition, stochastic epigenetic mutations increase exponentially during ageing [20]. Heyn et al. (2012) compared the CD4-T cells methylomes from newborns and nonagenarian/centenarians' individuals by microarray analyzing 450,000 CpG DNA sites and found an increased discordance between epigenomes with advanced age, consisting of a mean decrease in blood DNA methylation with increasing age in all gene compartments [21]. Nevertheless, the presence of hypermethylation at specific loci [21–31] has also been documented.

A research group compared CpG methylation changes with age across human blood, brain, kidney, and skeletal muscle samples using methylation arrays to identify tissue-specific age effects. They found age-related changes in DNA methylation that are both tissue specific and common across tissues. The tissue-specific changes are frequently located outside CpG islands with decreased methylation, and the common ones show the same distribution but the opposite trend [32]. This is in concordance with Christensen's group, who report an overall positive correlation between methylation and ageing for loci in the CpG islands, while for those that are not associated with CpG islands show significant loss of methylation with age in solid tissues [33]. In contrast, another study has suggested that most age-associated DNA methylation changes are tissue specific except for the *ELOVL2* gene promoter, which displays a consistent increase in DNA methylation with age in several tissues [34].

Some of the age-related DNA methylation changes may be explained by signatures in tissue composition (inflammation, fibrotic infiltration), and some other changes may also be explained by changes in chromatin structure. Regarding this last point, it has been observed the enrichment of some ageing-associated differentially methylated CpGs within lamina-associated domains (LADs) that are involved in the attachment of chromatin to the inner nuclear membrane; suggesting age-related epigenetic influences on chromatin boundary structure in relation to the nuclear membrane [21, 32]. However, further research is required to prove these hypotheses.

## Epigenetic Candidate Ageing Targets and Pathways

In a cohort study, more than half of ageing-associated differentially methylated regions showed age-related hypomethylation of coding genes for key regulatory proteins or specific chromatin modifiers (CTCF and EZH2, a member of

Polycomb-group family) [25]; thus, these epigenetic modifications may concomitantly contribute to phenotypic deterioration, such as age-related diseases.

Four different longevity pathways have been documented: decrease of insulin signaling; increase of AMPK (AMP-activated Protein Kinase); diminishing of TOR (Target of Rapamycin); and sirtuins [35]. Notably, researchers have identified informative age-associated differentially methylated regions in the promoter regions of specific genes with potential relevance for age-related diseases and longevity pathways. Some of these *loci* are: Sirtuin 5 (*SIRT5*), Sirtuin 7 (*SIRT7*), insulin-like growth factor binding protein 4 (*IGFBP4*), insulin-like growth factor-II (*IGF2*), estrogen receptor-1 (*ESR1*), hypermethylated in cancer 1 the transcriptional repressor 1 gene or Hypermethylated In Cancer 1 gene (*HIC1*), *p16/CDKN2A*, caspase-8 (*CASP8*) and others [21, 36, 37].

## Epigenetic Clock

Chronological age is the number of years a person has lived, and biological or physiological age refers to a measure of how well your body functions compared to your chronological age. Biological age is influenced by multiple factors (genes, lifestyle, behavior, environment, among others) and correlates with mortality and health status. The epigenetic clock is one potentially reliable predictor of biological age.

The dynamic DNA methylation throughout human lifetime exhibits a strong correlation with age and age-related outcomes. Since 2013, many researchers have built epigenetic clocks based on age-dependent methylation changes in certain CpG loci to track chronological age and predict biological age. Measures of accelerated age (when DNA methylation age>chronological age) have been developed to assess the health status of a person [38, 39]. The epigenetic drift and the epigenetic clock can modulate the phenomena associated to the ageing process. Genes with CpG sites predictive of age include genes associated with age-related diseases such as cancer and Alzheimer's disease (AD).

In the last years, several researchers have used commercial Bead Array technology, which provides quantitative array-based methylation measurement at the single-CpG-site level and offers high resolution for understanding epigenetic changes. Based on this technology, numerous CpG sites that are significantly correlated with age have been identified; some of them have been used to infer age with linear models using a selected set of DNA methylation markers in several tissues. These studies have demonstrated that DNA methylation patterns of nearly 30% of all CpG dinucleotides in the genome are influenced by age and that age-associated hypermethylation at CpG islands mainly targets genes that are not expressed in blood tissue, while age-associated hypomethylation targets more highly expressed genes [40].

For instance, Horvath's epigenetic clock consists of 353 CpG sites whose methylation levels can predict the chronological age in multiple human tissues [38]. Using a high-throughput bioinformatics pipeline, scientists have investigated the characteristics of the nucleotide's sequences surrounding the epigenetic clock

CpG´s, regarding the median methylation changes in different ages, the presence of CpG islands and its proximity to the transcription start sites of the genes. Common features of these sequences are G-quadruplexes and tentative splice site motifs. G-quadruplexes are non-canonical structures of GC-rich DNA and are recognition motifs for ageing-related proteins, such as the telomeric repeat binding factor 2 (TERF2) [41] and for polycomb repressive complex 2 (PRC2), which is responsible for histone H3K27 methylation during cell differentiation/proliferation [42]. PRC2 also shows a high affinity for RNA containing G-quadruplexes or loops [43]. There is evidence showing that CpG´s in epigenetic clock sequences, which possess G-quadruplexes (or potential PRC2 RNA target sites), undergo a methylation decrease during ageing [44].

So far, there are few studies with heterogeneous designs; thus, the association between DNA methylation age and age-related diseases is still controversial. A recent meta-analysis indicated that each 5-year increase in DNA methylation age was associated to an 8–15% increased risk of mortality. Future studies are required until we can use it as a clinical biomarker [45].

On the other hand, gender-related DNA methylation has been previously documented with a tendency towards higher methylation in males in repetitive DNA elements and differentially methylated regions, including imprinted genes [46]. An epigenome-wide association study (EWAS) in whole-blood samples taken from 1799 European men and women found that 1184 CpG sites were differentially methylated between men and women across all autosomes, including loci with differential gene expression and imprinted genes. These findings highlight the importance of considering gender in study designs of ageing and analyses [47, 48]. However, the exception to this global male hypermethylation is the X chromosome CpG islands hypermethylated among different tissues in females [49]. A recent study compared the effect of ageing on DNA methylation in male and female mice and humans and found that more than 95% of the age-related changes in DNA methylation in the hippocampus were sexually divergent, that is, there are sex divergences with ageing but these are not life-long sex differences [50].

The strongest evidence that the age-related changes in DNA methylation are involved in ageing comes from studies of anti-ageing interventions in mice, including caloric restriction, dwarfism and treatment with rapamycin. These interventions slow the epigenetic clock and prevent 20–40% of age-related changes in DNA methylation [50].

## Epigenetic Alterations in Some Age-Related Disorders

The epigenome of an aged person exhibits reduced plasticity of stem cells, limited stem cell pools, and deteriorated function of somatic cells. Therefore, most age-related disorders have an epigenetic component. It has been reported that alterations in epigenetic processes are risk factors in age-related pathologies, including AD, Parkinson's disease (PD), rheumatoid arthritis (RA), type 2 diabetes (T2D), and cancer (Table 8.1). Likewise, they are associated with disorders that exhibit premature ageing, such as Hutchinson-Gilford syndrome (HGS).

**Table 8.1** Epigenetic aberrations observed in some age-related diseases

| Age-related disease | Observed epigenetic aberration |
|---|---|
| Parkinson's disease | Elevated homocysteine levels and global DNA hypomethylation in the frontal cortex of PD patients, and in dementia with Lewy bodies [194] |
| | Epigenetic clock found accelerated epigenetic ageing in blood of PD patients [195] |
| | Decreased levels of histone acetylation by α-synuclein in dopaminergic neurons [196] |
| Alzheimer's disease | DNA hipomethylation in *INOS, IL-1, TNF-α* genes that are related to inflammation in the cerebral cortex of AD patients [197] |
| | Hypermethylation of *HTERT*, which is the catalytic unit of telomerase and allows that telomeres lengthen during cell replication. This causes a silencing of the gene and therefore an increase in cellular senescence [198] |
| | Reduction in the global DNA methylation in cells of the prefrontal cortex of AD patients [199, 200] |
| | Downregulation of acetylated histone marks such as H3K18/K23 in human temporal lobe tissue of 11 AD patients vs. 4 matched controls. In this regard, another research group found that enrichment of this histone acetylation mark determines transcription of genes encoding memory-related functions in rat neurons. Interconnections between acetylation of H3K14 and H3K18 and increased autophagy during ageing have also been revealed [201, 202] |
| | Increased levels of histone acetylation and H3K4me3 in frontal cortex, hippocampus, middle temporal gyrus, inferior temporal gyrus and occipital cortex of AD patients have been documented. On the other hand, decreased levels of H3K9me2 and histone acetylation have been reported in temporal lobe, occipital lobe and hippocampus of these patients [93] |
| | Increased serum levels of miR-125b have been proposed as a biomarker of AD as its content is correlated with the Mini Mental State Examination score that evaluates cognition impairment [144] |
| | Overexpression of miR-212 and miR-132 is observed in lymphoblastoid cell lines generated from AD patients compared with those generated from centenarians [141] |
| | miR-181 expression is downregulated in the brain and serum of AD patients [119] |
| | Decreased levels of ciRS-7 in CA1 region of hippocampus are observed in AD patients [179] |
| | Increased levels of lncRNAs BACEI-AS, 5IA, 17A, NDM29 and NAT-Rad18 are found in the brain of AD patients, which in turn are associated with high levels of amyloid β peptide [162] |
| Cardiovascular diseases | A hypermethylation trend with increasing replicative passage number in endothelial and vascular smooth muscle cells (SMCs) in estrogen receptor-genes (ER) which protect the cardiovascular system. SMCs protect against vascular injury. These epigenetic changes are similar to those occurring physiologically with ageing [203] |
| | A molecular mechanism that links age to overall disease risk is deregulation of CREB-regulated transcriptional coactivators, CRTCs. Epigenetic deregulation of CRTCs genes may contribute to the development of metabolic disorders. CRTCs genes also modulate organismal ageing, linking energy sensing to transcriptional regulation of longevity. As an example, CRTC2 modulates glucose homeostasis during fasting and diabetes by promoting histone H3 acetylation at lysine 9 (H3K9Ac) [204] |
| | miR-34a has been involved in the induction of ageing related processes and altered functions in cardiomyocytes and endothelial cells [136–138] |
| | miR-21 has been implicated in cell survival in cardiac fibroblasts, heart senescence and cardiac disease [131,139] |

In recent years, DNA methylation and histone acetylation and methylation have emerged as potential regulatory mechanisms that govern the transcription of several genes responsible for memory formation and behavior, through a link between environmental-lifestyle factors and variability in cognitive function during ageing.

Because epigenetic changes are mitotically and meiotically heritable, it has been postulated that various chromatin marks and DNA methylation status can be transmitted as an epigenetic memory to the next generation, the so-called transgenerational epigenetics. In this context, the interventions to modify epigenetics (diet or lifestyle) become relevant for healthy ageing and in patients with age-related disorders. For instance, studies in the rodent model for T2D, *Psammomys obesus*, have shown, parental diet regulates DNA and RNA methylation and the expression of genes implicated with the increased risk of obesity in offspring [51, 52].

## Histones and Post-translational Modifications (PTMs) in Ageing

Genomic DNA is packaged in a compact nuclear structure known as chromatin, which in turn is composed of nucleosomes. Each nucleosome is constituted by a histone octamer composed of four histone dimers (H2A, H2B, H3 and H4), wrapped into approximately 147 bp of DNA and separated from another nucleosome by linker DNA and histone H1 [53, 54].

Recent studies have proposed that histone loss is a hallmark of ageing, which is conserved in several species, including humans. A decrease in total levels of histones is observed in yeast and *Caenorhabditis elegans* ageing models [55]. Histone loss has been linked to a tumor suppression process probably associated with senescence in melanocytic neoplasia [56]. A decrease in H3 and H4 histone synthesis and levels of histone PTMs has been reported in human fibroblasts subjected to replicative ageing, which was attributed to telomere shortening. Interestingly, a decrease in those histone levels in primary fibroblasts was also found in cultures obtained from an old individual (92 years old) when compared with those of a young individual (9 years old), which were not subjected to replicative ageing, therefore, suggesting that histone loss is a physiological process in senescent cells [57]. It has been demonstrated that histone depletion is triggered by DNA damage response and mediated by proteolytic processing in lysosomes via autophagy [55, 56, 58]. The role of histone loss in the ageing process has been attributed to alterations in heterochromatin, which are characterized by a decrease in its distribution in the genome and the content of characteristic heterochromatin histone marks (such as H3K9me3 and H3K27me3) as evidenced in fibroblasts cells from a HGS patient and healthy aged individuals [59, 60]. Interestingly, it has been suggested that the increase in chromatin opening in T cells from aged people could be related to histone loss, which in part could explain the immunodeficiency observed in old people [61].

Histone variants are canonical histones paralogues whose expression is independent of DNA synthesis and have specific roles in several processes such as DNA repair and transcription. In general terms, the substitution of canonical histones with specific histone variants promotes changes in chromatin compaction by modifying the nucleosome composition or by recruiting specific epigenetic machinery [62]. Early studies have shown an increase in the content of H2A.2 (related to differentiation processes), H3.3 (commonly positioned in enhancers and heterochromatin, associated with development) and H2A.Z (participates in transcription initiation and maintenance of heterochromatin) in human lung fibroblasts subjected to replicative ageing, while H2A.1 (detected mainly in germ cells and zygotes), H3.1 (canonical H3) and H2A.X (participates in DNA damage response) were downregulated [55, 62, 63]. Although H2A.X was found decreased in human lung fibroblasts subjected to replicative ageing, it has been proposed that this histone variant is a typical hallmark of cellular senescence [64]. Interestingly, the accumulation and dynamic turnover of histone H3.3 with age have been reported in post-mortem glial and neuronal chromatin, which in turn is related to fundamental brain functions, such as neuronal plasticity and cognition [65].

It has been recently reported that histone variant H2A.J is accumulated in senescent human fibroblasts and ageing human skin, as well as it regulates the expression of genes associated with the senescent-associated secretory phenotype. This study highlighted histone H2A.J as a new possible therapeutic target against ageing-related diseases [66].

PTMs of histone tails, such as acetylation and methylation, are responsible for specific changes in gene expression [67]. Specific proteins are responsible for these enzymatic modifications of histones, which in turn participate in the establishment of an active or repressive transcriptional environment that promotes or inhibits transcription, respectively [68]. Generally, the transcriptional effect of a histone modification depends on the residue that is being modified, the type of modification and the combinatorial of other modifications in other residues and/or histones [69].

Histone acetylation is a typical hallmark of transcriptionally active chromatin, catalyzed by histone acetyl transferases (HATs) and removed by histone deacetylases (HDACs) [70, 71]. On the other hand, the transcriptional effect of histone methylation depends on the residue that is being modified and the genomic context. Regarding promoter regions, histone 3 methylated at lysine 4 (H3K4me) is a hallmark of transcriptional activation, whereas histone 3 methylated at lysine 9 and 27 (H3K9me and H3K27me) is related with transcriptional silencing [72–74].

The role of histone modifications in ageing has been highlighted in yeast, *C. elegans* and fly models [55]. Particularly, a decrease of Sir2 protein levels and activity, an enzyme that catalyzes H4K16 deacetylation, has been associated with ageing in yeast, whereas deficiencies of genes encoding proteins associated with H3K4 trimethylation (such as *WRD5, SETD-2* and *ASH2L*) increases lifespan in *C. elegans* [75, 76]. In flies, an increase of H3K4me3 levels has been associated with reduced lifespan, while increased longevity has been associated with H3K27me3 loss [77, 78]. It is important to note that the role of histone modifications in ageing is species specific since increased levels of H3K27me3 increase lifespan in *C. elegans*, which is contrary to flies [55, 79]. Physiological features of ageing have been associated with changes in acetylation or methylation levels of histones in several animal models [80, 81]; however, further studies are required to confirm these findings in human samples.

A decrease in the levels of H3K9me2, H3K9me3 and H4K20me3 (associated with heterochromatin) has been found in human fibroblasts subjected to replicative ageing [57, 82]. However, it has been found that senescent human fibroblasts also accumulate a specific heterochromatin structure (characterized by the enrichment of the histone marks H3K9me3, H3K27me3 and heterochromatin protein 1, HP1) defined as senescence-associated heterochromatic foci (SAHF, see later), which in turn may ensure the senescent phenotype and avoid cancer progression by controlling cell cycle progression [83, 84]. A recent study demonstrated that histone lysine methyltransferases members of the KMT1/Suv39 methyltransferase family, which catalyze H3K9me2 formation, are also able to methylate Lamin B1 to increase its stability and to promote heterochromatin binding to nuclear periphery, which is gradually lost in age-dependent manner in human dermal fibroblasts leading to altered heterochromatin organization [82]. Fibroblasts obtained from HGS patients present decreased levels of H3K27me3 and H3K9me3 histone marks, as well as increased levels of H4K20me3 [60]. A global decrease in H3K9me3 levels accompanied by alterations in heterochromatin structure is also observed in another progeroid syndrome, Werner syndrome, characterized by WRN protein deficiency, which is essential in DNA repair and heterochromatin stability [85]. On the other hand, a decrease in H3K4me3 along with an increase in H3K27me3 enrichment has been found in the promoters of *LEPRE1, LIMA1/EPLIN, MAGOHA* and *MAGOHB* genes in human senescent fibroblasts and associated with premature ageing [86].

The loss of histone acetylation in replicative senescence is important to avoid the expression of tumor-associated genes, such as the case of the tissue factor gene that promotes angiogenesis and cancer progression [87]. It has been recently demonstrated that cardiac ageing is accompanied by an accumulation of lysosphingolipid sphinganine, a potent HDAC1 inhibitor that leads to an increase in histone acetylation and DNA damage causing functional impairment of cardiac function. Surprisingly, the effects mediated by lysosphingolipid sphinganine can be partially prevented using acetyl transferase inhibitors [88]. A decrease in RB Binding Protein 4 (RBBP4), a chromatin remodeling factor that regulates histone acetylation, has been observed in ageing human post-mortem dentate gyrus of hippocampus. This finding was replicated in a mouse model with a dominant negative form of RBBP4, which presented hypoacetylation of histones H2BK20 and H4K12 in dentate gyrus, as well as memory deficiencies consistent with ageing [89]. SIRT1 is a NAD+-dependent HDAC that deacetylates histones (mainly H4K16) and non-histone proteins (such as NF-κB and PPARGC1A) and has been associated with longevity in several species [90]. SIRT1 also suppresses inflammatory responses, and its overexpression in microglia has been shown to protect against Aβ toxicity, by inhibiting NF-κB signaling. In contrast, its deficiency exacerbates ageing, or tau-associated cognitive deficits, and correlates with levels of IL-1β transcripts in mice. Interestingly, in humans, hypomethylation of IL-1β is associated with chronological age and with elevated IL-1β transcription. These findings reveal a novel epigenetic mechanism in ageing microglia that contributes to cognitive deficits in ageing and neurodegenerative diseases [91]. Thus, SIRT1 levels have been inversely correlated with typical neuropathologic changes in AD.

Decreased expression of SIRT6 (that removes acetyl group from lysine residues in histone H3) has also been associated with the pathogenesis of AD as well as with the classical hallmarks of ageing; therefore, it has also been proposed as a therapeutic target against this disease [92]. Several histone modifications have been described in the post-mortem brain of AD patients, suggesting that both transcriptionally active and repressed chromatin are altered in a region-dependent manner. In general terms, changes in histone modifications associated with transcriptional activation (such as increased levels of histone acetylation and H3K4me3) have been described in the frontal cortex, hippocampus, middle temporal gyrus, inferior temporal gyrus and occipital cortex of AD patients compared with respective controls (Table 8.1). On the other hand, alterations in histone modifications associated with transcriptional repression (such as increased levels of H3K9me2 and decreased levels of histone acetylation) have been reported in the temporal lobe, occipital lobe and hippocampus of these patients [93]. Modified levels of histone PTMs have also been found in other neurodegenerative diseases, such as increased levels of H3K4me3 in Huntington's disease and decreased levels of histone acetylation in PD and Huntington's disease [94] (Table 8.1).

On the other hand, epigenetic changes that occur during physiological ageing can increase the risk of tumour onset and progression [95, 96]. For instance, the epigenetic mark H3K18Ac associated with ageing plays an important role in driving progression of many types of cancer, including breast, colon, lung, hepatocellular, pancreatic, prostate and thyroid cancer [97]. HIRA is a histone chaperone complex that promotes healthy ageing and participates in the suppression of cancer [98]. In addition, there is a study which included normal tissues vs. primary tumours from breast, kidney, thyroid, skin and glia samples and demonstrated that DNA hypermethylation in ageing and cancer is associated with the same set of histone marks, including the repressive H3K27me3 and H3K9me3 marks, and the activating H3K4me1/3 PTMs [99].

The process of ageing in stem cells from different tissues is also accompanied by changes in the content of histone acetylation and methylation [100]. Particularly, an age-dependent and tissue-independent enrichment of H3K4me1 histone mark (associated with enhancers) has been associated with DNA hypomethylation in mesenchymal stem cells, suggesting that this epigenetic change could be associated with a differentiated phenotype and not with a pluripotent one [101]. Enrichment of bivalent chromatin domains (characterized by H3K4me3 and H3K27me3) in hematopoietic and embryonic stem cells correlates with differentially methylated regions that gain DNA methylation in aged differentiated cells, probably due to a loss of developmental potency since bivalent chromatin is a typical feature of pluripotent cells [31]. Interestingly, induced pluripotent stem cells obtained from HGS patients' fibroblasts display highly similar epigenomic (in regards of H3K4me3 and H3K27me3 histone marks) and transcriptomic profiles to normal embryonic stem cells, suggesting the possibility of reprogramming affected cells [102].

Osteoarthritis is a chronic musculoskeletal disorder highly associated with ageing and characterized by the altered function of chondrocytes, which produce increased amounts of proteolytic enzymes, leading to cartilage damage and loss of joint function [103]. It has been demonstrated that the induction of inducible nitric oxide synthase (NOS2) and cyclooxygenase 2 (PTGS2) expression by interleukin-1 in human osteoarthritis chondrocytes, involved in the initiation and progression of osteoarthritis, is mediated in part by the histone methyltransferase SET-1A-dependent increase in the levels of histone marks H3K4me2 and H3K4me3 at the respective *NOS2* and *PTGS2* promoters [104]. Leptin expression has also been associated with increased levels of H3K9 and H3K19 acetylation, leading to excessive nitric oxide production [105]. The expression of several HDACs is altered in osteoarthritis chondrocytes and cartilage, which in turn modifies the expression of key genes that maintain cartilage structure [106]. Furthermore, increased levels of H3K9me3 and H3K27me3 along with decreased levels of histone acetylation in several lysine residues of histone H3 have been found in osteoarthritis chondrocytes in the promoter of *SOX9*, an essential gene for the development and maintenance of chondrocyte phenotype [107].

To date, the studies assessing the role of histone loss, histone variants and histone modifications in ageing health and disease are increasing; however, more studies are required to complete the understanding of this process.

## Non-coding RNAs and Ageing

### MicroRNAs

MicroRNAs (miRNAs) are small RNAs (19 to 22 nucleotides in length) that regulate the expression of several mammalian genes involved in physiological and pathological processes, such as ageing [108–111]. These small RNAs are produced by the following process: synthesis of the primary miRNA by the transcription of a miRNA gene (mainly by RNA polymerase II), folding of the primary miRNA into a stem-loop of approximately 80 base pair long which is processed to generate the miRNA precursor (by the Drosha/Dgrc8 complex), miRNA precursor export to the cytoplasm (by the Exportin 5) and dissociation into a single miRNA that associates with the RNA-induced silencing complex (RISC) to inhibit translation via different mechanisms [112].

The relationship between miRNAs and ageing has been demonstrated in several studies [113]. Particularly, miRNAs have emerged as potential candidate biomarkers for diagnostic, prognostic and therapeutic purposes in physiological and pathological human ageing [114–116]. In extracellular body fluids, the content of specific miRNAs derived from peripheral blood and plasmatic exosomes shows a positive correlation with age and age-related diseases [117, 118]. For example, a diminution in the content of miR-181a has been detected in the circulation and the brain of aged people as compared with young people [119]. Interestingly, ageing-related miRNAs show distinct expression patterns in many cell types, including neurons, highlighting the importance of these small RNAs in ageing-associated diseases, such as neurodegenerative disorders [120]. Furthermore, it has been recently proposed that miRNAs can be secreted in the circulation by senescent cells to regulate inflammatory processes in other cells [119].

Studies performed in healthy long-lived individuals (which survive to the 95th percentile of life expectancy time) have identified several miRNAs associated with healthy ageing [121]. Interestingly, blood samples and different blood cell types from long-lived people show decreased levels of specific groups of miRNAs and pathways associated with disease processes (for example, cancer and AD), organismal ageing, inflammation, telomere shortening, metabolic disorders and replicative senescence, suggesting that centenarians have protection mechanisms against ageing deterioration [122–126]. The mechanisms involved in the increased expression of longevity-associated miRNAs in centenarians are unknown; however, it has been proposed that augmented miRNAs biogenesis in long-lived people could explain this upregulation [127]. Furthermore, it has been reported that several variants found in miRNAs binding sites of target mRNAs are associated with human longevity [128].

The identification of miRNAs associated with a senescent phenotype has demonstrated the role of these molecules in the regulation of signalling pathways by targeting essential genes for cell cycle, telomere maintenance, cytoskeletal remodelling, apoptosis survival, cell proliferation, mitochondrial functions and inflammation [119, 129, 130]. Mitochondrial functions are regulated by several ageing-associated miRNAs, which are involved in inflammatory processes, energy metabolism, mitochondrial transport and integrity, antioxidant response, mitochondrial respiration and apoptosis [131–133]. Regulation of autophagy by miRNAs is also a recognized mechanism associated with the induction of senescence, since autophagy plays a fundamental role in mitochondrial clearance and reactive oxygen species (ROS) production [134]. Induction of DNA lesions and accumulation of ROS have been associated with miR-494 in senescent fibroblasts [135].

Recent studies have highlighted miR-34a as an attractive molecular target against vascular senescence and cardiovascular diseases since it is involved in the induction of ageing-related processes and altered functions in cardiomyocytes and endothelial cells [136–138]. Other miRNAs, such as miR-21, have been associated with cell survival in cardiac fibroblasts, heart senescence and cardiac disease [131, 139]. In the liver, increased expression levels of miR-31-5p, miR-141-3p and miR-200c-3p has been associated with an age-dependent shortage of telomere length [140]. Cellular senescence in the skin has been associated with specific senescence-associated miRNAs identified in human dermal fibroblasts, keratinocytes, photoaged human skin and dermis from aged people [141].

In neurodegenerative diseases, the content of several miRNAs in brain tissues and circulation has been associated with AD [142, 143]. Particularly, miR-125b has been proposed as a non-invasive serum biomarker of AD since its content is correlated with the Mini Mental State Examination score, which evaluates cognition impairment [144]. Changes in the expression of ageing-associated miRNAs have been found in specific brain regions, whose altered expression has been also related to AD [119]. Interestingly, those miRNAs are involved in the myelination and c-myc pathways, the generation of Aβ and phosphorylated tau, regulation of brain inflammation, synaptic branching and connectivity, spine length, senile plaque density, mitochondria function, the induction of oxidative stress, the regulation of the expression of tumour suppressor genes and other ageing-associated molecular processes [119, 142]. It has been reported that miR-212 and miR-132 (that targets *SIRT1* mRNA) are decreased in lymphoblastoid cell lines generated from centenarians as compared with those of AD patients; therefore, proposing their involvement in the pathogenesis of AD [145]. Other diseases, including the chronic obstructive pulmonary disease, idiopathic fibrosis, osteoporosis, sarcopenia and diabetes, also show altered expression of miRNAs in the affected tissues and correlate with ageing processes [117, 146–148].

The study of ageing-associated miRNAs has also been performed in pluripotent stem cells, in which miRNAs are emerging as potential targets to rejuvenate old mesenchymal stem cells, as well as essential molecules in the regulation of self-renewal, activation of p53 pathway, decreased telomere length, inhibition of cell proliferation and differentiation and induced senescence in different somatic stem cell types [149, 150]. The role of miRNAs in the regulation of ageing-related processes has been reported in many cancer models as in the other epigenetic mechanisms. For a complete review about ageing-related miRNAs and cancer models, refer to [151, 152].

## Long Non-coding RNAs

Long Non-coding RNAs (lncRNAs) consist of RNA molecules with more than 200 nucleotides that do not translate into protein. There are more than 14,000 lncRNAs, which are generally transcribed by RNA pol II and are subjected to transcriptional modifications and splicing [153, 154]. They can be found in the nucleus, cytosol or mitochondria, and their biological function is to form different types of complexes by interacting with proteins and nucleic acids in order to regulate gene expression (by indirect epigenetic mechanisms or by direct mechanisms acting as antisense transcripts or transcriptional coactivators), nuclear location of transcription factors and stabilization of ribonucleoprotein complexes [155]. It has been reported that lncRNA´s are important in the regulation of ageing-associated mechanisms in humans and animal models, such as cell proliferation, differentiation, apoptosis and senescence [113]. Recent studies have identified several lncRNA´s differentially expressed in senescent and young fibroblasts, such as the senescence-associated lncRNA (SALNR) that maintains cellular senescence via inhibition of NF90 nucleolus translocation (which inhibits expression of senescence-associated mRNAs and miRNAs) and the SAL-RNA1 associated with the hallmarks of cellular senescence [156, 157].

Loss of imprinting of a well-known maternally expressed lncRNA, H19, is observed during ageing in normal and cancer tissues, in which it has tumour suppressor functions [158]. The expression of the X-inactive-specific transcript (*XIST*) is decreased in senescent fibroblasts [159]. In contrast, the HOX antisense intergenic RNA (*HOTAIR*) is highly expressed in senescent human fibroblasts and induces proteolysis via ubiquitination [160].

Premature ageing has been associated with altered expression of lncRNAs that participate in the regulation of the telomere length by modulating the TERT activity and synthesis of telomeric repeats [155, 161]. Furthermore, it has been reported that changes in the expression levels of some lncRNAs are associated with the development of AD [162].

## Circular RNAs and Ageing

Circular RNAs (circRNAs) are highly conserved covalently closed non-coding RNAs resistant to RNase R activity [163]. These circular molecules are more stable and abundant than their linear mRNA counterparts in many human cell types, and recent studies have demonstrated that some of these molecules translate into proteins [164, 165]. circRNAs regulate gene expression mainly by recruiting miRNAs in the cytoplasm and RNA binding proteins in the nucleus [166, 167]. circRNAs are generated by different splicing events from exonic, intronic and retained-intronic regions, which are distinct from canonical splicing of linear RNAs [168, 169].

The differential expression of circRNAs in specific tissues, developmental stages and physiological and pathological processes has attracted attention to study their potential as biomarkers and therapeutic targets [170]. In addition, circRNAs might regulate the senescence-associated phenotype in lung fibroblasts and non-cancer cell lines, the production of type I collagen in photoaged human dermal fibroblasts and apoptosis in vascular smooth cells and macrophages involved in atherosclerosis [113, 171–173]. Increased expression of specific circRNAs is associated with ageing in human granulosa cells and the heart [159, 174].

Interestingly, circRNAs are more distributed in the brain than in other tissues and are highly expressed in neural tissues during ageing [175, 176]. Furthermore, several brain-specific circRNAs are highly conserved between several species, including *Drosophila*. It has been proposed that circRNAs are necessary for normal brain function [177]. Furthermore, these circular molecules could have a role in synaptic function as they are differentially expressed during synaptogenesis and neuronal activity and are highly expressed in synapses [178]. Recent studies are elucidating the association between specific circRNAs and neurodegenerative disorders. Particularly, changes in the expression or signalling of the ciRS-7 have been associated with AD [179].

## Other Mechanisms

Multiple epigenetic changes are common to premature ageing in progeroid syndromes and natural ageing. Recent evidence showed that epigenetic systems could participate as drivers of both forms of ageing [180]. The nuclear lamina (NL) is a meshwork composed of the filamentous proteins A- and B-type lamins underneath the inner nuclear membrane. NL maintains the nuclear shape and forms independent but interacting networks [181], playing an important role in regulating chromatin organization and gene transcription through chromatin interactions [182].

HGS can also be defined within laminopathies with premature ageing, mainly caused by pathogenic variants in *LMNA* gene [183] and producing the mutant protein, progerin, which affects the nuclear morphology. Cells from HGS patients show a decrease in heterochromatin and are devoid of SAHF [59, 60]. Progerin-positive cells are present in cultured fibroblasts from aged normal donors (81–96 years). These cells display HGS-like defects in nuclear morphology, decreased H3K9me3 and HP1 and increased histone H2AX phosphorylation marks of the DNA damage loci. Interestingly, the inhibition of progerin showed the opposite effects. These experiments demonstrate that progerin acts in natural ageing. Progerin expression in normal human fibroblasts accelerates the loss of telomeres. Changes in lamina organization may directly affect telomere attrition, resulting in accelerated replicative senescence and progeroid phenotypes [180].

Telomeres are regions constituted by tandem repeats of non-coding DNA sequences 5′-(TTAGGG)n-3′ and a protein complex called shelterin, bound to them. This structure ensures the stability of the genome and protects the chromosomes from a wrong action of the DNA repair machinery [184] by allowing the formation of a chromatin loop called T-Loop [185].

Despite heterochromatin domains being established early during embryonic development, it has been shown that loss of constitutive heterochromatin (commonly at telomeres, centromeres, pericentromeres) occurs in senescence and ageing and is triggered by telomere shortening, transcription changes at boundaries and breakdown of the nuclear periphery [185].

Werner Syndrome and Dyskeratosis Congenita are genetic progeroid syndromes that mimic physiological ageing. There is evidence that loss of A-type lamins (lamins A and C) impact on telomere dynamics in these syndromes [186]. Thus, telomeres are also regulated by lamina-associated proteins such as LAP1, a protein involved in the positioning of lamins and chromatin and might also associate with telomere through interaction with two components of shelterin, TRF2 and RIF1 [187].

Chandra et al. (2015) demonstrated the mapping of architectural changes in the genome during cellular senescence using Hi-C (a technique to capture chromatin interactions in the nucleus). Their results revealed a loss of local interactions in heterochromatic regions within topologically associated domains (TADs); senescent cells seemed to gain cross-boundary interactions across TADs. Domains that lost boundary strength with ageing were enriched in H3K9me3 and LADs. Whereas the TAD boundaries that attained strength with age showed enrichment in H3K36me3 marks. The study also demonstrated that a LAD that drifted away from the nuclear periphery during senescence was near the *CDKN2A* locus, whose expression has been documented to be altered during ageing [188]. Their findings agreed with changes observed in HGS cells. Finally, it has been demonstrated that histone chaperones and components of the SWI/SNF ATP-dependent chromatin-remodelling complexes also participate in the process of normal and pathological ageing [189–192], and altogether, these findings add another layer of complexity to the mechanisms that alter gene expression in this process.

## Conclusions and Perspectives

We have attempted to summarize the emerging information about the diverse roles of epigenetics in healthy ageing and age-related diseases. However, it is not known if some of these changes are the cause or consequence of the ageing process; what is clear is that one must see the epigenetic modifications as a dynamic cross-talking process between genome and environment, where each modification influences the others (i.e. DNA methylation influences chromatin structures, histones PTMs).

Several important conclusions emerge from the presented findings: there are at least two ways to reverse or inhibit senescence by epigenetic mechanisms, whereby a healthy life expectancy could be prolonged. The first way involves rejuvenation through effective epigenetic reprogramming in cells undergoing senescence or cells derived from very aged patients or patients with progeroid syndromes, by which the induction of *in vitro*–induced pluripotent stem cells is effective. Although our lifespan is largely epigenetically determined; diet and other environmental factors can influence it by changing the epigenetic information. So, another opportunity to reverse ageing that concerns epigenetic modifications is the pharmacological/nutritional modulation of cell fate; for instance, modification of senescence signalling pathways such as by IGF-induced agents [119, 193]. This last point considers the reversible nature of epigenetic modifications, thus, research on epigenome opens new avenues for therapeutic interventions in ageing and age-associated diseases, including the devastating AD.

It is important to note that technology to study the epigenome is progressing rapidly, and this will facilitate an interesting perspective for performing longitudinal studies of epigenetic interventions in healthy aged individuals and in patients with age-related diseases, considering factors not included in most of the published studies, such as gender, circadian cycle and pharmacological treatment, among others.

## References

1. Brennan-Olsen SL, Cook S, Leech MT, Bowe SJ, Kowal P, Naidoo N, et al. Prevalence of arthritis according to age, sex and socioeconomic status in six low and middle income countries: analysis of data from the World Health Organization study on global AGEing and adult health (SAGE) Wave 1. BMC Musculoskelet Disord. 2017;18(1):271.
2. Andersen-Ranberg K, Christensen K, Jeune B, Skytthe A, Vasegaard L, Vaupel JW. Declining physical abilities with age: a cross-sectional study of older twins and centenarians in Denmark. Age Ageing. 1999;28(4):373–7.
3. Park DC, Lodi-Smith J, Drew L, Haber S, Hebrank A, Bischof GN, et al. The impact of sustained engagement on cognitive function in older adults: the Synapse Project. Psychol Sci. 2014;25(1):103–12.
4. López-Otín C, Blasco MA, Partridge L, Serrano M, Kroemer G. The hallmarks of aging. Cell. 2013;153(6):1194.
5. Mc Auley MT, Guimera AM, Hodgson D, Mcdonald N, Mooney KM, Morgan AE, et al. Modelling the molecular mechanisms of aging. Biosci Rep. 2017;37(1):BSR20160177.
6. Feil R, Fraga MF. Epigenetics and the environment: emerging patterns and implications. Nat Rev Genet. 2012;13(2):97–109.

7. Molina-Serrano D, Kyriakou D, Kirmizis A. Histone modifications as an intersection between diet and longevity. Front Gen. 2019;10:192.
8. Milagro FI, Mansego ML, De Miguel C, Martínez JA. Dietary factors, epigenetic modifications and obesity outcomes: progresses and perspectives. Mol Aspects Med. 2013;34(4):782–812.
9. Van Speybroeck L. From epigenesis to epigenetics: the case of C. H. Waddington. Ann N Y Acad Sci. 2002;981:61–81.
10. Smith ZD, Meissner A. DNA methylation: roles in mammalian development. Nat Rev Genet. 2013;14(3):204–20.
11. Bird A. DNA methylation patterns and epigenetic memory. Genes Dev. 2002;16(1):6–21.
12. Xiao FH, Wang HT, Kong QP. Dynamic DNA methylation during aging: a "prophet" of age-related outcomes. Front Genet. 2019;10:107.
13. Wilson VL, Jones PA. DNA methylation decreases in aging but not in immortal cells. Science. 1983;220(4601):1055–7.
14. Jintaridth P, Mutirangura A. Distinctive patterns of age-dependent hypomethylation in interspersed repetitive sequences. Physiol Genomics. 2010;41(2):194–200.
15. Bollati V, Tarantini L, Baccarelli A, Schwartz J, Wright R, Litonjua A, et al. Decline in genomic DNA methylation through aging in a cohort of elderly subjects. Mech Ageing Dev. 2009;130(4):234–9.
16. Xiao F-H, Kong Q-P, Perry B, He Y-H. Progress on the role of DNA methylation in aging and longevity. Brief Funct Genomics. 2016;15(6):454–9.
17. Jones MJ, Goodman SJ, Kobor MS. DNA methylation and healthy human aging. Aging Cell. 2015;14(6):924–32.
18. Ishimi Y, Kojima M, Takeuchi F, Miyamoto T, Yamada MA, Hanaoka F. Changes in chromatin structure during aging of human skin fibroblasts. Exp Cell Res. 1987;169(2):458–67.
19. Dell'Orco R. Research WW-B and biophysical, 1982 U. Micrococcal nuclease and DNase I digestion of DNA from aging human diploid cells. Biochem Biophys Res Commun. 1982;107(1):117–22.
20. Gentilini D, Garagnani P, Pisoni S, Bacalini MG, Calzari L, Mari D, et al. Stochastic epigenetic mutations (DNA methylation) increase exponentially in human aging and correlate with X chromosome inactivation skewing in females. Aging (Albany NY). 2015;7(8):568–78.
21. Heyn H, Li N, Ferreira HJ, Moran S, Pisano DG, Gomez A, et al. Distinct DNA methylomes of newborns and centenarians. Proc Natl Acad Sci. 2012;109(26):10522–7.
22. Bacalini MG, Boattini A, Gentilini D, Giampieri E, Pirazzini C, Giuliani C, et al. A meta-analysis on age-associated changes in blood DNA methylation: results from an original analysis pipeline for Infinium 450k data. Aging (Albany NY). 2015;7(2):97–109.
23. Maegawa S, Hinkal G, Kim HS, Shen L, Zhang L, Zhang J, et al. Widespread and tissue specific age-related DNA methylation changes in mice. Genome Res. 2010;20(3):332–40.
24. Reynolds LM, Taylor JR, Ding J, Lohman K, Johnson C, Siscovick D, et al. Age-related variations in the methylome associated with gene expression in human monocytes and T cells. Nat Commun. 2014;5:5366.
25. Mcclay JL, Aberg KA, Clark SL, Nerella S, Kumar G, Xie LY, et al. A methylome-wide study of aging using massively parallel sequencing of the methyl-CpG-enriched genomic fraction from blood in over 700 subjects. Hum Mol Genet. 2014;23(5):1175–85.
26. Beerman I, Bock C, Garrison BS, Smith ZD, Gu H, Meissner A, et al. Proliferation-dependent alterations of the DNA methylation landscape underlie hematopoietic stem cell aging. Cell Stem Cell. 2013;12(4):413–25.
27. Bell JT, Tsai PC, Yang TP, Pidsley R, Nisbet J, Glass D, et al. Epigenome-wide scans identify differentially methylated regions for age and age-related phenotypes in a healthy ageing population. PLoS Genet. 2012;8(4):e1002629.
28. Bocker MT, Hellwig I, Breiling A, Eckstein V, Ho AD, Lyko F. Genome-wide promoter DNA methylation dynamics of human hematopoietic progenitor cells during differentiation and aging. Blood. 2011;117(19):e182–9.
29. Longo DL, Traynor BJ, Cookson MR, Singleton AB, Hernandez DG, Gibbs JR, et al. Distinct DNA methylation changes highly correlated with chronological age in the human brain. Hum Mol Genet. 2011;20(6):1164–72.

30. Grönniger E, Weber B, Heil O, Peters N, Stäb F, Wenck H, et al. Aging and chronic sun exposure cause distinct epigenetic changes in human skin. PLoS Genet. 2010;6(5):6.
31. Rakyan VK, Down TA, Maslau S, Andrew T, Yang TP, Beyan H, et al. Human aging-associated DNA hypermethylation occurs preferentially at bivalent chromatin domains. Genome Res. 2010;20(4):434–9.
32. Day K, Waite LL, Thalacker-Mercer A, West A, Bamman MM, Brooks JD, et al. Differential DNA methylation with age displays both common and dynamic features across human tissues that are influenced by CpG landscape. Genome Biol. 2013;14(9):R102.
33. Christensen BC, Houseman EA, Marsit CJ, Zheng S, Wrensch MR, Wiemels JL, et al. Aging and environmental exposures alter tissue-specific DNA methylation dependent upon CPG island context. PLoS Genet. 2009;5(8):e1000602.
34. Slieker RC, Relton CL, Gaunt TR, Slagboom PE, Heijmans BT. Age-related DNA methylation changes are tissue-specific with ELOVL2 promoter methylation as exception. Epigenetics Chromatin. 2018;11(1):25.
35. Griñán-Ferré C, Izquierdo V, Otero E, Puigoriol-Illamola D, Corpas R, Sanfeliu C, et al. Environmental enrichment improves cognitive deficits, AD hallmarks and epigenetic alterations presented in 5xFAD mouse model. Front Cell Neurosci. 2018;12:224.
36. Jung M, Pfeifer GP. Aging and DNA methylation. BMC Biol. 2015 Jan;13:7.
37. Grabowska W, Sikora E, Bielak-Zmijewska A. Sirtuins, a promising target in slowing down the ageing process. Biogerontology. 2017;18(4):447–76.
38. Horvath S. DNA methylation age of human tissues and cell types. Genome Biol. 2013;14(10):R115.
39. Hannum G, Guinney J, Zhao L, Zhang L, Hughes G, Sadda SV, et al. Genome-wide methylation profiles reveal quantitative views of human aging rates. Mol Cell. 2013;49(2):359–67.
40. Bekaert B, Kamalandua A, Zapico SC, Van De Voorde W, Decorte R. Improved age determination of blood and teeth samples using a selected set of DNA methylation markers. Epigenetics. 2015;10(10):922–30.
41. Purohit G, Mukherjee AK, Sharma S, Chowdhury S. Extratelomeric binding of the telomere binding protein TRF2 at the PCGF3 promoter is G-quadruplex motif-dependent. Biochemistry. 2018;57(16):2317–24.
42. Mu W, Starmer J, Yee D, Magnuson T. EZH2 variants differentially regulate polycomb repressive complex 2 in histone methylation and cell differentiation. Epigenetics Chromatin. 2018;11(1):71.
43. Wang X, Goodrich KJ, Gooding AR, Naeem H, Archer S, Paucek RD, et al. Targeting of polycomb repressive complex 2 to RNA by short repeats of consecutive guanines. Mol Cell. 2017;65(6):1056–1067.e5.
44. Malousi A, Andreou AZ, Georgiou E, Tzimagiorgis G, Kovatsi L, Kouidou S. Age-dependent methylation in epigenetic clock CpGs is associated with G-quadruplex, co-transcriptionally formed RNA structures and tentative splice sites. Epigenetics. 2018;13(8):808–21.
45. Fransquet PD, Wrigglesworth J, Woods RL, Ernst ME, Ryan J. The epigenetic clock as a predictor of disease and mortality risk: a systematic review and meta-analysis. Clin Epigenetics. 2019;11(1):62.
46. El-Maarri O, Becker T, Junen J, Manzoor SS, Diaz-Lacava A, Schwaab R, et al. Gender specific differences in levels of DNA methylation at selected loci from human total blood: a tendency toward higher methylation levels in males. Hum Genet. 2007;122(5):505–14.
47. Peterson VS. Sex matters. Int Fem J Polit. 2014;16:389–409.
48. Singmann P, Shem-Tov D, Wahl S, Grallert H, Fiorito G, Shin SY, et al. Characterization of whole-genome autosomal differences of DNA methylation between men and women. Epigenetics Chromatin. 2015;8(1):43.
49. Cotton AM, Price EM, Jones MJ, Balaton BP, Kobor MS, Brown CJ. Landscape of DNA methylation on the X chromosome reflects CpG density, functional chromatin state and X-chromosome inactivation. Hum Mol Genet. 2015;24(6):1528–39.
50. Unnikrishnan A, Freeman WM, Jackson J, Wren JD, Porter H, Richardson A. The role of DNA methylation in epigenetics of aging. Pharmacol Ther. 2019;195:172–85.

51. Khurana I, Kaspi A, Ziemann M, Block T, Connor T, Spolding B, et al. DNA methylation regulates hypothalamic gene expression linking parental diet during pregnancy to the offspring's risk of obesity in Psammomys obesus. Int J Obes. 2016;40(7):1079–88.
52. Kaspi A, Khurana I, Ziemann M, Connor T, Spolding B, Zimmet P, et al. Diet during pregnancy is implicated in the regulation of hypothalamic RNA methylation and risk of obesity in offspring. Mol Nutr Food Res. 2018;62(14):e1800134.
53. Ramaswamy A, Ioshikhes I. Dynamics of modeled oligonucleosomes and the role of histone variant proteins in nucleosome organization. Adv Protein Chem Struct Biol. 2013;90:119–49.
54. Cutter AR, Hayes JJ. A brief review of nucleosome structure. FEBS Lett. 2015;589:2914–22.
55. Song S, Johnson FB. Epigenetic mechanisms impacting aging: a focus on histone levels and telomeres. Genes (Basel). 2018;9(4):E201.
56. Adams PD, Ivanov A, Pawlikowski J, Manoharan I, Van TJ, Nelson DM, et al. Lysosome-mediated processing of chromatin in senescence. J Cell Biol. 2013;202(1):129–43.
57. O'Sullivan RJ, Kubicek S, Schreiber SL, Karlseder J. Reduced histone biosynthesis and chromatin changes arising from a damage signal at telomeres. Nat Struct Mol Biol. 2010;17(10):1218–25.
58. Hauer MH, Seeber A, Singh V, Thierry R, Sack R, Amitai A, et al. Histone degradation in response to DNA damage enhances chromatin dynamics and recombination rates. Nat Struct Mol Biol. 2017;24(2):99–107.
59. Scaffidi P, Misteli T. Lamin A-dependent nuclear defects in human aging. Science (80). 2006;312(5776):1059–63.
60. Shumaker DK, Dechat T, Kohlmaier A, Adam SA, Bozovsky MR, Erdos MR, et al. Mutant nuclear lamin A leads to progressive alterations of epigenetic control in premature aging. Proc Natl Acad Sci. 2006;103(23):8703–8.
61. Ucar D, Márquez EJ, Chung C-H, Marches R, Rossi RJ, Uyar A, et al. The chromatin accessibility signature of human immune aging stems from CD8+ T cells. J Exp Med. 2017;214(10):3123–44.
62. Talbert PB, Henikoff S. Histone variants on the move: substrates for chromatin dynamics. Nat Rev Mol Cell Biol. 2017;18(2):115–26.
63. Rogakou EP, Sekeri-Pataryas KE. Histone variants of H2A and H3 families are regulated during in vitro aging in the same manner as during differentiation. Exp Gerontol. 1999;34(6):741–54.
64. Correia-Melo C, Jurk D, Passos JF. Robust multiparametric assessment of cellular senescence. Methods Mol Biol. 2013;965:409–19.
65. Maze I, Wenderski W, Noh K-M, Bagot RC, Tzavaras N, Purushothaman I, et al. Critical role of histone turnover in neuronal transcription and plasticity. Neuron. 2015;87(1):77–94.
66. Contrepois K, Coudereau C, Benayoun BA, Schuler N, Roux PF, Bischof O, et al. Histone variant H2A. J accumulates in senescent cells and promotes inflammatory gene expression. Nat Commun. 2017;8:14995.
67. Jenuwein T, Allis CD. Translating the histone code. Science. 2001;293(5532):1074–80.
68. Glass CK, Rosenfeld MG. The coregulator exchange in transcriptional functions of nuclear receptors. Genes Dev. 2000;14(2):121–41.
69. Kouzarides T. Chromatin modifications and their function. Cell. 2007;128(4):693–705.
70. Lander ES, Linton LM, Birren B, Nusbaum C, Zody MC, Baldwin J, et al. Initial sequencing and analysis of the human genome. Nature. 2001;409(6822):860–921.
71. Oñate SA, Tsai SY, Tsai MJ, O'Malley BW. Sequence and characterization of a coactivator for the steroid hormone receptor superfamily. Science. 1995;270(5240):1354–7.
72. Benevolenskaya EV. Histone H3K4 demethylases are essential in development and differentiation. Biochem Cell Biol. 2007;85(4):435–43.
73. Klose RJ, Zhang Y. Regulation of histone methylation by demethylimination and demethylation. Nat Rev Mol Cell Biol. 2007;8(4):307–18.
74. Barski A, Cuddapah S, Cui K, Roh TY, Schones DE, Wang Z, et al. High-resolution profiling of histone methylations in the human genome. Cell. 2007;129(4):823–37.

75. Dang W, Steffen KK, Perry R, Dorsey JA, Johnson FB, Shilatifard A, et al. Histone H4 lysine 16 acetylation regulates cellular lifespan. Nature. 2009;459(7248):802–7.
76. Greer EL, Maures TJ, Hauswirth AG, Green EM, Leeman DS, Maro GS, et al. Members of the H3K4 trimethylation complex regulate lifespan in a germline-dependent manner in C. elegans. Nature. 2010;466(7304):383–7.
77. Li L, Greer C, Eisenman RN, Secombe J. Essential functions of the histone demethylase Lid. PLoS Genet. 2010;6(11):e1001221.
78. Siebold AP, Banerjee R, Tie F, Kiss DL, Moskowitz J, Harte PJ. Polycomb repressive complex 2 and trithorax modulate drosophila longevity and stress resistance. Proc Natl Acad Sci. 2010;107(1):169–74.
79. Maures TJ, Greer EL, Hauswirth AG, Brunet A. The H3K27 demethylase UTX-1 regulates C. elegans lifespan in a germline-independent, insulin-dependent manner. Aging Cell. 2011;10(6):980–90.
80. Ryder DJ, Judge SM, Beharry AW, Farnsworth CL, Silva JC, Judge AR. Identification of the acetylation and ubiquitin-modified proteome during the progression of skeletal muscle atrophy. PLoS One. 2015;10(8):e0136247.
81. Rodova M, Lu Q, Li Y, Woodbury BG, Crist JD, Gardner BM, et al. Nfat1 regulates adult articular chondrocyte function through its age-dependent expression mediated by epigenetic histone methylation. J Bone Miner Res. 2011;26(8):1974–86.
82. Rao RA, Ketkar AA, Kedia N, Krishnamoorthy VK, Lakshmanan V, Kumar P, et al. KMT1 family methyltransferases regulate heterochromatin–nuclear periphery tethering via histone and non-histone protein methylation. EMBO Rep. 2019;20(5):e43260.
83. Narita M, Nũnez S, Heard E, Narita M, Lin AW, Hearn SA, et al. Rb-mediated heterochromatin formation and silencing of E2F target genes during cellular senescence. Cell. 2003;113(6):703–16.
84. Chandra T, Kirschner K, Thuret J-Y, Pope BD, Ryba T, Newman S, et al. Independence of repressive histone marks and chromatin compaction during senescent heterochromatic layer formation. Mol Cell. 2012;47(2):203–14.
85. Zhang W, Li J, Suzuki K, Qu J, Wang P, Zhou J, et al. A Werner syndrome stem cell model unveils heterochromatin alterations as a driver of human aging. Science. 2015;348(6239):1160–3.
86. Succoio M, Comegna M, D'Ambrosio C, Scaloni A, Cimino F, Faraonio R. Proteomic analysis reveals novel common genes modulated in both replicative and stress-induced senescence. J Proteomics. 2015;128:18–29.
87. Kurz DJ, Payeli S, Greutert H, Briand Schumacher S, Lüscher TF, Tanner FC. Epigenetic regulation of tissue factor inducibility in endothelial cell senescence. Mech Ageing Dev. 2014;140:1–9.
88. Ahuja G, Bartsch D, Yao W, Geissen S, Frank S, Aguirre A, et al. Loss of genomic integrity induced by lysosphingolipid imbalance drives ageing in the heart. EMBO Rep. 2019;20(4):e47407.
89. Pavlopoulos E, Jones S, Kosmidis S, Close M, Kim C, Kovalerchik O, et al. Molecular mechanism for age-related memory loss: the histone-binding protein RbAp48. Sci Transl Med. 2013;5(200):200ra115.
90. Engel N, Mahlknecht U. Aging and anti-aging: unexpected side effects of everyday medication through sirtuin1 modulation. Int J Mol Med. 2008;21(2):223–32.
91. Cho S-H, Chen JA, Sayed F, Ward ME, Gao F, Nguyen TA, et al. SIRT1 deficiency in microglia contributes to cognitive decline in aging and neurodegeneration via epigenetic regulation of IL-1β. J Neurosci. 2015;35(2):807–18.
92. Mohamad Nasir NF, Zainuddin A, Shamsuddin S. Emerging roles of sirtuin 6 in Alzheimer's disease. J Mol Neurosci. 2018;64(2):157–61.
93. Narayan P, Dragunow M. Alzheimer's disease and histone code alterations. Adv Exp Med Biol. 2017;978:321–36.
94. Portela A, Esteller M. Epigenetic modifications and human disease. Nat Biotechnol. 2010;28(10):1057–68.
95. Klutstein M, Nejman D, Greenfield R, Cedar H. DNA methylation in cancer and aging. Cancer Res. 2016;76(12):3446–50.

96. Lin RK, Wang YC. Dysregulated transcriptional and post-translational control of DNA methyltransferases in cancer. Cell Biosci. 2014;4(1):46.
97. Hałasa M, Wawruszak A, Przybyszewska A, Jaruga A, Guz M, Kałafut J, et al. H3K18Ac as a marker of cancer progression and potential target of anti-cancer therapy. Cells. 2019;8(5):485.
98. Rai TS, Cole JJ, Nelson DM, Dikovskaya D, Faller WJ, Vizioli MG, et al. HIRA orchestrates a dynamic chromatin landscape in senescence and is required for suppression of Neoplasia. Genes Dev. 2014;28(24):2712–25.
99. Pérez RF, Tejedor JR, Bayón GF, Fernández AF, Fraga MF. Distinct chromatin signatures of DNA hypomethylation in aging and cancer. Aging Cell. 2018;17(3):e12744.
100. Chen D, Kerr C. The epigenetics of stem cell aging comes of age. Trends Cell Biol. 2019;29(7):563–8.
101. Fernández AF, Bayón GF, Urdinguio RG, Toraño EG, García MG, Carella A, et al. H3K4me1 marks DNA regions hypomethylated during aging in human stem and differentiated cells. Genome Res. 2015;25(1):27–40.
102. Chen Z, Chang WY, Etheridge A, Strickfaden H, Jin Z, Palidwor G, et al. Reprogramming progeria fibroblasts re-establishes a normal epigenetic landscape. Aging Cell. 2017;16(4):870–87.
103. Van der Kraan PM, Van den Berg WB. Chondrocyte hypertrophy and osteoarthritis: role in initiation and progression of cartilage degeneration? Osteoarthr Cartil. 2012;20(3):223–32.
104. El Mansouri FE, Chabane N, Zayed N, Kapoor M, Benderdour M, Martel-Pelletier J, et al. Contribution of H3K4 methylation by SET-1A to interleukin-1-induced cyclooxygenase 2 and inducible nitric oxide synthase expression in human osteoarthritis chondrocytes. Arthritis Rheum. 2011;63(1):168–79.
105. Iliopoulos D, Malizos KN, Tsezou A. Epigenetic regulation of leptin affects MMP-13 expression in osteoarthritic chondrocytes: possible molecular target for osteoarthritis therapeutic intervention. Ann Rheum Dis. 2007;66(12):1616–21.
106. Portal-Núñez S, Esbrit P, Alcaraz MJ, Largo R. Oxidative stress, autophagy, epigenetic changes and regulation by miRNAs as potential therapeutic targets in osteoarthritis. Biochem Pharmacol. 2016;108:1–10.
107. Kim K, Park YS, Im GI. Changes in the epigenetic status of the SOX-9 promoter in human osteoarthritic cartilage. J Bone Miner Res. 2013;28(5):1050–60.
108. Bartel DP. MicroRNAs: genomics, biogenesis, mechanism, and function. Cell. 2004;116:281–97.
109. Danka Mohammed CP, Park JS, Nam HG, Kim K. MicroRNAs in brain aging. Mech Ageing Dev. 2017;168:3–9.
110. Lin X, Zhan J-K, Wang Y-J, Tan P, Chen Y-Y, Deng H-Q, et al. Function, role, and clinical application of microRNAs in vascular aging. Biomed Res Int. 2016;2016:6021394.
111. Victoria B, Nunez Lopez YO, Masternak MM. MicroRNAs and the metabolic hallmarks of aging. Mol Cell Endocrinol. 2017;455:131–47.
112. Iwakawa H, Tomari Y. The functions of microRNAs: mRNA decay and translational repression. Trends Cell Biol. 2015;25(11):651–65.
113. Gomez-Verjan JC, Vazquez-Martinez ER, Rivero-Segura NA, Medina-Campos RH. The RNA world of human ageing. Hum Genet. 2018;137(11–12):865–79.
114. Cardoso AL, Fernandes A, Aguilar-Pimentel JA, de Angelis MH, Guedes JR, Brito MA, et al. Towards frailty biomarkers: candidates from genes and pathways regulated in aging and age-related diseases. Ageing Res Rev. 2018;47:214–77.
115. Kumar S, Vijayan M, Bhatti JS, Reddy PH. MicroRNAs as peripheral biomarkers in aging and age-related diseases. Prog Mol Biol Transl Sci. 2017;146:47–94.
116. Smith-Vikos T, Liu Z, Parsons C, Gorospe M, Ferrucci L, Gill TM, et al. A serum miRNA profile of human longevity: findings from the Baltimore Longitudinal Study of Aging (BLSA). Aging (Albany NY). 2016;8(11):2971–87.
117. Olivieri F, Albertini MC, Orciani M, Ceka A, Cricca M, Procopio AD, et al. DNA damage response (DDR) and senescence: shuttled inflamma-miRNAs on the stage of inflamm-aging. Oncotarget. 2015;6(34):35509–21.

118. Rani A, O'Shea A, Ianov L, Cohen RA, Woods AJ, Foster TC. miRNA in circulating microvesicles as biomarkers for age-related cognitive decline. Front Aging Neurosci. 2017;9:323.
119. Hekmatimoghaddam S, Dehghani Firoozabadi A, Zare-Khormizi MR, Pourrajab F. Sirt1 and Parp1 as epigenome safeguards and microRNAs as SASP-associated signals, in cellular senescence and aging. Ageing Res Rev. 2017;40:120–41.
120. Huh CJ, Zhang B, Victor MB, Dahiya S, Batista LF, Horvath S, et al. Maintenance of age in human neurons generated by microRNA-based neuronal conversion of fibroblasts. Elife. 2016;5:e18648.
121. Gudmundsson H, Gudbjartsson DF, Kong A, Gudbjartsson H, Frigge M, Gulcher JR, et al. Inheritance of human longevity in Iceland. Eur J Hum Genet. 2000;8(10):743–9.
122. ElSharawy A, Keller A, Flachsbart F, Wendschlag A, Jacobs G, Kefer N, et al. Genome-wide miRNA signatures of human longevity. Aging Cell. 2012;11(4):607–16.
123. Noren Hooten N, Abdelmohsen K, Gorospe M, Ejiogu N, Zonderman AB, Evans MK. microRNA expression patterns reveal differential expression of target genes with age. PLoS One. 2010;5(5):e10724. Blagosklonny MV, editor
124. Gombar S, Jung H, Dong F, Calder B, Atzmon G, Barzilai N, et al. Comprehensive microRNA profiling in B-cells of human centenarians by massively parallel sequencing. BMC Genomics. 2012;13(1):353.
125. Serna E, Gambini J, Borras C, Abdelaziz KM, Belenguer A, Sanchis P, et al. Centenarians, but not octogenarians, up-regulate the expression of microRNAs. Sci Rep. 2012;2(1):961.
126. Balzano F, Deiana M, Dei Giudici S, Oggiano A, Pasella S, Pinna S, et al. MicroRNA expression analysis of centenarians and rheumatoid arthritis patients reveals a common expression pattern. Int J Med Sci. 2017;14(7):622–8.
127. Borrás C, Serna E, Gambini J, Inglés M, Vina J. Centenarians maintain miRNA biogenesis pathway while it is impaired in octogenarians. Mech Ageing Dev. 2017;168:54–7.
128. Crocco P, Montesanto A, Passarino G, Rose G. Polymorphisms falling within putative miRNA target sites in the 3′UTR region of *SIRT2* and *DRD2* genes are correlated with human longevity. J Gerontol Ser A Biol Sci Med Sci. 2016;71(5):586–92.
129. Lafferty-Whyte K, Cairney CJ, Jamieson NB, Oien KA, Keith WN. Pathway analysis of senescence-associated miRNA targets reveals common processes to different senescence induction mechanisms. Biochim Biophys Acta. 2009;1792(4):341–52.
130. Noren Hooten N, Fitzpatrick M, Wood WH, De S, Ejiogu N, Zhang Y, et al. Age-related changes in microRNA levels in serum. Aging (Albany NY). 2013;5(10):725–40.
131. Pourrajab F, Vakili Zarch A, Hekmatimoghaddam S, Zare-Khormizi MR. The master switchers in the aging of cardiovascular system, reverse senescence by microRNA signatures; as highly conserved molecules. Prog Biophys Mol Biol. 2015;119(2):111–28.
132. Rippo MR, Olivieri F, Monsurrò V, Prattichizzo F, Albertini MC, Procopio AD. MitomiRs in human inflamm-aging: a hypothesis involving miR-181a, miR-34a and miR-146a. Exp Gerontol. 2014;56:154–63.
133. Chan SY, Zhang Y-Y, Hemann C, Mahoney CE, Zweier JL, Loscalzo J. MicroRNA-210 controls mitochondrial metabolism during hypoxia by repressing the iron-sulfur cluster assembly proteins ISCU1/2. Cell Metab. 2009;10(4):273–84.
134. Lauri A, Pompilio G, Capogrossi MC. The mitochondrial genome in aging and senescence. Ageing Res Rev. 2014;18:1–15.
135. Bandiera S, Rüberg S, Girard M, Cagnard N, Hanein S, Chrétien D, et al. Nuclear outsourcing of RNA interference components to human mitochondria. Pfeffer S, editor. PLoS One. 2011;6(6):e20746.
136. Boon RA, Iekushi K, Lechner S, Seeger T, Fischer A, Heydt S, et al. MicroRNA-34a regulates cardiac ageing and function. Nature. 2013;495(7439):107–10.
137. Zhao T, Li J, Chen AF. MicroRNA-34a induces endothelial progenitor cell senescence and impedes its angiogenesis via suppressing silent information regulator 1. Am J Physiol Endocrinol Metab. 2010;299(1):E110–6.
138. Guo Y, Li P, Gao L, Zhang J, Yang Z, Bledsoe G, et al. Kallistatin reduces vascular senescence and aging by regulating microRNA-34a-SIRT1 pathway. Aging Cell. 2017;16(4):837–46.

139. Thum T, Gross C, Fiedler J, Fischer T, Kissler S, Bussen M, et al. MicroRNA-21 contributes to myocardial disease by stimulating MAP kinase signalling in fibroblasts. Nature. 2008;456(7224):980–4.
140. Capri M, Olivieri F, Lanzarini C, Remondini D, Borelli V, Lazzarini R, et al. Identification of miR-31-5p, miR-141-3p, miR-200c-3p, and GLT1 as human liver aging markers sensitive to donor-recipient age-mismatch in transplants. Aging Cell. 2017;16(2):262–72.
141. Toutfaire M, Bauwens E, Debacq-Chainiaux F. The impact of cellular senescence in skin ageing: a notion of mosaic and therapeutic strategies. Biochem Pharmacol. 2017;142:1–12.
142. Reddy PH, Williams J, Smith F, Bhatti JS, Kumar S, Vijayan M, et al. MicroRNAs, aging, cellular senescence, and Alzheimer's disease. Prog Mol Biol Transl Sci. 2017;146:127–71.
143. Geekiyanage H, Jicha GA, Nelson PT, Chan C. Blood serum miRNA: non-invasive biomarkers for Alzheimer's disease. Exp Neurol. 2012;235(2):491–6.
144. Tan L, Yu J-T, Liu Q-Y, Tan M-S, Zhang W, Hu N, et al. Circulating miR-125b as a biomarker of Alzheimer's disease. J Neurol Sci. 2014;336(1–2):52–6.
145. Hadar A, Milanesi E, Walczak M, Puzianowska-Kuźnicka M, Kuźnicki J, Squassina A, et al. SIRT1, miR-132 and miR-212 link human longevity to Alzheimer's disease. Sci Rep. 2018;8(1):8465.
146. Barnes PJ. Senescence in COPD and its comorbidities. Annu Rev Physiol. 2017;79(1):517–39.
147. Brown DM, Goljanek-Whysall K. microRNAs: modulators of the underlying pathophysiology of sarcopenia? Ageing Res Rev. 2015;24(Pt B):263–73.
148. Marini F, Cianferotti L, Brandi M. Epigenetic mechanisms in bone biology and osteoporosis: can they drive therapeutic choices? Int J Mol Sci. 2016;17(8):1329.
149. Choi SW, Lee JY, Kang K-S. miRNAs in stem cell aging and age-related disease. Mech Ageing Dev. 2017;168:20–9.
150. Okada M, Kim HW, Matsu-ura K, Wang Y-G, Xu M, Ashraf M. Abrogation of age-induced microRNA-195 rejuvenates the senescent mesenchymal stem cells by reactivating telomerase. Stem Cells. 2016;34(1):148–59.
151. Neault M, Couteau F, Bonneau É, De Guire V, Mallette FA. Molecular regulation of cellular senescence by microRNAs: implications in cancer and age-related diseases. Int Rev Cell Mol Biol. 2017;334:27–98.
152. Saeidimehr S, Ebrahimi A, Saki N, Goodarzi P, Rahim F. MicroRNA-based linkage between aging and cancer: from Epigenetics View Point. Cell J. 2016;18(2):117–26.
153. Derrien T, Johnson R, Bussotti G, Tanzer A, Djebali S, Tilgner H, et al. The GENCODE v7 catalog of human long noncoding RNAs: analysis of their gene structure, evolution, and expression. Genome Res. 2012;22(9):1775–89.
154. Ulitsky I, Bartel DP. lincRNAs: genomics, evolution, and mechanisms. Cell. 2013;154(1):26–46.
155. Jain S, Thakkar N, Chhatai J, Pal Bhadra M, Bhadra U. Long non-coding RNA: functional agent for disease traits. RNA Biol. 2017;14(5):522–35.
156. Wu C-L, Wang Y, Jin B, Chen H, Xie B-S, Mao Z-B. Senescence-associated long non-coding RNA (SALNR) delays oncogene-induced senescence through NF90 regulation. J Biol Chem. 2015;290(50):30175–92.
157. Abdelmohsen K, Panda A, Kang M-J, Xu J, Selimyan R, Yoon J-H, et al. Senescence-associated lncRNAs: senescence-associated long noncoding RNAs. Aging Cell. 2013;12(5):890–900.
158. Fu VX, Dobosy JR, Desotelle JA, Almassi N, Ewald JA, Srinivasan R, et al. Aging and cancer-related loss of insulin-like growth factor 2 imprinting in the mouse and human prostate. Cancer Res. 2008;68(16):6797–802.
159. Abdelmohsen K, Panda AC, De S, Grammatikakis I, Kim J, Ding J, et al. Circular RNAs in monkey muscle: age-dependent changes. Aging (Albany NY). 2015;7(11):903–10.
160. Yoon J-H, Abdelmohsen K, Kim J, Yang X, Martindale JL, Tominaga-Yamanaka K, et al. Scaffold function of long non-coding RNA HOTAIR in protein ubiquitination. Nat Commun. 2013;4:2939.
161. Grammatikakis I, Panda AC, Abdelmohsen K, Gorospe M. Long noncoding RNAs(lncRNAs) and the molecular hallmarks of aging. Aging (Albany NY). 2014;6(12):992–1009.

162. Luo Q, Chen Y. Long noncoding RNAs and Alzheimer's disease. Clin Interv Aging. 2016;11:867–72.
163. Chen L-L, Yang L. Regulation of circRNA biogenesis. RNA Biol. 2015;12(4):381–8.
164. Yang Y, Fan X, Mao M, Song X, Wu P, Zhang Y, et al. Extensive translation of circular RNAs driven by N6-methyladenosine. Cell Res. 2017;27(5):626–41.
165. Salzman J, Gawad C, Wang PL, Lacayo N, Brown PO. Circular RNAs are the predominant transcript isoform from hundreds of human genes in diverse cell types. Preiss T, editor. PLoS One. 2012;7(2):e30733.
166. Cortés-López M, Miura P. Emerging functions of circular RNAs. Yale J Biol Med. 2016;89(4):527–37.
167. Zhang Y, Zhang X-O, Chen T, Xiang J-F, Yin Q-F, Xing Y-H, et al. Circular intronic long noncoding RNAs. Mol Cell. 2013;51(6):792–806.
168. Salzman J, Chen RE, Olsen MN, Wang PL, Brown PO. Cell-type specific features of circular RNA expression. PLoS Genet. 2013;9(9):e1003777.
169. Han Y-N, Xia S-Q, Zhang Y-Y, Zheng J-H, Li W. Circular RNAs: a novel type of biomarker and genetic tools in cancer. Oncotarget. 2017;8(38):64551–63.
170. Qu S, Zhong Y, Shang R, Zhang X, Song W, Kjems J, et al. The emerging landscape of circular RNA in life processes. RNA Biol. 2017;14(8):992–9.
171. Du WW, Yang W, Liu E, Yang Z, Dhaliwal P, Yang BB. Foxo3 circular RNA retards cell cycle progression via forming ternary complexes with p21 and CDK2. Nucleic Acids Res. 2016;44(6):2846–58.
172. Panda AC, Grammatikakis I, Kim KM, De S, Martindale JL, Munk R, et al. Identification of senescence-associated circular RNAs (SAC-RNAs) reveals senescence suppressor CircPVT1. Nucleic Acids Res. 2017;45(7):4021–35.
173. Holdt LM, Stahringer A, Sass K, Pichler G, Kulak NA, Wilfert W, et al. Circular non-coding RNA ANRIL modulates ribosomal RNA maturation and atherosclerosis in humans. Nat Commun. 2016;7:12429.
174. Cheng J, Huang J, Yuan S, Zhou S, Yan W, Shen W, et al. Circular RNA expression profiling of human granulosa cells during maternal aging reveals novel transcripts associated with assisted reproductive technology outcomes. Yu Y, editor. PLoS One. 2017;12(6):e0177888.
175. Knupp D, Miura P. CircRNA accumulation: a new hallmark of aging? Mech Ageing Dev. 2018;173:71–9.
176. Gruner H, Cortés-López M, Cooper DA, Bauer M, Miura P. CircRNA accumulation in the aging mouse brain. Sci Rep. 2016;6(1):38907.
177. Piwecka M, Glažar P, Hernandez-Miranda LR, Memczak S, Wolf SA, Rybak-Wolf A, et al. Loss of a mammalian circular RNA locus causes miRNA deregulation and affects brain function. Science (80). 2017;357(6357):eaam8526.
178. Rybak-Wolf A, Stottmeister C, Glažar P, Jens M, Pino N, Giusti S, et al. Circular RNAs in the mammalian brain are highly abundant, conserved, and dynamically expressed. Mol Cell. 2015;58(5):870–85.
179. Lukiw WJ, Circular RNA. (circRNA) in Alzheimer's disease (AD). Front Genet. 2013;4:307.
180. Ashapkin VV, Kutueva LI, Kurchashova SY, Kireev II. Are there common mechanisms between the Hutchinson-Gilford progeria syndrome and natural aging? Front Genet. 2019;10:455.
181. Nmezi B, Xu J, Fu R, Armiger TJ, Rodriguez-Bey G, Powell JS, et al. Concentric organization of A- and B-type lamins predicts their distinct roles in the spatial organization and stability of the nuclear lamina. Proc Natl Acad Sci. 2019;116(10):4307–15.
182. Crasto S, Di Pasquale E. Induced pluripotent stem cells to study mechanisms of laminopathies: focus on epigenetics. Front Cell Dev Biol. 2018;6:172.
183. Bertrand AT, Chikhaoui K, Yaou RB, Bonne G. Clinical and genetic heterogeneity in laminopathies. Biochem Soc Trans. 2011;39(6):1687–92.
184. Palm W, de Lange T. How shelterin protects mammalian telomeres. Annu Rev Genet. 2008;42(1):301–34.

185. Doksani Y, Wu JY, de Lange T, Zhuang X. Super-resolution fluorescence imaging of telomeres reveals TRF2-dependent T-loop formation. Cell. 2013;155(2):345–56.
186. Decker ML, Chavez E, Vulto I, Lansdorp PM. Telomere length in Hutchinson-Gilford progeria syndrome. Mech Ageing Dev. 2009;130(6):377–83.
187. Chojnowski A, Ong PF, Wong ES, Lim JS, Mutalif RA, Navasankari R, et al. Progerin reduces LAP2α-telomere association in hutchinson-gilford progeria. Elife. 2015;4:1–21.
188. Chandra T, Ewels PA, Schoenfelder S, Furlan-Magaril M, Wingett SW, Kirschner K, et al. Global reorganization of the nuclear landscape in senescent cells. Cell Rep. 2015;10(4):471–83.
189. Zhang R, Poustovoitov MV, Ye X, Santos HA, Chen W, Daganzo SM, et al. Formation of macroH2A-containing senescence-associated heterochromatin foci and senescence driven by ASF1a and HIRA. Dev Cell. 2005;8(1):19–30.
190. Burrows AE, Smogorzewska A, Elledge SJ. Polybromo-associated BRG1-associated factor components BRD7 and BAF180 are critical regulators of p53 required for induction of replicative senescence. Proc Natl Acad Sci U S A. 2010;107(32):14280–5.
191. Pegoraro G, Kubben N, Wickert U, Göhler H, Hoffmann K, Misteli T. Ageing-related chromatin defects through loss of the NURD complex. Nat Cell Biol. 2009;11(10):1261–7.
192. Cho I, Tsai P-F, Lake RJ, Basheer A, Fan H-Y. ATP-dependent chromatin remodeling by Cockayne syndrome protein B and NAP1-like histone chaperones is required for efficient transcription-coupled DNA repair. PLoS Genet. 2013;9(4):e1003407.
193. Sikora E. Rejuvenation of senescent cells-The road to postponing human aging and age-related disease? Exp Gerontol. 2013;48(7):661–6.
194. Obeid R, Schadt A, Dillmann U, Kostopoulos P, Fassbender K, Herrmann W. Methylation status and neurodegenerative markers in Parkinson disease. Clin Chem. 2009;55(10):1852–60.
195. Horvath S, Ritz BR. Increased epigenetic age and granulocyte counts in the blood of Parkinson's disease patients. Aging (Albany NY). 2015;7(12):1130–42.
196. Kontopoulos E, Parvin JD, Feany MB. α-synuclein acts in the nucleus to inhibit histone acetylation and promote neurotoxicity. Hum Mol Genet. 2006;15(20):3012–23.
197. Lee J-H, Ryu H. Epigenetic modification is linked to Alzheimer's disease: is it a maker or a marker? BMB Rep. 2010;43(10):649–55.
198. Silva PNO, Gigek CO, Leal MF, Bertolucci PHF, De Labio RW, Payão SLM, et al. Promoter methylation analysis of SIRT3, SMARCA5, HTERT and CDH1 genes in aging and Alzheimer's disease. J Alzheimer's Dis. 2008;13(2):173–6.
199. Bennett DA, Yu L, Yang J, Srivastava GP, Aubin C, De Jager PL. Epigenomics of Alzheimer's disease. Transl Res. 2015;165(1):200–20.
200. Furuya TK, Da Silva PNO, Payão SLM, Rasmussen LT, De Labio RW, Bertolucci PHF, et al. SORL1 and SIRT1 mRNA expression and promoter methylation levels in aging and Alzheimer's Disease. Neurochem Int. 2012;61(7):973–5.
201. Borodinova AA, Kuznetsova MA, Alekseeva VS, Balaban PM. Histone acetylation determines transcription of atypical protein kinases in rat neurons. Sci Rep. 2019;9(1):4332.
202. Zhang K, Schrag M, Crofton A, Trivedi R, Vinters H, Kirsch W. Targeted proteomics for quantification of histone acetylation in Alzheimer's disease. Proteomics. 2012;12(8):1261–8.
203. Gensous N, Bacalini MG, Pirazzini C, Marasco E, Giuliani C, Ravaioli F, et al. The epigenetic landscape of age-related diseases: the geroscience perspective. Biogerontology. 2017;18(4):549–59.
204. Escoubas CC, Silva-García CG, Mair WB. Deregulation of CRTCs in aging and age-related disease risk. Trends Genet. 2017;33(5):303–21.

# Microbiome Research and Aging

# 9

B. P. Chávez-Elizalde, O. S. Barrera-Vázquez, and M. F. Carrillo-Vega

*"We are born 100% human but we die 90% microbial."*

—Mändar Reet

## Abbreviations

| | |
|---|---|
| ARAP2 | ArfGAP and RhoGAP domain with ankyrin repeat and PH domain 2 |
| CCL2 | C-C motif chemokine ligand 2 |
| CMV | Cytomegalovirus |
| CXCR4 | C-X-C chemokine receptor type 4 |
| DAP2 | Dipeptidyl aminopeptidase 2 |
| DNA | Deoxyribonucleic acid |
| EBV | Epstein-Barr virus |
| FOS | Fructo-oligosaccharide |
| Fut-2 | Fucosyltransferase 2 |
| GWAS | Genome-wide association study |
| HHV | Human herpesvirus |
| HSV-1 | Herpes simplex virus 1 |
| HSV-2 | Herpes simplex virus 2 |
| IBD | Inflammatory bowel disease |
| IgA | Immunoglobulin A |

B. P. Chávez-Elizalde · M. F. Carrillo-Vega (✉)
Department of Clinical Epidemiological Research, Instituto Nacional de Geriatría (INGER), Mexico City, Mexico
e-mail: mcarrillo@inger.gob.mx

O. S. Barrera-Vázquez
División de Ciencias Básicas, Instituto Nacional de Geriatría (INGER), Mexico City, Mexico



J. C. Gomez-Verjan, N. A. Rivero-Segura (eds.), *Clinical Genetics and Genomics of Aging*, https://doi.org/10.1007/978-3-030-40955-5_9

| | |
|---|---|
| IgG | Immunoglobulin G |
| IL-12 | Interleukin 12 |
| IL12RA | Interleukin 12 receptor A |
| IL-17 | Interleukin 17 |
| IL23R | Interleukin 23 receptor |
| JAK/Stat | Janus kinase/*signal* transducer and activator of transcription |
| KEGG | Kyoto Encyclopedia of Genes and Genomes |
| LDL | Low density level |
| LINGO2 | Leucine rich repeat and Ig domain containing *2* |
| MHC | C-type lectin (CLEC), major histocompatibility complex |
| NOD1 | Nucleotide-binding oligomerization domain-containing protein 1 |
| NOD2 | Nucleotide-binding oligomerization domain-containing protein 2 |
| PLD1 | Phospholipase D1 |
| PUFAs | *Polyunsaturated fatty acids* |
| RNA | Ribonucleic acid |
| SCFAs | *Short-chain fatty acids* |
| SLIT3 | Slit homolog 3 |
| Stat 5A | Signal transducer and activator of transcription 5 A |
| Stat 5B | Signal transducer and activator of transcription 5 B |
| TCR | *T-cell receptor* |
| TGF-β | Transforming growth factor beta |
| UBR3 | Ubiquitin protein ligase E3 component n-recognin 3 |
| VDR | Vitamin D receptor |
| VPLs | Virus-like particles |
| VSCs | Volatile sulfur compounds |

## Introduction

The human microbiome represents a growing area of research that integrates the biomedical and clinical sciences. Through the first, depth understanding of the molecular characteristics of the host and the microbiota has arisen. The clinical and epidemiological research allows the understanding of the interactions between the host and the microbiota over time.

Integration of the knowledge that arises from different fields allows an optimal understanding of the nature and function of the human microbiome. Through this union, some mechanisms by which the microbiome acts in the health-disease process had been identified. The positive results from studies on the subject place the microbiome as a promising element in the medical area, specifically for geriatrics.

## Microbiome: A General Overview

The microbiota is understood as the collection of microbial taxa in a given environment. The microbiome, on the other hand, is the collection of genes and genomes encoded by the microbiota [1].

Since the first publication of the first human genome took place in 2001, the study of the microbiome had increased. The early studies were carried out based on cultures of the oral cavity and intestine. Subsequently, the molecular profiles on microbial biochemistry of all niches of the human body came to light [2].

Recent studies show that microbial communities differ from each other according to the ecological niche where they are found. It is known that microbial communities have greater taxonomic complexity and diversity in the oral cavity and the gastrointestinal tract [3, 4].

Presently it is known that each human hosts roughly 100 trillion microbes with genetic and phenotypic implications for the human body [5]. With this quantity in mind, it is easy to think that the dysfunction, also called dysbiosis, is strongly related to the presence of various diseases. In this respect, not only the quantity but the diversity of microorganisms are strongly associated with an unhealthy state [6].

All this information has been possible to elucidate by high-throughput sequencing technology that allows describing the genetic and functional (transcriptomic, proteomic, and metabolic) characteristics of the microbiome [7]. Through these novel techniques, it has been established that the human microbiome encompasses different kingdoms as bacteria, archaea, viruses, protozoa, and fungi [8]. The first three are the most studied in the field of human health.

Regarding bacteria, it has been proposed that they mediate phenotypic differences between individuals, much like gene variants in the host genome [9]. By means of symbiotic processes, this kingdom might impact human biology as they are numerous, are diverse, differ between individuals, and interact with the host and each other over a long period of time [9, 10].

Concerning the abundance and diversity of human-associated archaea, knowledge is minimal as the bacteria-targeting protocols are unsuitable for characterizing the full spectrum of archaea. As a consequence, little is known about their function and their overall role in human health.

The virome is defined as the set of total viruses that are present in a particular environment. Within the human organism, several types of viromes are considered, as the human body has several compartments where different virus communities are found. The virome is integrated into the microbiome and classified into two groups: prokaryotic virus or bacteriophages and eukaryotic viruses [11]. Several factors, such as age, diet, and the presence of other components of the microbiome, influence the composition of the virome [11].

The virome and bacterial microbiome are essential determinants of human health and disease. However, the human virome has been challenging to quantify. Moreover, it is likely different between individuals and beyond tissues in each person. The limitations in the quantification of the virome have been resolved with the development of the next-generation sequencing. This technique has allowed the discovery of new viruses and the characterization of the virome in healthy and sick individuals, finding the association of viruses with certain diseases. Among the different functions of the virome, it was found that viruses can interact with other components of the microbiome, such as bacteria, induced modulation of the antiviral immune response [11], and also bacterial and archaea infections due to genetic content of virus-like particle (VLP) bacteriophages [12].

On the other hand, microbiome bacteria have been largely studied. In fact, through the 16S ribosomal RNA gene sequencing technique [13, 14], bacterial phyla had been classified into four groups: *Firmicutes*, *Actinobacteria*, *Proteobacteria*, and *Bacteroidetes* [15].

## Human Microbiota Composition

The composition of the human microbiota depends on the specific properties of the local environment [16]. In this respect, it has been established that the micro-environment depends on the molecular components of the mucosal layer, intestinal peristalsis, contractility, and epithelial integrity [17–19]. See Fig. 9.1.

Figure 9.1 depicts a visual representation of the gut microbiota composition throughout the lifespan. Variations between individuals and within an individual throughout the lifespan can be seen. In this respect, it can be said that the concentration of *Bacteroidetes* grows as an individual does, from 12.6% for newborns to 57% for older adults. Conversely, *Actinobacteria* composition reduces with age until it reaches 0.4%, and the *Firmicutes*, *Proteobacteria*, and other microbial are maintained relatively stable throughout life in healthy adults and decay at old age [20–22].

Several factors such as diet, drug use, and social environment, as well as the ecological heterogeneity, such as host genetics, influence variations between the

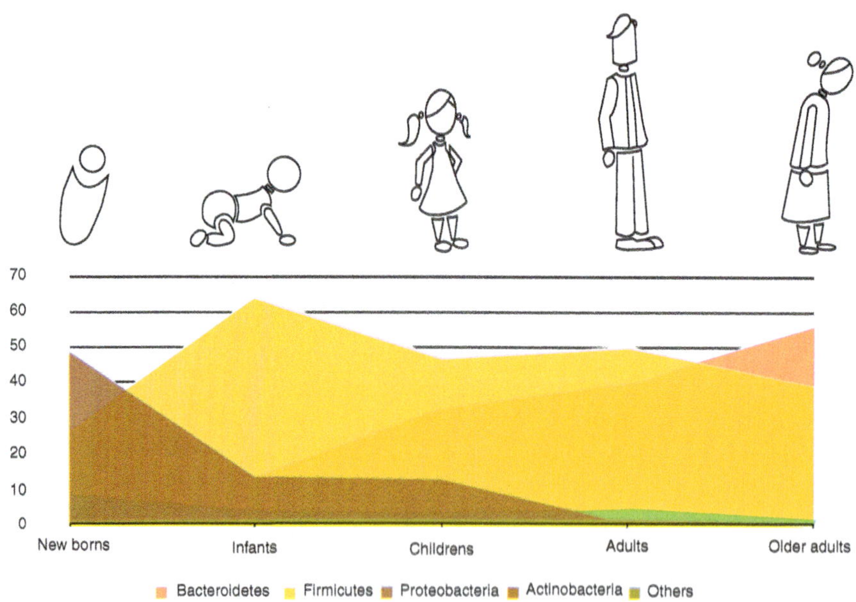


Fig. 9.1 Gut microbiota throughout lifespan

microbiota compositions from one human to another [23]. On these aspects, some examples are listed below.

It is known that the microbial composition in the intestine of newborns is strongly influenced by the type of milk received, that is, the introduction of breast milk or formula creates a differential environment at this age [24, 25]. During the first years of life, the microbiota is unstable. Later, during adulthood, it reaches its stability [26], but at advanced ages, dramatic changes in its composition are associated with various diseases and frailty [27, 28].

Regarding pathological processes, it is known that cancer, obesity, diabetes, and inflammatory bowel disease (IBD) are associated with specific microbial alterations [29, 30]. In older ages, a burden of intrinsic and extrinsic factors affects the composition of the microbiome and plays a determining role in every tract and tissue. Such mentioned factors can be seen in Fig. 9.2.

| Intrinsic | | Extrinsic |
|---|---|---|
| Age<br>Ethnic group<br>Genetics<br>Hormones<br>In utero environment | **Oral** | Denture use<br>Diet<br>Diseases (Gingivitis, Pediodontitis, Xerostomy)<br>Hygiene<br>Smoking |
| Age<br>Ethnic group<br>Genetics<br>Hormones<br>In utero environment | **Respiratory** | Antibiotics<br>Diseases (Asthma, COPD, Pneumonia)<br>Environment<br>Smoking |
| Age<br>Ethnic group<br>Genetics<br>Hormones<br>In utero environment | **Gastrointestinal** | Antibiotics<br>Diet<br>Diseases (Constipation, Obesity, Diverticulosis)<br>Exercise<br>Stress |
| Age<br>Ethnic group<br>Genetics<br>Hormones<br>In utero environment<br>Sex (Menopause/Andropause) | **Genitourinary** | Anatomy<br>Diseases (Infections, Urinary incontinence, Urolithiasis)<br>Hygiene<br>Voiding habits<br>Vasectomy/Salpingoclasy |
| Age<br>Ethnic group<br>Cutaneous structure<br>Chemical composition<br>Genetics<br>Hormones<br>Immune system<br>Location on the body | **Skin** | Chemical<br>Commercial products<br>Diseases<br>Hidratation<br>Hygiene<br>Makeup<br>Sun exposure |

**Fig. 9.2** Factors that affect microbiome composition in different tracts and tissues in older adults

## Microbiome Research and Aging: A Clinical Perspective

Aging is characterized by the accumulation of damage at the molecular level (DNA and proteins) and dysfunction of the organelles [31–33]. In addition to senescent cells and compositional changes in the extracellular compartment, these changes are determinants of the organic and systemic decline [34–36]. The microbiota reacts dynamically to these environment changes by altering the metabolic function and composition of individual bacterial species.

The immune system also has an essential role in commensal microbial communities by selectively eliminating pathogens and allowing only the development of commensal agents. However, during aging, progressive or sudden immune dysfunction is generated. Besides, inflammation is a normal process that induces inadequate surveillance among the host and the microbiota, leading to the appearance of dysbiosis, an imbalance in the composition of the bacterial community [37].

Therefore, research in the field has demonstrated that aging is a potential modifier of the composition and function of the human microbiome. Figure 9.3 shows the local composition of the microbiome in an average older adult. It can be seen that *Bacteroidetes* and *Firmicutes* species are the most prevalent in this age.

Recent data has shown that older people hide a microbiota that differs in the type and number of microorganisms from that of younger adults [38]. Young people are enriched with bacterial taxa that possess immunomodulatory activities, such as *Clostridium* and *Bifidobacterium*. On the other hand, the bacterial communities associated with older individuals are found enriched with pathobionts such as

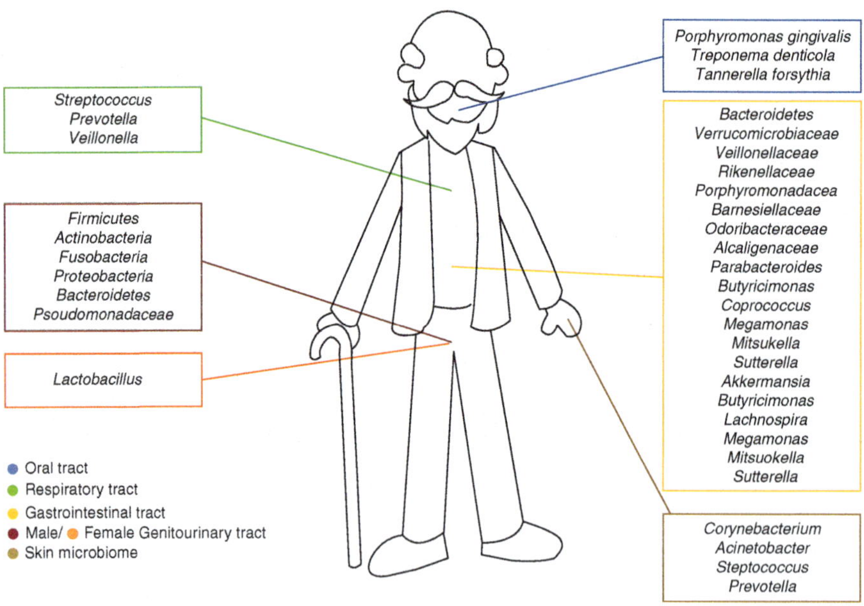


**Fig. 9.3** Composition of the microbiota in older adults

*Enterobacteriaceae* and *Proteobacteria* [39, 40]. This information suggests that age-dependent immune deterioration could allow the evolution of bacterial strains that are responsible for specific bacterial infections in this population.

Research on microbiome and aging also helps to generate information that allows calculating the age of an individual. This project has been called the "aging clock of the human microbiome." It aims to predict the age of the host with an accuracy of approximately 4 years [41].

All the information given by the aging research allows knowing that the microbial composition has an essential role in the establishment of cellular and tissue homeostasis. Additionally, it is known that age-dependent changes in the microbial composition can contribute to increasing of frailty and development of diseases during the late stages of life [42, 43].

On the other hand, studies on centenarians and supercentenarians have evidenced the adaptation of the microbiota to the physiological changes of the long aging process. It has been demonstrated that the microbiota on this population maintains the health and promotes the survival. Additionally, a relationship between a healthy microbiota and longevity had been proposed [44]. A possible pathway is an immunological and metabolic regulation linked to the increase of bacterial compounds like *Christensenellaceae*, *Akkermansia*, and *Bifidobacterium* [44, 45].

Although the causes that lead to changes in the composition and function of the microbiota during aging are still unknown, the evidence has established that the local microbiome plays an essential role in human health.

## Oral Microbiome

Both bacteria and viruses are the main components of the oral microbiome that is located in the tooth surfaces (supragingival and subgingival regions), cheeks, palate, saliva, and the tongue coating.

An average person has 700 bacterial species in their mouth interacting with the virome [46]. In this respect, it has been found that the human oral virome is mainly composed of bacteriophages belonging to the *Siphoviridae* family and a lesser extent by the families *Myoviridae* and *Podoviridae*. The oral virome seems to be also different between individuals and stable in time without suffering external disturbances [11].

As for eukaryotic viruses, most studies have focused solely on DNA viruses. The presence of human herpesvirus (HHV) in saliva such as herpes simplex virus 1 and 2 (HSV-1, HSV-2), cytomegalovirus (CMV), and Epstein-Barr virus (EBV) has been found. Besides, these viruses have a relationship with oral diseases such as periodontitis. A recent study has identified herpesviruses, phytoviruses, poxviruses, mimiviruses, baculoviruses, and papillomaviruses in the saliva of individuals with antibiotic therapy, where papillomavirus was the most abundant viral population, even considering the most extensive viral population: phages [11].

As can be seen, saliva is the fluid with the highest count of microorganisms. It is typically integrated by *Neisseria flavescens*, *Rothia mucilaginosa*, *Prevotella melaninogenica*, *Streptococcus mitis*, *Streptococcus*, *Streptococcus salivarius*, *Actinomyces*, *Granulicatella adiacens*, *Porphyromonas pasteri*, and *Veillonella atypical* [47].

The type and concentration of species change throughout life as a consequence of different intrinsic and extrinsic mechanisms. In older ages, the altered immune responses, reduced salivary flow, or denture can be important determinants of the characteristic dysbiosis that leads to oral health problems. Periodontal disease, for example, is caused by the proliferation of *Eubacterium nodatum* and *P. intermedia* [48]. Other studies demonstrated that *Porphyromonas gingivalis* is associated with the presence of periodontitis [49].

The microbiome can be modified to reduce the impact of such alterations. Following Terai et al. [50], oral probiotics contribute to oral health across the inhibition of volatile sulfur compounds (VSCs), which play an antibacterial role against pathogenic bacteria that cause periodontal disease and dental caries.

In this sense, it is known that in the supragingival plaque, which is responsible for caries formation, *Candida* species are the predominant pathogens, especially in adults >70 years [51].

## Respiratory Tract

Few studies have focused on the virome of the lung and respiratory tract. However, a population of bacteriophages as well as bacteria have been found in the lungs.

It has been suggested that there is a population of 19 different types of phages in the human respiratory tract. With regard to eukaryotic viruses, members of the *Paramyxoviridae*, *Orthomyxoviridae*, and *Picornaviridae* families have been found in patients with lower respiratory tract infections. In nasal and nasopharyngeal samples, pathogenic viruses of the families *Paramyxoviridae*, *Coronaviridae*, *Adenoviridae*, *Parvoviridae*, *Picornaviridae*, and *Orthomyxoviridae* were found [11]. These viruses are commonly seen as being part of the viral community in healthy individuals. However, it is not yet clarified if they are linked with persistent asymptomatic infections [11].

According to previous reports, *Streptococcus*, *Prevotella*, and *Veillonella* are the most common genera in the mouth. *Pseudomonas*, *Streptococcus*, *Prevotella*, *Fusobacterium*, *Haemophilus*, *Veillonella*, and *Porphyromonas* are essential organisms in the lungs.

Some authors have postulated a division of the respiratory tract according to their microorganism concentration [52]. The nasopharyngeal communities include *Streptococcus*, *Shigella*, *Acinetobacter*, and *Corynebacterium* spp. Even though, oropharyngeal communities are composed by *Prevotella*, *Fusobacterium*, *Neisseria*, *Leptotrichia*, and *Veillonella* spp.

This specific configuration plays an important role in the presence of diseases at older ages. The presence of *M.* or *C. pneumoniae* as well as *Proteobacteria*

(*Haemophilus*), *Pseudomonadaceae*, *Enterobacteriaceae*, *Burkholderiaceae*, and *Neisseriaceae* is associated with asthma disease at older ages [42].

Some extrinsic factors can be determinants of such local dysbiosis. Smoking, for example, promotes pathogenic colonization in the mouth, with no consequences in the microbiome of the lungs [53].

## Gastrointestinal Tract

Plenty of information can be found about the topic as during decades the gut microbiota has been the most studied field. Large evidence shows that the gut microbiome is essential for the health of the host due to its metabolic and trophic functions.

About the human gastrointestinal virome, it is known that the phages are the most abundant entities in this tract. Specifically, the double-stranded DNA phages *Myoviridae*, *Podoviridae*, and *Siphoviridae* are the most abundant. The members of the *Corticoviridae*, *Inoviridae*, *Leviviridae*, and *Tectiviridae* families have been identified less frequently. Interestingly the presence of eukaryotic viruses in the intestinal tract is much less characterized. However, some studies have shown at least 16 different viral DNA families and 10 RNA families. In pathological processes, viruses belonging to the *Reoviridae*, *Caliciviridae*, *Picornaviridae*, *Picobirnaviridae*, *Astroviridae*, and *Parvoviridae* families have been found [11].

It is known that the most prevalent organisms in the gut are bacteria. This group is composed of 40% *Firmicutes* and 57% *Bacteroidetes*, followed by *Actinobacteria* and *Proteobacteria* [54, 55]. Recent research has reclassified the gut composition of *Bacteroides* in *Alistipes*, *Prevotella*, *Paraprevotella*, *Parabacteroides*, and *Odoribacter* [56]. This composition also includes the archaea group and *Methanobrevibacter smithii* and *Methanosphaera stadtmaniae*, this two being the most present ones in the gut microbiome [38].

As shown by Biagi et al. [44], older adults, especially the centenarians, experience a reduction in the diversity of microorganisms. Additionally, an increased colonization by opportunistic species and pathobionts can be seen in this group. It has been found that the most predominant phylum, family, and genus in centenarians are *Bacteroidetes*, *Verrucomicrobiaceae*, *Veillonellaceae*, *Rikenellaceae*, *Porphyromonadaceae*, *Barnesiellaceae*, *Odoribacteraceae*, *Alcaligenaceae*, *Parabacteroides*, *Butyricimonas*, *Coprococcus*, *Akkermansia*, *Lachnospira*, *Megamonas*, *Mitsuokella*, and *Sutterella* such as *Methanobacteriaceae* that appears more in the centenarians [57].

These changes can be associated with endogenous factors like genetics, in utero environment, age, and hormones. Some exogenous factors, like diet, exercise, obesity, stress, and antibiotics, among others, can also contribute to the configuration [58].

It cannot be challenging to think that diet is the most influential determinant of gut microbiome. Extensive research has been published around the subject.

A study by Singh et al. [8] showed that a high-unsaturated fat diet increases *Streptococcus*, *Lactobacillus*, *Bifidobacterium*, and *Akkermansia muciniphila*. This configuration is associated with a decrease in total cholesterol, specifically LDL cholesterol. On the other hand, a high-saturated fat diet increases *Bacteroides*, *Bilophila*, and *Faecalibacterium prausnitzii*, which leads to increases in inflammation processes and less insulin sensitivity.

Different types of proteins influence gut microbiome; for example, plant protein increases *Bifidobacterium* and *Lactobacillus* and decreases *Bacteroides* and *Clostridium perfringens*. This configuration increases high short-chain fatty acids that inhibit inflammation. Animal protein, on the other hand, increases *Bacteroides*, *Alistipes*, *Bilophila*, and *Ruminococcus* and decreases *Bifidobacterium* that elevates trimethylamine N-oxide and reduces short-chain fatty acids (SCFAs). Results mentioned above are related to cardiovascular and inflammatory bowel diseases.

Diet can be a potent gut microbiome modifier. For this reason, numerous studies have been conducted to demonstrate the impact of specific diet components on the diversity of the gut microbiota [8]. The results of many of these studies have proved that probiotics and prebiotics consumption are a feasible alternative, especially for specific population groups such as older adults [59].

Although mycobiota has not yet been evaluated in older adults, metagenomic studies have shown that alterations of the intestine mycobiota are frequent. It was found greater diversity in the intestine of infants (0–2 years) and children (3–10 years) than in adults (≥18 years). The suppression of the bacterial microbiota induced by the treatment of antibiotics results in the growth of the intestinal mycobiota, possibly due to the reduction of ecological competition [60].

## Genitourinary Tract

The microbiome of the genitourinary tract encompasses from genitals, bladder, and the urinary tract. Regarding the virome, it remains mostly unexplored. Phages constitute more than 99% of all the viruses of the tract. Notwithstanding, there is no evidence about its impact on health status. About eukaryotic viruses, only DNA viruses have been characterized. In urine and vaginal samples, the most common species are *Papillomaviridae*, *Herpesviridae*, *Anelloviridae*, and *Polyomaviridae* [11].

*Lactobacillus* and *Streptococcus*, on the other hand, are the main bacteria of the region. Some others, as *Alloscardovia*, *Burkholderia*, *Jonquetella*, *Klebsiella*, *Saccharofermentans*, *Rhodanobacter*, and *Veillonella*, have been recognized but in less quantity.

Some studies have shown that variations in the urinary microbiome depend on sex and age. The type of urinary metabolites, the anatomic structures, hormones, and histology are the most important determinants of such variations [61].

In respect to extrinsic factors, D-mannose, a substance present in cranberry, apple, or pineapple juices, suppresses the union between bacterial type 1 fimbriae and cell surfaces. The consequent effect is the reduce colonization of pathogens of the urinary tract and further infections [62]. Also, vitamin D has a protective factor against urinary incontinence [63]. Conversely, a high sodium, calcium, and animal protein diet increases the risk of urolithiasis [64].

Specifically, for the vagina, the evidence shows that there are at least five major types of vaginal microbiota called community state types [65]. The most abundant species in this habitat is *Lactobacillus*, as the vaginal epithelium is rich in glycogen, the key nutrient for vaginal lactobacilli. After menopause, the amount of *Lactobacillus* decreases as a consequence of reduced availability of glycogen driven by estrogen levels. The reduction in estrogens also influences the bacterial diversity of the vagina [16].

In this respect, Petricevic et al. [66] demonstrated that the consumption of probiotics improved the vaginal flora of postmenopausal.

The microbiome of the male genital tract is less studied, but it is known that the tract has different types of species. For example, the penis microbiome is composed of aerobic, microaerophilic, and anaerobic bacteria [67]. Some differences in the composition are attributable to the age, but circumcision, sexual activity, and vasectomy also influence. Nelson et al. [68] showed that 52.6% of the microorganisms in the penis are *Firmicutes*, while the remaining percentage is composed by *Actinobacteria*, *Fusobacteria*, *Proteobacteria*, and *Bacteroidetes*.

Some studies have proved the connection between the gut microbiota and that from the genitourinary tract. Poutahidis et al. [69] postulated that changes in the gut microbiota might improve the immune system with a consequent improvement in the tissue homeostasis and health in general. To prove their theory, *L. reuteri* was administered to aged mice that increased testicular weight, seminiferous tubule, and conspicuous Leydig cell areas before the administration. The explanation is that *L. reuteri* increases levels of circulating testosterone as a consequence of the aging process, across blocking pro-inflammatory IL-17 signaling that recapitulates the beneficial effects of probiotics.

## Skin

Skin microbiome depends on the cutaneous structure and its chemical composition. Thus, the location on the body, skin constitution, and topographical skin variability are also important. The fatty tissue and the level of hydration are further essential determinants of the type of organisms.

Due to the low biomass obtained from the skin samples, it has been challenging to study viral groups. On phage populations, recent studies show that up to 94% of viral sequences did not match a known viral genome in databases of reference [11]. The *Caudovirales* and those in the families *Myoviridae* and *Siphoviridae* have been found in the skin. On the other hand, the skin of healthy people can harbor several eukaryotic viruses for periods, such as those of the viruses belonging to *Adenoviridae*, *Anelloviridae*, *Circoviridae*, *Herpesviridae*, *Papillomaviridae*, *Phycodnaviridae*, *Poxviridae*, and *Polyomaviridae* families. However, studies on the search for characterization of RNA virus populations in the skin are missing [11].

In skin, it has been identified that *Propionibacterium* and *Staphylococcus* are found in sebaceous skin sites and *Corynebacterium*, *Staphylococcus*, and *Betaproteobacteria* in moist areas, while *Betaproteobacteria*, *Corynebacterium*, and *Flavobacteriales* are found in dry sites [70].

Other factors linked with the composition of the microbiome are the immune system, sex, and age. In this regard, specifically, the age-dependent changes that the skin experiment in the structure and appearance, are caused by molecular alterations like increase in pH, decreased ability to quench reactive oxygen species, and increased matrix metalloproteinase activity. Those variables play an essential role in the skin microbiome configuration [71]. In this respect, Shibagaki et al. [72] reported that in older adults *Corynebacterium*, *Acinetobacter*, *Streptococcus*, and *Prevotella* are the bacteria with the highest presence.

As well as for the other cavities, oral treatments are an effective alternative to improve the current state of the microbiome in the skin. It was shown by Maguire and Maguire [71] that the oral supplementation of *L. paracasei* increased the serum concentration of TGF-beta, an indispensable factor for skin integrity. Besides, this group showed that the use of probiotics restores the pH of the skin and returns protease activity levels.

It can be seen that diet has a strong relationship with the composition of the microbiota in all the tracts. Table 9.1 resumes some dietary interventions that recently prove a positive effect on the human microbiome.

Table 9.1 describes that diet directly affects the microbiota composition, especially from the gut. This is because the tract has a malleable ecosystem that improves the adaptation to intrinsic and extrinsic factors. This flexibility optimizes the metabolic and immune performance in response to environmental and physiological changes, improving health status [45]. Besides, the majority of dietary interventions had demonstrated a positive effect on the reduction of inflammatory status.

Additional information has shown that fermentation activity carried out by the gut microbiome results in reduced hunger and increased satiety levels, which reduces energy intake [81, 82]. Moreover, changes in the gut microbiome of obese patients induced by prebiotics decrease the circulation of lenomorelin or ghrelin and increase the peptide tyrosine tyrosine or PYY [74].

**Table 9.1** Research on the effect of dietary interventions on the human microbiome

| Intervention | Decreases | Increases | Health impact |
|---|---|---|---|
| Fiber (non-digestible carbohydrates) | – | *Bifidobacterium* spp., *Lactobacillus* spp., *Akkermansia muciniphila* | Reduces inflammatory diseases like obesity [73, 74] |
| Fermentable substrates | *Bacteroidetes* | *Lactobacillus*, *Faecalibacterium prausnitzii*, *Akkermansia muciniphila* | Alteration in the storage of lipids and reduction in the production of inflammatory cytokines in obese people [75]. Gut barrier [76] |
| Prebiotics (inulin and FOS) | *Faecalibacterium prausnitzii* and *Lactobacilli* spp. | *Enterobacteriaceae* | Improved exhaustion and handgrip strength (phenotypic criteria of frailty) [77] |
| SCFA | *F. Prausnitzii* | – | Loss of butyrate-producing commensals with inflammation |
| Anti-inflammatory peptides | *F. Prausnitzii* | – | Reduced anti-inflammatory effects |
| Polyphenols | – | *A. muciniphila*, *Bifidobacterium* sp., *Lactobacillus* sp., *Bacteroidetes* sp., *Eubacterium* sp., and *Escherichia coli* | Maintenance of the barrier function and proglucagon levels [78] |
| | | | Regulate learning and memory, prevent neuroinflammation, and modulate neurotransmitter levels |
| Western diet | | *Collinsella* | Promotes obesity |
| Mediterranean diet | *Proteobacteria* and *Bacillaceae* | *Bacteroides* and *Clostridium* | Anti-inflammatory effects [79] |
| FOS | – | *Bifidobacterium* | Reduction of carcinogenicity, improvement of mineral absorption, and decrease in levels of serum cholesterol and levels of serum glucose [80] |
| Inulin | – | *Bifidobacterium adolescentis*, *Bifidobacterium longum*, and *Faecalibacterium prausnitzii* | Relieve constipation, improve mineral absorption, and control of lipid and glucose metabolism [77] |
| PUFAs (omega-3) | – | *Roseburia*, *Bifidobacterium*, and *Lactobacillus* sp. | Metabolic disorder and chronic inflammation associated with early life exposure to antibiotics |
| Vitamin D3 | *Proteobacteria* and *Helicobacter* sp. | – | Deficiency is associated with neuropsychiatric, inflammatory, and metabolic disorders [79] |

*Abbreviations*: *FOS* fructo-oligosaccharide, *PUFAs* polyunsaturated fatty acids, *SCFA* short-chain fatty acids

## The Microbiological Attributes of Tissues, Pathways, and Genes

The genome-wide association study (GWAS) and other studies in the field have helped to understand and analyze in greater depth the association of tissues, pathways, and genes with microbiome attributes. There is evidence where specific human genes are repeatedly associated with the microbiome. Also, it is shown that there is a genetic influence on the abundance of different microbial pathways and functions [83].

A relationship of the different variants of the microbiome with genes related to immunity has been described. Enrichment analyses show that the genes involved in signaling of factors, as leptin, JAK/Stat, melatonin, chemokine, and CXCR4, among others, had an impact on the microbiome [84]. A study of the nasal microbiota showed that factors involved in the modulation of mucosal immunity, such as IgA, IgG, IL12/IL12RA, TCR, and STAT5A/B, have an important role in structuring the microbiome of the aerial pathway.

Significant associations of microbial and functional abundance have been found with genes involved in the immune response [85], such as CCL2, DAP2, and IL23R (in turn involved in inflammatory), as well as genes of the nucleotide-binding oligomerization domain NOD1 and NOD2, two CLEC loci, and two genetic variants in the MHC region. Additionally, the association between the abundance of the *Rikenellaceae* family and a locus containing the UBR3 gene has been described. This gene codes for a protein involved in ubiquitination [86], thus playing a crucial role in the immune system. Also, genetic variants of the PLD1 and LINGO2 genes, which have been involved with obesity, have an association with *Akkermansia* and *Blautia*. Interestingly, both have been associated with related phenotypes with obesity [83].

## Human Genes and Proteins Involved in Microbiome

In this respect, the association of the SLIT3 gene with the abundance of unclassified *Clostridiaceae* [87] and *Dermacoccus* in the nasal vestibule has been described [88]. In addition, there is a relationship between the gene coding for the vitamin D receptor (VDR) with *Parabacteroides*, because its abundance was significantly higher when VDR is downregulated [89]. On the other hand, the Fut2 gene, which is associated with Crohn's disease, interacts with the intestinal microbiota [90]. There is also an enrichment of genes associated with the microbiome by the KEGG pathway, responsible for the biosynthesis of primary bile acids [84]. Similarly, there is an association between the MetaCyc bacterial bile acid metabolism pathway and the ARAP2 gene [85]. This information evidence the existence of an interaction between the genetics of the host and the microbiome through the regulation of bile acid metabolism.

## Conclusions

During the last years, significant advances in the field of microbiome and aging research have been carried out; new approaches for its study have allowed the understanding of the genomic nature of the microbiota. In this regard, the introduction of metagenomics had increased knowledge of the genes that potentially allow microbes to influence their hosts in unexpected ways. Thanks to these advances, it is well known that microbiota constitutes an essential determinant of the health and longevity of humans.

Notwithstanding these advances, several gaps in knowledge remain unsolved. For example, full characterization of the microbiome and its related products and metabolites is challenging work, because trillions of microbes host the human body. The diverse nature of microbial communities had forced to focus the efforts on cataloguing the microorganisms and describing their characteristics. On the other hand, their interaction with each other, and tendency to form intricate networks, makes it difficult to predict their behavior. This limitation is a challenging element to identify correlations between microbial species and disease. Additionally, several aspects of the human virome still remain unknown. This is because studies in the field are limited as a consequence of the number of patients required. The available studies have been performed only in certain human populations, and therefore no general conclusions have been made.

These limitations need to be solved, and new research on the field is required to provide functional insights into the microbiome and its mechanisms of action. There is a special necessity to develop knowledge that allows the use of microbiome as a potential method of disease diagnosis, prognosis, and treatment.

Some advances have been proposed in this area, for example, personalized therapeutics. This novel approach arises from the knowledge about the influence of the microbiome on multiple clinical outcomes. Available findings in the field suggest that interactions of the bacteria with the immune system improve drug efficacy.

Several researchers have postulated that information based on extensive, standardized, longitudinal human microbiome studies need to be carried out to establish normal and disease-specific microbiome patterns. Additionally, well-designed clinical trials need to be designed to prove novel techniques to modulate the human microbiome in specific health conditions.

Many areas of opportunity can be mentioned. However, modulation of the microbiome by extrinsic factors can be a way to apply the actual knowledge in the clinical setting. Nowadays, it is possible to ensure that lifestyle and diet play a significant role in determining the microbiome. In this respect, novel therapies, as fecal transplantation adds to the traditional dietary interventions, both demonstrated to be a potential therapeutic approach for the aging population.

**Acknowledgments** Special thanks to Pamela Tella-Vega for the awesome images for this work.

## References


1. Lu M, Wang Z. Linking gut microbiota to aging process: a new target for anti-aging. Food Sci Human Wellness. 2018;7(2):111–9.
2. Integrative H. The integrative human microbiome project. Nature. 2019;569(7758):641.
3. Human Microbiome Project C. Structure, function and diversity of the healthy human microbiome. Nature. 2012;486(7402):207–14.
4. Clemente J, Pehrsson E, Blaser M, Sandhu K, Gao Z, Wang B, et al. The microbiome of uncontacted Amerindians. Sci Adv. 2015;1(3):e1500183.
5. Wang B, et al. The human microbiota in health and disease. Engineering. 2017;3(1):71–82.
6. Sommer F, Anderson J, Bharti R, Raes J, Rosenstiel P. The resilience of the intestinal microbiota influences health and disease. Nat Rev Microbiol. 2017;15(10):630–8.
7. Arnold J, Roach J, Azcarate-Peril A. Emerging Technologies for gut microbiome research. Trends Microbiol. 2016;24(11):887–901.
8. Singh R, Chang H, Yan D, Lee K, Ucmak D, Wong K, et al. Influence of diet in the gut microbiome and implications for human health. J Transl Med. 2017;15(1):73.
9. Hooper LV, Gordon JI. Commensal host-bacterial relationships in the gut. Science. 2001;292(5519):1115–8.
10. Cadwell K. The virome in host health and disease. Immunity. 2015;42(5):805–13.
11. Zarate S, et al. Human Virome Arch Med Res. 2017;48(8):701–16.
12. Carding S, Davis N, Hoyles L. Review article: the human intestinal virome in health and disease. Aliment Pharmacol Ther. 2017;46(9):800–15.
13. Sanschagrin S, Yergeau E. Next-generation sequencing of 16s ribosomal RNA gene amplicons. J Vis Exp. 2014;90:e51709.
14. Almonacid D, Kraal L, Ossandon F, Budovskaya Y, Cardenas JP, Bik E, et al. 16S rRNA gene sequencing and health reference ranges for 28 clinically relevant microbial taxa from the human gut microbiome. PLoS One. 2017;12(5):e0176555.
15. Costello EK, Lauber CL, Hamady M, Fierer N, Gordon JI, Knight R. Bacterial community variation in human body habitats across space and time. Science. 2009;326(5960):1694–7.
16. Zapata H, Quagliarello V. The microbiota and Microbiomein aging: potential implications in health and age-related diseases. J Am Geriatr Soc. 2015;63(4):776–81.
17. Donaldson G, Lee S, Mazmanian S. Gut biogeography of the bacterial microbiota. Nat Rev Microbiol. 2016;14(1):20–32.
18. Rolig A, Mittge E, Ganz J, Troll J, Melancon E, Wiles T, et al. The enteric nervous system promotes intestinal health by constraining microbiota composition. PLoS Biol. 2017;15(2):e2000689.
19. Sommer F, Backhed F. Know your neighbor: microbiota and host epithelial cells interact locally to control intestinal function and physiology. BioEssays. 2016;38(5):455–64.
20. Odamaki T, Kato K, Sugahara H, Hashikura N, Takahashi S, Xiao JZ, et al. Age-related changes in gut microbiota composition from newborn to centenarian: a cross-sectional study. BMC Microbiol. 2016;16:90.
21. Flores GE, Caporaso JG, Henley JB, Rideout JR, Domogala D, Chase J, et al. Temporal variability is a personalized feature of the human microbiome. Genome Biol. 2014;15(12):531.
22. Davenport E, Sanders J, Song SJ, Amato K, Clark A, Knight R. The human microbiome in evolution. BMC Biol. 2017;15(1):127.
23. Rothschild D, Weissbrod O, Barkan E, Kurilshikov A, Korem T, Zeevi D, et al. Environment dominates over host genetics in shaping human gut microbiota. Nature. 2018;555:210–5.
24. Stewart C, Ajami N, O'Brien J, Hutchinson D, Smith D, Wong M, et al. Temporal development of the gut microbiome in early childhood from the TEDDY study. Nature. 2018;562(7728):583–8.
25. Forbes J, Azad M, Vehling L, Tun H, Konya T, Guttman D, et al. Association of Exposure to formula in the hospital and subsequent infant feeding practices with gut microbiota and risk of overweight in the first year of life. JAMA Pediatr. 2018;172(7):e181161.

26. Bokulich N, Chung J, Battaglia T, Henderson N, Jay M, Li H, et al. Antibiotics, birth mode, and diet shape microbiome maturation during early life. Sci Transl Med. 2016;8(343):343ra82.
27. O'Toole P, Jeffery I. Gut microbiota and aging. Science. 2015;350(6265):1214–5.
28. Bodogai M, O'Connell J, Kim K, Kim Y, Moritoh K, Chen C, et al. Commensal bacteria contribute to insulin resistance in aging by activating innate B1a cells. Sci Transl Med. 2018;10(467):eaat4271.
29. Fulbright L, Ellermann M, Arthur J. The microbiome and the hallmarks of cancer. PLoS Pathog. 2017;13(9):e1006480.
30. Ni J, Wu G, Albenberg L, Tomov V. Gut microbiota and IBD: causation or correlation? Nat Rev Gastroenterol Hepatol. 2017;14(10):573–84.
31. Morimoto R, Cuervo A. Protein homeostasis and aging: taking care of proteins from the cradle to the grave. J Gerontol A Biol Sci Med Sci. 2009;64A(2):167–70.
32. Vaidya A, Mao Z, Tian X, Spencer B, Seluanov A, Gorbunova V. Knock-in reporter mice demonstrate that DNA repair by non-homologous end joining declines with age. PLoS Genet. 2014;10(7):e1004511.
33. Zhou C, Slaughter B, Unruh J, Guo F, Yu Z, Mickey K, et al. Organelle-based aggregation and retention of damaged proteins in asymmetrically dividing cells. Cell. 2014;159(3):530–42.
34. Ewald C, Landis J, Porter-Abate J, Murphy C, Blackwell T. Dauer-independent insulin/IGF-1-signalling implicates collagen remodelling in longevity. Nature. 2015;519(7541):97–101.
35. Elderman M, Sovran B, Hugenholtz F, Graversen K, Huijskes M, Houtsma E, et al. The effect of age on the intestinal mucus thickness, microbiota composition and immunity in relation to sex in mice. PLoS One. 2017;12(9):e0184274.
36. Childs B, Durik M, Baker D, van Deursen J. Cellular senescence in aging and age-related disease: from mechanisms to therapy. Nat Med. 2015;21(12):1424–35.
37. Li H, Qi Y, Jasper H. Preventing age-related decline of gut compartmentalization limits microbiota Dysbiosis and extends lifespan. Cell Host Microbe. 2016;19(2):240–53.
38. Mihajlovski A, Doré J, Levenez F, Alric M, Brugére J. Molecular evaluation of the human gut methanogenic archaeal microbiota reveals an age-associated increase of the diversity. Environ Microbiol Rep. 2010;2(2):272–80.
39. Quercia S, Candela M, Giuliani C, Turroni S, Luiselli D, Rampelli S, et al. From lifetime to evolution: timescales of human gut microbiota adaptation. Front Microbiol. 2014;5:587.
40. Smith P, Willemsen D, Popkes M, Metge F, Gandiwa E, Reichard M, et al. Regulation of life span by the gut microbiota in the short-lived African turquoise killifish. elife. 2017;6:e27014.
41. Galkin F, Aliper A, Putin E, Kuznetsov I, Gladyshev V, Zhavoronkov A. Human microbiome aging clocks based on deep learning and tandem of permutation feature importance and accumulated local effects. bioRxiv. 2019. https://doi.org/10.1101/507780.
42. Chotirmall S, Burke C. Aging and the microbiome: implications for asthma in the elderly? Expert Rev Respir Med. 2015;9(2):125–8.
43. Yamashita Y, Takeshita T. The oral microbiome and human health. J Oral Sci. 2017;59(2):201–6.
44. Biagi E, Rampelli S, Turroni S, Quercia S, Candela M, Brigidi P. The gut microbiota of centenarians: signatures of longevity in the gut microbiota profile. Mech Ageing Dev. 2017;165(Pt B):180–4.
45. Santoro A, Ostan R, Candela M, Biagi E, Brigidi P, Capri M, et al. Gut microbiota changes in the extreme decades of human life: a focus on centenarians. Cell Mol Life Sci. 2018;75(1):129–48.
46. Aas J, Paster B, Stokes L, Olsen I, Dewhirst F. Defining the normal bacterial flora of the oral cavity. J Clin Microbiol. 2005;43(11):5721–32.
47. Bek-Thomsen M, Tettelin H, Hance I, Nelson K, Kilian M. Population diversity and dynamics of Streptococcus mitis, Streptococcus oralis, and Streptococcus infantis in the upper respiratory tracts of adults, determined by a nonculture strategy. Infect Immun. 2008;76(5):1889–96.
48. Feres M, Teles F, Teles R, Figueiredo L, Faveri M. The subgingival periodontal microbiota in the aging mouth. Periodontol 2000. 2016;72(1):30–53.
49. Zakaria M, Futura M, Takeshita T, Shibata Y, Sundari R, Eshima N, et al. Oral microbiome in community-dwelling elderly and its relation to oral and general health conditions. Oral Dis. 2017;23(7):973–82.

50. Terai T, Okumura T, Imai S, Nakao M, Yamaji K, Ito M, et al. Screening of probiotic candidates in human oral bacteria for the prevention of dental disease. PLoS One. 2015;10(6):e128657.
51. Flevari A, Theodorakopoulou M, Armaganidis A, Dimopoulos G. Treatment of invasive candidiasis in the elderly: a review. Clin Interv Aging. 2013;8:1199–208.
52. Charlson E, Chen J, Custers-Allen R, Bittinger K, Li H, Sinha R, et al. Disordered microbial communities in the upper respiratory tract of cigarette smokers. PLoS One. 2010;5(12):e15216.
53. Morris A, Beck J, Schloss P, Campbell T, Crothers K, Curtis J, et al. Comparison of the respiratory microbiome in healthy nonsmokers and smokers. Am J Respir Crit Care Med. 2013;187(10):1067–75.
54. Arumugam M, Raes J, Pelletier E, Le Paslier D, Yamada T, Mende D, et al. Enterotypes of the human gut microbiome. Nature. 2011;473(7346):174–80.
55. Icaza-Chávez M. Microbiota intestinal en la salud y la enfermedad. Rev Gastroenterol Mex. 2013;78(4):240–8.
56. Price-Lloyd J, Abu-Ali G, Huttenhower C. The healthy human microbiome. Genome Med. 2016;8(1):51.
57. Wang F, Yu T, Huang G, Cai D, Liang X, Su H, et al. Gut microbiota community and its assembly associated with age and diet in Chinese centenarians. J Microbiol Biotechnol. 2015;25(8):1195–204.
58. Maruvada P, Leone V, Kaplan LM, Chang EB. The human microbiome and obesity: moving beyond associations. Cell Host Microbe. 2017;22(5):589–99.
59. Matsumoto K, Takada T, Shimizu K, Moriyama K, Kawakami K, Hirano K, et al. Effects of a probiotic fermented milk beverage containing lactobacillus casei strain Shirota on defecation frequency, intestinal microbiota, and the intestinal environment of health individuals with soft stools. J Biosci Bioeng. 2010;110(5):547–52.
60. Strati F, Di Paola M, Stefanini I, Albanese D, Rizzetto L, Lionetti P, et al. Age and gender affect the composition of fungal population of the human gastrointestinal tract. Front Microbiol. 2016;7:1227.
61. Aragón I, Herrera-Imbroda B, Queipo-Ortuño M, Castillo E, Del Moral J, Gómez-Millán J, et al. The urinary tract microbiome in health and disease. Eur Urol Focus. 2018;4(1):128–38.
62. Whiteside SA, Razvi H, Dave S, Reid G, Burton JP. The microbiome of the urinary tract-a role beyond infection. Nature. 2015;12(2):81–90.
63. Robinson D, Giarenis I, Cardozo L. You are what you eat: the impact of diet on overactive bladder and lower urinary tract symptoms. Maturitas. 2014;79(1):8–13.
64. Marckmann P, Osther P, Pedersen AN, Jespersen B. High-protein diets and renal health. J Ren Nutr. 2015;25(1):1–5.
65. Smith S, Ravel J. The vaginal microbiota, host defence and reproductive physiology. J Physiol. 2017;595(2):451–63.
66. Petricevic L, Unger F, Viernstein H, Kiss H. Randomized, double-blind, placebo-controlled study of oral lactobacilli to improve the vaginal flora of postmenopausal women. Eur J Obstet Gynecol Reprod Biol. 2008;141(1):54–7.
67. Mändar R. Microbiota of male genital tract: impact on the health of man and his partner. Pharmacol Res. 2013;69(1):32–41.
68. Nelson D, Van Der Pol B, Dong Q, Revanna K, Fan B, Easwaran S, et al. Characteristic male urine microbiomes associate with asymptomatic sexually transmitted infection. PLoS One. 2010;5(11):e14116.
69. Poutahidis T, Springer A, Levkovich T, Qi P, Varian B, Lakritz J, et al. Probiotic microbes sustain youthful serum testosterone levels and testicular size in aging mice. PLoS One. 2014;9(1):e84877.
70. Moissl-Eichinger C, Probst A, Birarda G, Auerbach A, Koskinen K, et al. Human age and skin physiology shape diversity and abundance of archaea on skin. Sci Rep. 2017;7(1):4039.
71. Maguire M, Maguire G. The role of microbiota, and probiotics and prebiotics in skin health. Arch Dermatol Res. 2017;309(6):411–21.

72. Shibagaki N, Suda W, Clavaud C, Bastien P, Takayasu L, Iioka E, et al. Aging-related changes in the diversity of women's skin microbiomes associated with oral bacteria. Sci Rep. 2017;7(1):10567.
73. Makki K, Deehan E, Walter J, Backhed F. The impact of dietary Fiber on gut microbiota in host health and disease. Cell Host Microbe. 2018;23(6):705–15.
74. So D, Whelan K, Rossi M, Morrison M, Holtmann G, Kelly J, et al. Dietary fiber intervention on gut microbiota composition in healthy adults: a systematic review and meta-analysis. Am J Clin Nutr. 2018;107(6):965–83.
75. Tavares Da Silva S, Araújo dos Santos C, Bressan J. Intestinal microbiota; relevance to obesity and modulation by prebiotics and probiotics. Nutr Hosp. 2013;28(4):1039–48.
76. Holscher H. Dietary fiber and prebiotics and the gastrointestinal microbiota. Gut Microbes. 2017;8(2):172–84.
77. Theou O, Jayanama K, Fernández-Garrido J, Buigues C, Pruiboom L, Hoogland AJ, et al. Can a prebiotic formulation reduce frailty levels in older people? J Frailty Aging. 2019;8(1):48–52.
78. Murtaza N, Ó Cuív P, Morrison M. Diet and the microbiome. Gastroenterol Clin N Am. 2017;46(1):49–60.
79. Sandhu KV, Sherwin E, Schellekens H, Stanton C, Dinan T, Cryan J. Feeding the microbiota-gut-brain Axis: diet, microbiome and neuropsychiatry. Transl Res. 2017;179:223–44.
80. Kolida S, Tuohy K, Gibson GR. Prebiotic effects of inulin and oligofructose. Br J Nutr. 2002;87(Suppl 2):S193–7.
81. Roberfroid M, Gibson G, Hoyles L, McCartney A, Rastall R, Rowland I, et al. Prebiotic effects: metabolic and health benefits. Br J Nutr. 2010;104(Suppl 2):S1–63.
82. Cani P, Bibiloni R, Knauf C, Waget A, Neyrinck A, Delzenne N, et al. Changes in gut microbiota control metabolic endotoxemia-induced inflammation in high-fat diet-induced obesity and diabetes in mice. Diabetes. 2008;57(6):1470–81.
83. Goodrich J, Davenport E, Clark A, Ley R. The relationship between the human genome and microbiome comes into view. Annu Rev Genet. 2017;51:413–33.
84. Blekhman R, Goodrich J, Huang K, Sun Q, Bukowski R, Bell J, et al. Host genetic variation impacts microbiome composition across human body sites. Genome Biol. 2015;16:191.
85. Bonder M, Kurilshikov A, Tigchelaar E, Mujagic Z, Imhann F, et al. The effect of host genetics on the gut microbiome. Nat Genet. 2016;48(11):1407–12.
86. Turpin W, Espin-Garcia O, Xu W, Silverberg M, Kevans D, et al. Association of host genome with intestinal microbial composition in a large healthy cohort. Nat Genet. 2016;48(11):1413–7.
87. Goodrich J, Davenport E, Beaumont M, Jackson M, Knight R, et al. Genetic determinants of the gut microbiome in UK twins. Cell Host Microbe. 2016;19(5):731–43.
88. Igartua C, Davenport E, Gilad Y, Nicolae D, Pinto J, Ober C. Host genetic variation in mucosal immunity pathways influences the upper airway microbiome. Microbiome. 2017;5(1):16.
89. Wang J, Thingholm L, Skiecevičienė J, Rausch P, Kummen M, et al. Genome-wide association analysis identifies variation in vitamin d receptor and other host factors influencing the gut microbiota. Nat Genet. 2016;48(11):1396–406.
90. Xie H, Guo R, Zhong H, Feng Q, Lan Z, et al. Shotgun metagenomics of 250 adult twins reveals genetic and environmental impacts on the gut microbiome. Cell Syst. 2016;3(6):572–84.

# Molecular Basis of Progeroid Diseases

# 10

Ian García-Aguirre, Feliciano Monterrubio-Ledezma, Alma Alamillo-Iniesta, Susana Castro-Obregón, and Bulmaro Cisneros

## Abbreviations

| | |
|---|---|
| APS | Atypical Progeria Syndromes |
| ASO | Antisense Oligonucleotides |
| BAC | Bacterial Artificial Chromosome |
| BS | Bloom Syndrome |
| CRM1 | Chromosomal Region Maintenance 1 |
| CS | Cockayne Syndrome |
| CSA | Cockayne Syndrome protein A |
| CSB | Cockayne Syndrome protein B |
| DSB | Double-Strand Break |
| FTI | Farnesyltransferase Inhibitors |
| HGPS | Hutchinson-Gilford Progeria Syndrome |
| iPSCs | induced Pluripotent Stem Cells |
| MAD | Mandibuloacral Dysplasia |
| mTOR | mammalian Target of Rapamycin |
| NE | Nuclear Envelope |
| NER | Nucleotide Excision Repair |
| NES | Nuclear Export Signal |
| NGPS | Nestor-Guillermo Progeria Syndrome |

I. García-Aguirre · F. Monterrubio-Ledezma · A. Alamillo-Iniesta · B. Cisneros (✉)
Department of Genetics and Molecular Biology, Center of Research and Advanced Studies (CINVESTAV-IPN), Mexico City, Mexico
e-mail: ian.garcia@cinvestav.mx; eduardo.monterrubio@cinvestav.mx; bcisnero@cinvestav.mx

S. Castro-Obregón
Department of Neurodevelopment and Physiology, Institute of Cellular Physiology, National Autonomous University of Mexico (UNAM), Mexico City, Mexico
e-mail: scastro@ifc.unam.mx



J. C. Gomez-Verjan, N. A. Rivero-Segura (eds.), *Clinical Genetics and Genomics of Aging*, https://doi.org/10.1007/978-3-030-40955-5_10

| | |
|---|---|
| NPC | Nuclear Pore Complexes |
| Prx1 | Paired related homeobox 1 |
| RD | Restrictive Dermopathy |
| ROS | Reactive Oxygen Species |
| RTS | Rothmund-Thomson Syndrome |
| TCR | Transcription-Coupled Repair |
| TTD | Trichothiodystrophy |
| WS | Werner Syndrome |
| WT | Wild Type |
| XP | Xeroderma Pigmentosum |
| XPO1 | Exportin-1 |

## Introduction

Aging is a universal process that occurs across all living species. In humans, aging is characterized by a gradual decline of physical and psychological capacities that cause in turn metabolic and cognitive alterations, resulting in increasing vulnerability to environmental challenge and a growing risk for disease and death [1]. Since aging comprises the greatest risk factor for a variety of chronic diseases, including cancer, cardiovascular disorders, and neurodegenerative diseases [2], one of the goals of biomedical research is to decipher the molecular mechanism underlying aging, which in turn might facilitate the development of treatments aimed at delaying the onset of age-related diseases and to extend the human life span.

The use of humans in aging studies is complicated due to several factors, including ethical, environmental, and social issues, and even economic reasons, and more importantly, due to the human long natural life span. The human aging process takes decades to develop, making it virtually impossible to perform longitudinal studies by following subjects throughout their lives. Thus, the most widely employed models of aging are short-lived organisms, including yeast, roundworm, fruit fly, and mice. Indeed, large-scale genetic screenings have identified numerous genes and drugs that significantly lengthen life span in these organisms; however, the biological relevance of such longevity genes to human aging remains not fully established [3].

An alternative strategy to the investigation of aging using the humans themselves is the study of progeroid syndromes, a group of very rare genetic disorders characterized by accelerated aging and the presence of clinical features that resemble physiological aging, including osteoarthritis and osteoporosis, loss of muscle mass, hair loss, short stature, skin tightness, and cardiovascular diseases [4]. In addition to the genuine medical interest in improving the quality of life of these patients, the study of progeroid syndromes has attracted great interest in the past 10 years, in that they constitute an invaluable source of information for understanding the molecular basis of human aging.

The present chapter provides an overview of the most common progeroid syndromes affecting humans, offering an updated review of clinical features and the genetic bases and molecular mechanisms underlying these. In addition, current evidence and future perspectives for developing therapeutic strategies aimed at alleviating physiological impairment in these devastating pathologies are discussed, with special emphasis placed on Hutchinson-Gilford progeria syndrome, for which the development of therapeutic approaches has already begun.

## Classification of Human Progeroid Syndromes

To date, more than 20 progeroid syndromes have been described in the literature, and the fact that the majority of these disorders derive from alterations in genome stability highlights the crucial role of DNA in aging [5]. Genome maintenance implicates both DNA repair and nuclear integrity systems, which together defend the human genome from abrasion across time. Thus, although progeroid syndromes are genetically heterogeneous, they can be classified in two main categories, according to the pathway/mechanism affected in the disease: the first group clusters together progeroid syndromes caused by mutations that affect the structure or posttranslational maturation of lamin A, a main compound of nuclear lamin, while the second group includes syndromes caused by mutations that alter DNA repair mechanisms.

### Lamin A-linked Progeroid Syndromes

Eukaryotic cells organize their genome within the nucleus, which is outlined by the nuclear envelope (NE). The NE physically divides the nuclear and cytoplasmic compartments; it consists of the inner and outer nuclear membranes and the nuclear pore complexes (NPC). Transport of macromolecules between the nuclear and cytoplasmic occurs through NPC, which span the double membrane of the NE. Directly beneath the inner nuclear membrane lies the nuclear lamina, a proteinaceous meshwork comprising the type V intermediate filaments termed A-type lamins and B-type lamins, which preserve the nuclear structure and connect the cytoskeleton to the intranuclear chromatin via its binding with both NE integral proteins and the DNA itself [6]. The LMNA gene encodes A-type lamins (lamins A and C) by alternative mRNA splicing, while B-type lamins (lamin B1 and B2) are encoded by LMNB1 and LMNB2 genes, respectively. Lamins C2 and B3, which are exclusively expressed in germ cells, derive from the alternative splicing of LMNA and LMNB1 genes, respectively [7]. Expression of A-type lamins A occurs after tissue differentiation, while that of B-type lamins emerges during embryonic development, to continue in a ubiquitous manner throughout adult life [8]. The nuclear lamina is involved in many nuclear activities, including DNA repair and replication, gene expression, epigenetic regulation, chromatin organization, cell-cycle regulation, cell differentiation, and cellular senescence [9]. Therefore, it is not surprising that mutations in lamin genes, which impair the function of the nuclear lamina function, result in severe disorders-denominated laminopathies. In particular, mutations in the LMNA gene (located in the long arm of chromosome 1 [1q21-q22]) or mutations in the ZMP24 gene (encoding a metalloprotease specifically involved in lamin A posttranslational processing) give rise to a variety of premature aging disorders, including HGPS, mandibuloacral dysplasia (MAD), restrictive dermopathy (RD), Nestor-Guillermo progeria syndrome (NGPS), and other atypical progeria syndromes (APS).

### Hutchinson-Gilford Progeria Syndrome

The Hutchinson-Gilford progeria syndrome (HGPS) was first described by Jonathan Hutchinson in 1886 and for the second time by Hastings Gilford in 1897. Although HGPS is a very rare autosomal-dominant premature aging disorder, with an incidence rate estimated at one per 4-8 million live births, its study has become a topic of great interest because the disease recapitulates distinctive features of physiological aging. Therefore, its study might allow identification of the genetic/molecular mechanisms underlying aging. The symptomatology of HGPS includes bone (osteopenia and osteoporosis), muscle (sarcopenia), skin (lipodystrophy), metabolic (high energy expenditure), and cardiovascular (atherosclerosis) alterations [10]. Patients with HGPS exhibit a complex phenotype characterized by short stature, large skull, alopecia, prominent eyes, and thin skin [11]. This disorder is lethal and patients die at around 13 years of age due to myocardial attack or stroke. In 2003, the genetic basis of HGPS was identified; the majority of typical patients with HGPS (approximately 90%) have a spontaneous single nucleotide substitution (1824 C > T) in the LMNA gene [11]. Although this mutation is silent (the altered triplet codon corresponds to the same amino-acid residue), it activates a cryptic splicing site within exon 11, resulting in the synthesis of prelamin A mRNA, which contains an internal deletion of 150 base pairs. Consequently, this leads to the translation of a mutant lamin A termed progerin, which harbors a deletion of 50 amino acids within its C-terminus. Progerin is permanently farnesylated because the deletion eliminates the cleavage site for Zmpste24, the enzyme that removes the last 15 amino acids from pre-lamin A, including its farnesylated cysteine, rendering mature lamin A [11–13].

***Molecular mechanism of HGPS*** Progerin acts in a dominant gain-of-function manner by aberrantly anchoring to the NE and disturbing nuclear lamin function. Since lamins and their protein partners modulate different nuclear processes, acting as a hub gathering different signaling pathways, the presence of progerin might affect central regulatory mechanism [12]. Consistent with this notion, HGPS cells show a plethora of cellular defects, including aberrant nuclear morphology, loss of peripheral heterochromatin, altered DNA repair, gene expression, and telomere instability (Fig. 10.1).

The cascade of noxious effects exerted by progerin ultimately causes physiological impairment during development of tissues and organs. Progerin action occurs at different levels; it has been demonstrated that progerin directly binds to lamin A, preventing normal lamin A function to take place. Alternatively, progerin gains in affinity for nuclear proteins, which are commonly not partners of lamin A; for instance, the increased binding of progerin with a transcriptional co-activator

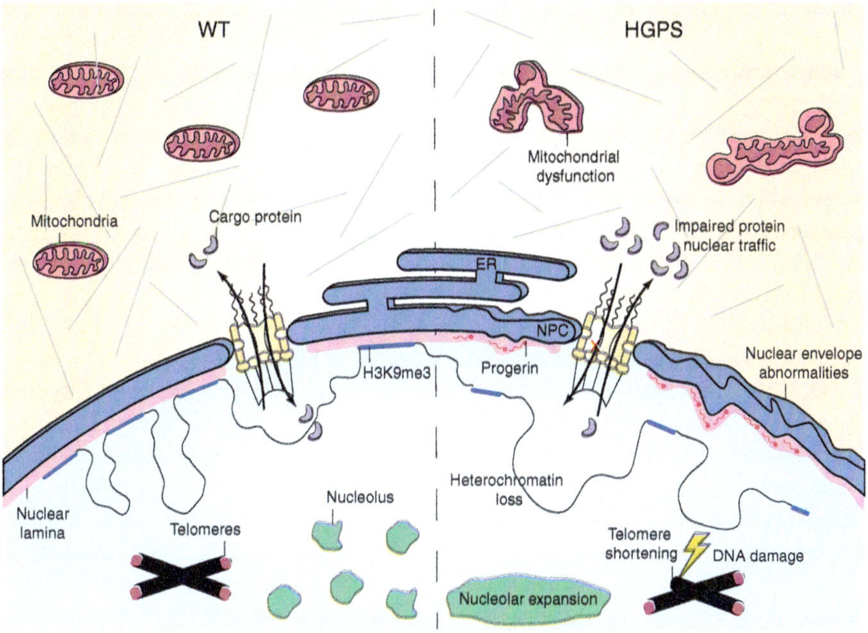


**Fig. 10.1** Schematic model showing the molecular and cellular aging marks of Hutchinson Gilford progeria syndrome (HGPS) cells. *Left. Illustration of a wild type* (WT) cell, showing proper organization of the nuclear envelope (NE), nuclear lamina, and the heterochromatin marker H3K9m3, as well as normal morphology of mitochondria, telomeres, and nucleoli. *Right.* The expression of progerin, the dominant negative mutant variant of lamin A, disturbs the structure of the NE, thereby inducing mitochondrial dysfunction, heterochromatin loss, nucleolar expansion, telomere shortening and impaired nuclear traffic of proteins

involved in skeletogenesis and vasculogenesis termed Prx1 (paired related homeobox 1) was previously observed [14]. Progerin can also perturb cellular functions in an indirect manner; for instance, progerin-induced damage to the NE structure alters in turn the nuclear-cytoplasmic trafficking of proteins, giving rise to imbalance in the partition of proteins between cytoplasm and nucleus [15–17], as well as the functional link between cytoskeleton and NE, then disturbing cell polarity and migration [18].

## Mandibuloacral Dysplasia

MAD is a hereditable autosomal recessive disease, of which the first causative mutation was identified in 2002 in the LMNA gene [19], implying for the first time a central role for the nuclear lamina in aging. To date, two different variants of MAD have been described: MADA is caused by mutations in the LMNA gene, while MADB originates due to ZMPSTE24 gene mutations, encoding for the zinc metallopeptidase STE24 [20]. Interestingly, some individuals with MAD have no mutations in either of these genes, implying that additional, as-yet-unidentified gene(s) may also cause the disorder [21].

Affected individuals display skeletal abnormalities including underdevelopment of the jaw bone and the collarbone, bone loss at the ends of the fingers and toes, joint deformities, mottled or patchy skin pigmentation, and partial lipodystrophy. Lipodystrophy appears to be associated with the metabolic syndrome because patients exhibited insulin resistance, glucose intolerance, and diabetes. Additional symptoms included dental abnormalities, growth retardation, and short stature in adulthood. However, symptomatology and the onset of the disease varies between patients; MADA symptomatology starts in adulthood, but children aged 4–5 years can be affected, while symptoms in subjects with MDAB appear earlier, commonly by 2 years of age [20].

***Molecular basis of MAD*** The homozygous R527H mutation in exon 9 of the LMNA gene has been commonly reported in patients with MAD [19, 20]; this mutation is located on the external surface of the lamin A domain involved in the formation of salt bridges [19]. Thus, the substitution of a basic residue (arginine) with a neutral one (cysteine) might disrupt the surface structure of the protein, with consequent effects on lamin A structure/function. Since lamin A governs multiple nuclear functions, including the maintenance of nuclear integrity, DNA repair, and gene expression, it is expected that MAD mutations disturb chromatin structure and/or gene regulation. On the other hand, because the zinc metalloproteinase enzyme ZMPSTE24 is involved in removing the C-terminal tail of prelamin A during lamin A maturation, it is thought that the compound heterozygous mutations in the ZMPSTE24 gene interrupt lamin A maturation, which results in prelamin A accumulation [22]. The immature protein aberrantly localizes at the NE and fails to interact properly with lamin A partners, causing a cascade of toxic effects in nuclear processes.

Regardless of the type of MAD, the presence of defective lamin A results in tissue-specific pathology, for instance, impaired adipocytes differentiation, might give rise to lipodystrophy and disrupted osteoclast differentiation might provoke altered turnover of bone [23].

### Restrictive Dermopathy

RD is a very rare and severe congenital disorder characterized by intrauterine growth retardation and fetal hypokinesia. Symptomatology after birth includes epidermal hyperkeratosis, decreased bone density, and pulmonary deficiency, the latter commonly leading to perinatal death. Patients with RD display a phenotype characterized by microstomia, small pinched nose, and sparse or absent eyelashes and eyebrows [24]. RD is commonly caused by a composition of heterozygous or homozygous mutations in the ZMPSTE24 gene [22].

***Molecular basis of RD*** The presence of mutations in both alleles of the ZMPSTE24 gene renders virtually no detectable levels of ZMPSTE24 in patients; thus, the least amount of residual enzyme activity correlates with the most severe disease symptomatology. As mentioned previously, the deficiency in ZMPSTE24 activity prevents lamin A maturation, which ultimately results in pre-lamin A accumulation in different tissues/organs, affecting a plethora of cellular functions modulated by mature lamin A [22].

### Nestor-Guillermo Progeria Syndrome

NGPS is a relatively new hereditary progeroid syndrome, characterized by an aged appearance (alopecia and skin wrinkling) and premature-aging physiological features, including growth retardation, decreased subcutaneous fat, skeletal abnormalities, osteoporosis, insulin resistance, and cardiovascular disease. Recently the genetic basis of NGPS was ascribed to the BANF1 gene (also known as BAF1), via the identification of a homozygous point mutation (c.34G >A [p.Ala12Thr]) in patients with NGPS [25]. The BANF1 gene encodes for the barrier-to-auto integration factor 1 (BAF1).

***Molecular mechanisms of NGPS*** BAF1 protein binds to chromatin and nuclear lamins, including pre-lamin A, which confers on it the ability to functionally link chromatin to the inner NE. Consistent with this, BAF1 has been involved in different nuclear functions, such as postmitotic nuclear assembly, chromatin remodeling, gene expression, and DNA replication and repair [26, 27]. Thus, it is expected that mutations in the BANF1 gene causing NGPS affect one or several of the aforementioned cellular processes. Interestingly, mutant protein BAF1 is unable to bind pre-lamin A, which in turn impairs chromatin organization [28]. However, it has been postulated that the NGPS cellular phenotype is caused by the inability of mutant protein BAF1 to bind DNA, instead of an effect on nuclear lamina, because mutant BAF1 protein preserves its interaction with lamins and histone H3 [29].

### Atypical Progeria Syndromes

Several APS that involved 28 different heterozygous, homozygous, or compound heterozygous mutant variants in the LMNA gene have been reported [30], which are distributed along the 12 exons of this gene [31–34] Patients with APS exhibit clinical features that resemble HGPS, including growth retardation, skeletal anomalies, alopecia, lipodystrophy, diabetes, and, in some cases, atherosclerosis. Faces with prominent eyes, a pointed nose, and mandibular hypoplasia are characteristic in these patients.

***Molecular mechanism of APS*** The correlation between the phenotypes of patients with APS and the localization of lamin A mutations remain elusive. It is thought that APS mutations mapping in lamin A domains involved in key protein-protein interactions might result in a more severe phenotype. For instance, lamin A variants affecting the Ig-like domain are predicted to disrupt protein folding, disturbing protein–protein interactions more globally than mutations in surface residues [35].

## DNA Repair-Related Progeroid Syndromes

As mentioned previously, premature aging syndromes are often caused by mutations in genes whose function is to preserve genomic integrity. In this respect, the RecQ family of DNA helicases has been found to function in DNA damage repair, including base excision repair and in DNA double-strand break (DBS) repair, as well as in DNA replication subjected to a normal or stressed state [36]. Mutations in three RecQ genes (WRN, BLM, and RECQL4) give rise to the Werner syndrome (WS), Bloom syndrome (BS), and Rothmund-Thomson syndrome (RTS), respectively [37]. Additional genetic defects in the DNA damage repair system also cause the following disorders: Cockayne syndrome (CS), xeroderma pigmentosum (XP), and trichothiodystrophy (TTD).

### Werner Syndrome

WS is a rare autosomal recessive disorder characterized by features compatible with accelerated aging, including short stature, skin atrophy, loss of subcutaneous fat, graying and scarce hair, cataracts, diabetes mellitus, hypogonadism, osteoporosis, atherosclerosis, and cancer [38, 39]. Interestingly, symptoms begin to appear early in the third decade of life and patients commonly die in their 50s due to myocardial infarction and cancer [40]. WS was originally described in 1904, and the causative gene was identified in 1996 by positional cloning [41]. WS is caused by homozygous or compound heterozygous mutations in the WRN gene, which encodes RecQ helicase, a protein with both helicase and exonuclease activities. The latter activity confers on this enzyme the ability to function in DNA metabolism, including DNA repair (double-strand breaks [DBS] during DNA replication), transcription, and telomere maintenance [42].

***Molecular mechanisms of WS*** The majority of WS mutations result in the loss of RecQ helicase activity, with few amino-acid substitutions that abolish enzyme activity or provoke protein instability [42]. Perturbation of WS helicase activity might result in a failure to repair DBS by homologous recombination or error-prone non-homologous end joining, and ultimately, in genomic instability. Consistent with this notion, primary fibroblasts from patients with WS exhibit chromosomal aberrations and very limited replicative capacity [43, 44]. Likewise, altered telomere maintenance due to WRN protein dysfunction may explain, at least in part, the distinctive range of tumors affecting patients with WS [45].

### Bloom Syndrome (BS)

BS, a very rare autosomal recessive disorder, was first described in 1954 by David Bloom. BS is characterized by growth and immune deficiencies, skin photosensitivity, insulin resistance, and telangiectasia (multiple small dilated blood vessels). Unlike patients with WS, patients with BS do not exhibit a progeria phenotype but instead are prone to develop multiple types of cancer, including breast, prostate, and lung [46]. The genetic basis of BS is the presence of biallelic loss-of-function mutations in the BLM gene, which encodes for DNA helicase RecQ, also denominated

Bloom syndrome (BLM) protein. BLM uses the energy of ATP hydrolysis to unwind DNA from the 3′ to 5′ direction.

***Molecular mechanisms of BS*** BLM protein, together with topoisomerase III alpha (TopIIIα) and RMI1 and RMI2 (RecQ-mediated genome instability proteins 1 and 2, respectively), are involved in regulating multiple steps of DNA repair machinery, including the repair of DBS during DNA synthesis [47, 48]; therefore, in the absence of BLM protein, patients with BS accumulate a broad range of DNA damage, including high rates of sister chromatid exchanges, leading to their greatly increased incidence of cancer [36, 47].

### Rothmund-Thomson Syndrome (RTS)

RTS is a rare autosomal recessive disorder that displays clinical characteristics of premature aging, including small stature, poikiloderma, alopecia, osteopenia, cataracts, and increased risk of cancer [49]. Homozygous or compound heterozygous mutations in RECQL4 gene, which encodes for an ATP-dependent DNA helicase, have been found in approximately two-thirds of patients with RTS, and the gene responsible for the remaining cases of RTS is unknown [50, 51]. RECQL4 has been found involved in different DNA repair mechanisms, including homologous recombination and non-homologous end-joining for DSB, nucleotide excision repair for UV DNA damage, and base excision repair [52].

***Molecular mechanisms of RTS*** Owing to the role of RECQL4 in DNA replication, DNA damage repair, and in the maintenance of both telomere and mitochondrial DNA integrity [53, 54], the aging-related clinical features and the predisposition to cancer observed in RTS patients could be attributed to the defective function of RECQL4 on these various processes [55]. Supporting this idea that chromosomal instability may be the underlying cause of cancer predisposition in patients with RTS, high frequencies of premature centromere separation and aneuploidy were found in cells from an RTS mouse model [56].

### Cockayne Syndrome

The Cockayne syndrome (CS) was first described by Edward Alfred Cockayne in 1936. CS is a rare genetic disorder with an incidence of 2–3 per million newborns, which is characterized by short stature, wrinkled and aging-appearing skin, photosensitivity, hearing and hair loss, and retinal atrophy. Progressive neurological dysfunction, microcephaly, and intellectual deficit have also been reported [57].

***Molecular mechanism of CS*** It is considered as a DNA repair disorder, because patient's cells exhibit defective transcription-coupled repair (TCR), a subclass of the nucleotide excision repair system (NER). CS is caused by mutations in the ERCC6 and ERCC8 genes, which encode for Cockayne syndrome protein B (CSB) and A (CSA) [58]. Both CSB and CSA proteins interact with pol II and act not only in the TCR mechanism but in RNA synthesis as well. The latter causes that CS cells undergo transcription repression in response to UV irradiation. CSB has the ability to remodel chromatin, while CSB is component of an E3 ubiquitin ligase complex. Thus, CSB is necessary to TCR initiation, while CSA promotes proteasome-mediated elimination of CSB at the end of the repair process, enabling transcription to continue [59]. CS cells also display mitochondrial dysfunction, which could be explained by the function of CSB in mitochondrial DNA transcription [60, 61].

#### Xeroderma Pigmentosum

Xeroderma pigmentosum (XP) is an autosomal recessive disorder that was first reported by Moriz Kaposi in 1874 [62]. XP is characterized by photosensitivity, wrinkled-dried aged skin, plaid pigmentation, skin tumors, and progressive neurologic alterations [62, 63].

***Molecular mechanism of XP*** The disease is caused by mutations in various genes that participate in DNA repair, including XPE and XPC proteins, which participate in the recognition of damaged DNA during global genome repair. Other XP causative genes are: XPA, whose function is to corroborate DNA damage; XPB and XPD, proteins with 3´-5´ and 5´-3´ helicase activities, respectively; XPG, an enzyme with 3´and 5´ nuclease activity; and XPV, which is a bypass polymerase implicated in postreplicative DNA repair after UV stress [60, 64]. Thus, altered activity of the aforementioned enzymes are consistent with the appearance of XP clinical manifestations.

#### Trichothiodystrophy

TTD is a rare autosomal recessive disorder, whose main characteristic is a deficiency of sulfur/cysteine levels in hair. Clinically, TTD is distinguished by developmental delay, intellectual deficit, ichthyosis, photosensitivity in most cases, frequent infections, and brittle and shortened hair [65].

***Molecular mechanism of TTD*** This disorder is caused by mutations in different genes involved in DNA repair and transcription, with the majority of patients harboring mutations in the XPD gene. Additional mutations associated with TTD involve the following genes: XPB, TDA, and TTDN1 [64, 66], the latter with unknown function.

## Cellular and Animal Models in HGPS

As mentioned previously, research on aging has been mainly approached employing cellular and animal models due to the inherent difficulties in conducting experimental studies on human beings themselves, including ethical principles, environmental and social factors, and the long natural life span of humans [67].

### Cellular Models

The use of primary cell cultures has provided valuable mechanistic information about the aging process, because it allows a more controlled manipulation of cellular processes, compared with that of tissues or whole organisms. Specifically, primary dermal fibroblasts and their derivative induced pluripotent stem cells (iPSCs) have been extensively utilized in the study of HGPS.

### Dermal Primary Fibroblasts

The skin is the most external tissue of the body and consequently undergoes the impact of environmental exposure to UV radiation and pollution, resulting in physiological alterations that resemble aging [1]. It is thought that dermal fibroblast cultures consolidate the chronic individual state of exogenous aging mechanisms; in keeping with this notion, dermal fibroblasts display a majority of the established characteristics of aging, such as genome instability, telomere attrition, mitochondrial dysfunction, cellular senescence, and loss of proteostasis [68]. Therefore, skin fibroblast cultures derived from biopsy samples obtained from healthy donors or from individuals affected by any premature aging syndrome have been a preferred model for aging at the cellular level, representing a faithful in vitro system to investigate the molecular mechanisms/signaling pathways that accompany aging [1, 68].

In particular, the study of HGPS dermal fibroblasts in conjunction with the overexpression of progerin in genotypically normal human cells has allowed for the elucidation of the different molecular mechanism/signaling pathways underlying premature aging, including defects in the NE structure/function, DNA repair, epigenetic regulation, heterochromatin organization, gene expression, and mitochondrial function (Fig. 10.1) [7, 11, 69–71]. Because HGPS fibroblasts undoubtedly reveal the disease phenotype, they provide a relevant tool for testing chemical compounds/drugs with therapeutic potential, by monitoring the alleviation of aging hallmarks in response to a given treatment (see later).

### Patient-Derived induced Pluripotent Stem Cells

The unique feature of iPSCs is their capability for unlimited self-renewal and reproduction of all adult cell types in the course of their differentiation. Thus, generation of patient-derived iPSCs offers a precious instrument for studying HGPS pathogenesis in a tissue-specific fashion, for instance, vascular cells become atherosclerotic and are responsible for the cardiovascular dysfunction observed in patients. Furthermore, longitudinal studies on HGPS iPSCs will permit the analysis of disease progression, from progerin expression to its downstream toxic effects. In fact, HGPS iPSCs cells have already been used to correct the HGPS mutation throughout homologous recombination [72] and to screen therapeutic drugs and would provide in the future the basis for cell replacement therapies [4].

## Animal Models for HGPS

In recent years, animal models have been at the forefront of aging research, making important contributions to a better understanding of this process at the organismal level. Some animals have been preferred in aging research, ranging from invertebrate (Caenorhabditis elegans and Drosophila melanogaster) to mammal species (murine and primate species). Nonetheless, scientists preferably chose mouse models for the study of age-related diseases for various reasons: (a) mice are closely related to humans, with nearly 99% of human orthologous in mice; (b) their relatively short lifespan and small size allow surveillance of the aging process within a pertinent time frame and make their housing less expensive; (c) the feasibility of performing genetic manipulations facilitates the engineering of transgenic strains (gain- and loss-of function mice) that model premature aging disorders. In this section, we describe the major HGPS mouse models previously developed (see Table 10.1 for details).

### Zmpste24$^{-/-}$ Knock-Out Mice

Curiously, two different Zmpste24−/− knock-out mice were the first murine models created for studying HGPS [73, 74]. Since ZMPSTE24 cuts off the last 15 amino acids of the protein (including the farnesylcysteine), thereby rendering mature lamin A [75], these Zmpste24-null mice accumulate farnesylated prelamin A. The mice originated by Bergo et al. appear to be normal at birth but later display HGPS features, including growth retardation, muscle weakness, alopecia, and numerous spontaneous bone fractures [73], while the Zmpste24 knock-out mice generated by Pendas et al. exhibited growth retardation, dilated cardiomyopathy, muscular alterations, lipodystrophy, and premature death [74]. At the molecular level, the farnesylated prelamin A perturbs the NE, induces cellular senescence, and impairs stem cell function and DNA repair [76].

### LMNA Knock-in Mice

On the other hand, a knock-in mutant mouse (LMNAHG), harboring a lamin A allele lacking introns 10 and 11 and the last 150 nucleotides of exon 11, expressed progerin solely from the mutant allele [77–79]. With the exception of cardiovascular dysfunction, homozygous and heterozygous LMNAHG mice exhibit HGPS features, including loss of subcutaneous fat, alopecia, osteoporosis, and premature death [77, 80, 81]. An alternative HGPS mouse was created (BAC-G608G mice),

**Table 10.1** Mice models for HGPS and other progeroid syndromes

| Mouse model | Gene defect | Human disease | References |
|---|---|---|---|
| *Lmna*$^{HG/+}$ | *Lmna* | HGPS | [77, 80] |
| *Lmna*$^{HG/HG}$ | *Lmna* | HGPS | [77, 80] |
| *Lmna*$^{G609G/+}$ | *Lmna* | HGPS | [84, 85] |
| *Lmna*$^{G609G/G609G}$ | *Lmna* | HGPS | [84] |
| *BAC-G608G* | Tg(*LMNA G608G*) | HGPS | [78] |
| *Zmpste24*$^{-/-}$ | *Zmpste24* | HGPS | [73, 74] |
| *Wrn*$^{-/-}$ | *Wrn* | WS | [86, 87] |
| *Wrn*$^{-/-}$*Terc*$^{-/-}$ | *Wrn, Terc* | WS | [88] |
| *Ercc6*$^{m/m}$/*Xpa*$^{-/-}$ | Double *Ercc6/Xpa* knockout | CS | [89] |
| *Csa*$^{-/-}$ (*ERCC8*$^{-/-}$) | *Csa* (*ERCC8*) | CS | [90–92] |
| *Csb*$^{m/m}$ (*ERCC6* $^{m/m}$) | *Csb* (*ERCC6*) | CS | [89, 91, 93] |
| CKO Blm$^{tm1Ches/tm4Ches;\ Hs\text{-}cre}$ | Blm | BS | [94] |

*HGPS* Hutchinson-Gilford Progeria Syndrome, *WS* Werner Syndrome, *CS* Cockayne Syndrome, *BS* Bloom Syndrome which carries a 164-kb bacterial artificial chromosome containing the G608G mutated human LMNA gene, flanked by regulatory DNA regions, for proper expression and splicing. Unexpectedly, these mice showed no HGPS hallmarks, but developed progressive loss of vascular smooth muscle cells, a characteristic found in patient biopsies [78]. An inducible transgenic mouse was generated with the aim of avoiding progerin toxicity during development, and specifically, to analyze its effect on epidermal keratinocyte biology. These mice demonstrated loss of subcutaneous fat, fibrosis of the dermis, and incomplete maturation of the sebaceous glands.

#### LMNA$^{G609G}$ Mice

Finally, the group of López-Otín generated a transgenic mouse-denominated LMNAG609G [82], which faithfully recreates the natural human HGPS mutation that drives the expression of progerin in patients due to an aberrant splicing event (G608G). These mice accumulate progerin and mimic the main clinical manifestations of human HGPS, including growth retardation, bone and cardiovascular alterations, curvature of the spine, and premature death, with nuclear morphology defects and defective DNA repair exhibited at cellular level. This mouse model has been extensively employed to develop therapeutic strategies against HGPS (see later). Other mouse models with various LMNA gene mutations have been developed to clarify the role of lamina A in premature aging [83]. Finally, additional mice models that have been developed for the study of other progeroid syndromes are shown in Table 10.1

## Therapeutic Perspective in HGPS

To date, there is no medicine to halt or delay the progression of HGPS, and patients receive only palliative medication to prevent/ameliorate chronic manifestations of old age (high cholesterol levels, blood clots, and potential heart attacks). Nevertheless, recent advances in aging research employing cellular and animal models have paved the way for developing therapeutic strategies against HGPS. A broad spectrum of treatments has been addressed, which could be grouped into two main categories: a) progerin-targeting strategies and b) strategies aimed at alleviating the downstream toxic effects driven by progerin (see Fig. 10.2 for details). This section offers an updated description and discussion of experimental approaches toward the establishment of therapeutic procedures for HGPS (see Fig. 10.2 and Table 10.2 for details).

### Progerin-Targeting Strategies

In that progerin exerts its action by a gain-of-function mechanism, the majority of strategies have been designed to prevent/reduce progerin toxicity by removing it, impeding its isoprenylation, or diminishing its expression using approaches acting at DNA, mRNA, and protein levels.

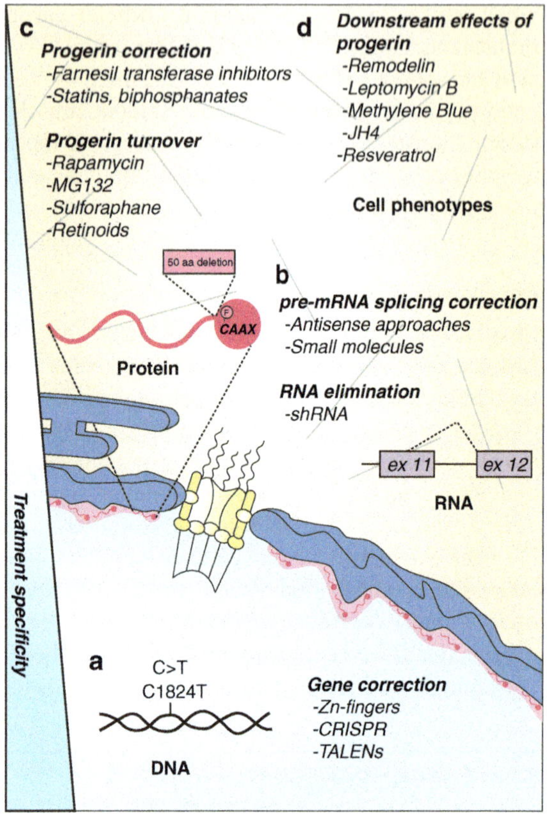


**Fig. 10.2** Therapeutic strategies to treat Hutchinson Gilford progeria syndrome (HGPS). Treatments aimed to alleviate HGPS can be targeted at different levels: (**a**) DNA level, correction of the HGPS mutation using CRISPER/Cas technology. (**b**) RNA level, modulation of splicing by exon skipping using antisense technology. (**c**) Protein level, clearance of progerin using drugs that induced autophagy (Rapamycin and MG132) or prevention of progerin farnesylation using farnesyl transferase inhibitors (FTI). (**d**) Cellular level, alleviation of noxious downstream effects driving by progerin using different drugs/compounds; JH4 avoids the aberrant interaction between progerin and lamin A; remodelin and leptomycin B normalize nuclear import of proteins and nuclear export of proteins, respectively; and methylene blue ameliorates mitochondrial dysfunction

**Table 10.2** Therapeutic drugs for HGPS

| Compound | Mechanism of action | Study model | Therapeutic effects | References |
|---|---|---|---|---|
| FTI | Farnesyltransferase inhibitor | Patient's fibroblasts | Alleviates nuclear morphology | [80, 114–117] |
| | | | Alleviates nucleolar abnormalities | |
| | | HGPS mice | Increases adipose tissue mass | |
| | | | Improves body weight curves | |
| | | | Reduces rib fractures | |
| | | | Improves bone mineralization | |
| | | | Improves cortical bone thickness | |
| | | | Improves the survival | |
| | | Clinical trails | Weight gain | |
| | | | Improves cardiovascular status | |
| | | | Improves bone geometry | |

Table 10.2 (continued)

| Compound | Mechanism of action | Study model | Therapeutic effects | References |
|---|---|---|---|---|
| Remodelin | Acetyl-transferase (NAT10) inhibitor | Patient's fibroblasts | Alleviates nuclear morphology<br>Reduces DNA damage<br>Alleviates heterochromatin loss<br>Prevents senescence | [118–120] |
| | | HGPS mice | Reduces DNA damage<br>Alleviates nuclear morphology<br>Enhances health span<br>Decreases weight loss<br>Ameliorates cardiac pathology | |
| Blue methylene | Antioxidant agent | Patient's fibroblasts | Alleviates mitochondrial dysfunction<br>Reduces oxidative stress<br>Prevents senescence | [111] |
| MG132 | Proteasome inhibitor | Patient's fibroblasts | Alleviates nuclear morphology<br>Prevents senescence<br>Reduces DNA damage | [103] |
| | | HGPS mice | Reduces progerin levels | |
| JH4 | Interruption of progerin-lamin A/C binding | Patient's fibroblasts | Prevents senescence<br>Alleviates heterochromatin loss | [121] |
| | | HGPS mice | Body mass gain<br>Increases horizontal force<br>Increases organ size<br>Alleviates nuclear morphology<br>Extents lifespan | |
| LMB | CRM1 (Exportin-1) inhibitor | Patient's fibroblasts | Alleviates nuclear morphology<br>Alleviates nucleolar abnormalities<br>Alleviates heterochromatin loss<br>Prevents senescence | [17] |
| Rapamycin | mTOR inhibitor | Patient's fibroblasts | Reduces DNA damage<br>Reduces progerin levels<br>Alleviates heterochromatin loss | [122] |

## Correction of the HGPS Mutation by Genome Editing

The most direct and theoretically possible therapy is to permanently correct the genomic DNA of the lamin A locus by homologous recombination, utilizing the CRISPR/CAS system (Fig. 10.2) [95]. However, application of this technology currently is unfeasible because of the low efficiency of such procedures, even in tissue-cultured cells. Furthermore, scientists should be cautious before propelling this tool into the clinical area, because of potential issues, including off-target effects and ethical concerns.

### Splicing Modulation

Exon skipping technology using antisense oligonucleotides (ASO) to modify pathological mRNA splicing events has been successfully employed for treating Duchenne muscular dystrophy [96]. Owing to the aberrant LMNA splicing event, which is the HGPS molecular basis, this approach appears feasible to avoid progerin expression by shifting the output of lamin A toward lamin C (Fig. 10.2). Supporting this idea, the use of an antisense oligonucleotide target at exon 11 of the LMNA gene was effective to decrease progerin levels in fibroblasts of patients with HGPS and in the HGPS mouse model; consequently, this treatment reduced the frequency of nuclear shape abnormalities [97, 98]. Although this splicing modulation strategy could be useful to treat HGPS, administration of ASO to humans requires the overcoming of some obstacles, including the use of harmless and effective ASO and a precise method of delivery to target tissue.

### Progerin Clearance

Enhancing of progerin degradation through the autophagic–lysosomal pathway is a recently proposed strategy to treat HGPS. It has been shown that treatment of patient-derived fibroblasts with Rapamycin, an immunosuppressive agent used in organ transplantation, accelerates progerin turnover, which in turn results in improvement of both nuclear morphology and chromatin organization, as well as in delayed cellular senescence (Fig. 10.2 and Table 10.2) [99, 100]. At organismal level, administration of Rapamycin to lamin A/C-deficient mice recovers cardiac and skeletal muscle function and extends lifespan [101, 102]. Because Rapamycin is a potent inhibitor of mTOR (mammalian target of Rapamycin), a signaling pathway involved in multiple cellular processes (cytoskeleton remodeling, translation, cell growth, and autophagy itself), its use in patients may have nontrivial adverse effects. Despite this, a clinical trial (NCT02579044) using a Rapamycin-derivative agent (Everolimusan) in combination with Ionafarnib is currently being conducted in subjects with progeria. Alternatively, treatment with proteasome inhibitor MG132 promotes progerin clearance by autophagy in primary fibroblasts and iPSC stem cells derived from patients with HGPS (Fig. 10.2) [103]. The therapeutic effects of MG132 include enhanced cell viability and proliferation and decreased cellular senescence (Table 10.2). The efficacy of MG132 in reducing progerin levels was replicated in skeletal muscle from an HGPS mouse model (Table 10.2) [87]. It is expected that chronic treatment with MG132 will exert a generalized effect on protein turnover, which might limit its use in clinical studies.

### Blocking of Progerin Farnesylation

The first therapy to be addressed was the administration of farnesyltransferase inhibitors (FTI), with the presumption that progerin toxicity is mainly provided by the farnesyl moiety. FTI reversibly bind to the farnesyltransferase CAAX binding site in progerin [104]. Hence, blocking of progerin farnesylation would prevent progerin-mediated damage in HGPS-associated cellular processes (Fig. 10.2). In human HGPS fibroblasts, this therapy improved nuclear and nucleolar morphology but failed to alleviate cellular senescence, DNA damage, or mitochondrial function (Table 10.2) [105], while in a HGPS mouse model, defects in bone mineralization and cardiac tissue vascularization were alleviated and lifespan was extended (Table 10.2), as reviewed in [106]. A clinical trial to administer an FTI (lonafarnib) to a cohort of 25 patients was conducted in 2007 (NCT00425607). After 2 years of treatment, only some patients showed improvement in body weight, bone mineral density, and/or cardiac vasculature; unfortunately, the lifespan of the patients was extended by only 1.6 years (Table 10.2) [4]. It was recently shown that progerin becomes alternatively prenylated when FTI action is blocked. This could explain the limited efficiency of FTI in progeroid mouse models and in patients with HGPS. To solve this problem, combinatory therapy using Zoledronate (N-bisphosphonate) and Pravastatin (statin), to block both protein farnesylation and geranylgeranylation, has been tested. This treatment rescues the HGPS phenotype in human HGPS fibroblasts, while in the progeroid mouse Zmpste24$^{-/-}$, various physiological traits were improved, including growth, weight, and longevity (Table 10.2), as reviewed in [106]. A clinical trial treating 12 patients with HGPS with a combination of Zoledronate and a statin (ClinicalTrials.gov, NCT00731016) was initiated in 2013. Nevertheless, it is noteworthy that long-term outcomes of this therapy are unknown; researchers must be cautious because inhibition of protein prenylation affects numerous CaaX motif-contained proteins, including type B lamins and all the membrane-bound small GTPases (e.g., Ras).

#### Alleviation of Progerin-Induced Pathogenic Mechanisms

Progerin exerts downstream toxic effects on a plethora of cellular processes, including nuclear and nucleolar structure, mitochondrial function, heterochromatin organization, protein nuclear trafficking, and cellular senescence. Thus, some alternative treatments aimed at ameliorating the ulterior negative impact of progerin have been proposed.

#### Normalization of Nuclear Trafficking of Proteins

Owing to the harmful effect exerted by progerin on nuclear envelope structure/function, it is expected that nucleocytoplasmic transport of proteins through the nuclear pore complex (NPC), a highly regulated process related to proteostasis and cellular signaling [107], could be disturbed by progerin, thereby altering nucleocytoplasmic partitioning of critical proteins (transcription factors, enzymes, and structural proteins) (Fig. 10.2). Thus, it is plausible to speculate that altered nuclear trafficking of proteins might be part of the molecular basis underlying HGPS. Supporting this hypothesis, perturbation of the Ran GTPase gradient affecting nuclear import of some proteins with high molecular weights (Ubc9, and nucleoporin TPR) was previously reported in human HGPS fibroblasts [15, 108]. Furthermore, the nonclassical transport pathway mediated by Transportin-1 (TNPO1) is impaired in human HGPS fibroblasts, due to cytoplasmic sequestration of TNPO1 by the microtubule network [16]. Interestingly, treatment of human HGPS fibroblasts with remodelin (acetyltransferase NAT10 inhibitor) releases TNPO1 from the cytoplasm of HGPS cells, restoring the TNPO1-dependent nuclear import pathway, which in turn improves chromatin organization and prevents premature senescence of these cells in a progerin-independent fashion (Table 10.2) [16].

Based on the previous results, our laboratory was prompted to analyze whether nuclear protein export is impaired in HGPS as well. Exportin-1 (XPO1), also known as chromosomal region maintenance 1 (CRM1), is the major transport receptor that exports proteins across the nuclear membrane to the cytoplasm, via recognition of the hydrophobic-rich nuclear export signal(s) (NES) present in the cargo molecules [109]. We show, to our knowledge for the first time, that the CRM1-driven nuclear protein export mechanism is abnormally enhanced in HGPS fibroblasts, due to the overexpression of CRM1 [17]. We provide evidence that CRM1 is a primary target of progerin and that dysregulation of the nuclear protein export system is critically involved in the disease, because pharmacological inhibition of CRM1 using Leptomycin B alleviates virtually all the HGPS hallmarks analyzed, including aberrant nuclear morphology, nucleolar expansion, cellular senescence, loss of peripheral heterochromatin, and lamin B1 downregulation (Table 10.2). Furthermore, ectopic overexpression of CRM1 enabled normal fibroblasts to acquire HGPS hallmarks, namely, cellular senescence, depleted lamin B1 levels, and the loss of peripheral chromatin [17]. Thus, pharmacological modulation of CRM1 clearly provides a viable and promising therapy against HGPS, and in vivo evaluation of this therapy in HGPS animal models comprises the next logical step.

### Neutralization of Progerin Aberrant Interactions

Another alternative strategy to fight HGPS is the use of compounds that bind specifically to progerin, impeding its aberrant interaction with nuclear regulatory proteins, thereby correcting the altered processes of HGPS cells. Following this notion, a chemical (JH4) with the ability to block the harmful interaction between progerin and lamin A was recently identified [97] (Fig. 10.2). Remarkably, treatment of human HGPS fibroblasts with JH4 ameliorated nuclear morphology defects and prevented both premature senescence and growth arrest (Table 10.2) Moreover, administration of JH4 to Lmna$^{G609G/G609G}$ mice resulted in the alleviation of various physical and physiological traits altered in this mouse, including body mass, organ size, and lifespan extension (Table 10.2).

### Correction of Mitochondrial Dysfunction

Mitochondria are involved in energy production and cellular metabolism, and dysfunction of this key organelle results in increased levels of reactive oxygen species (ROS), DNA, and protein damage, and consequently in cellular aging [110]. Accordingly, increased ROS and mitochondrial dysfunction have been observed in HGPS fibroblasts and in LMNA$^{G609G/+}$ mice; while HGPS fibroblasts exhibit swollen and fragmented mitochondria with altered mobility [111], murine cells showed diminished ATP synthesis [85]. Interestingly, treatment of HGPS fibroblasts with the antioxidant compound methylene blue rescued not only mitochondrial morphology and function but also nuclear morphology and the loss of heterochromatin (Table 10.2)

[111]. Likewise, administration of ROCK inhibitor Y-27632 decreases ROS levels and improves mitochondrial function, together with amelioration of nuclear morphology defects [112]. Furthermore, restoration of NRF2 transcriptional activity in HGPS cells prevents both oxidative stress and increased ROS levels [113].

## Conclusions

Recent advances in the study of progeroid syndromes, especially HGPS, have provided novel insights into our understanding of the aging process in humans. The main progeroid syndromes revised in this chapter are caused by mutations in genes encoding for DNA repair enzymes or the nuclear lamina protein lamin A, which reinforces the notion that genome instability is a critical determinant of aging. The study models that recapitulate progeroid syndromes have dramatically stimulated aging research; while cellular models have allowed the dissection of basic cellular and molecular processes linked to aging, mice models have facilitated screening of therapeutic drugs. It is expected that upcoming technologies and the design of novel optimized animal models will help to accomplish a translational medicine approach in aging research, with HGPS being the ideal model for such a goal.

**Funding** Bilateral Agreement CNR (Italy)/CINVESTAV (Mexico), Grant/Award Number: CNR2018/4. Geriatric National Institute, Mexico, Grant/Award Number: INGER-DICRECITES-008-2018.

## References

1. Lopez-Otin C, Blasco MA, Partridge L, Serrano M, Kroemer G. The hallmarks of aging. Cell. 2013;153(6):1194–217.
2. Kennedy BK, Berger SL, Brunet A, Campisi J, Cuervo AM, Epel ES, et al. Geroscience: linking aging to chronic disease. Cell. 2014;159(4):709–13.
3. Valenzano DR, Aboobaker A, Seluanov A, Gorbunova V. Non-canonical aging model systems and why we need them. EMBO J. 2017;36(8):959–63.
4. Gordon LB, Rothman FG, Lopez-Otin C, Misteli T. Progeria: a paradigm for translational medicine. Cell. 2014;156(3):400–7.
5. Carrero D, Soria-Valles C, Lopez-Otin C. Hallmarks of progeroid syndromes: lessons from mice and reprogrammed cells. Dis Model Mech. 2016;9(7):719–35.
6. Hetzer MW. The nuclear envelope. Cold Spring Harb Perspect Biol. 2010;2(3):a000539.
7. Dechat T, Pfleghaar K, Sengupta K, Shimi T, Shumaker DK, Solimando L, et al. Nuclear lamins: major factors in the structural organization and function of the nucleus and chromatin. Genes Dev. 2008;22(7):832–53.
8. Schreiber KH, Kennedy BK. When lamins go bad: nuclear structure and disease. Cell. 2013;152(6):1365–75.
9. Prokocimer M, Davidovich M, Nissim-Rafinia M, Wiesel-Motiuk N, Bar DZ, Barkan R, et al. Nuclear lamins: key regulators of nuclear structure and activities. J Cell Mol Med. 2009;13(6):1059–85.
10. Dorado B, Andres V. A-type lamins and cardiovascular disease in premature aging syndromes. Curr Opin Cell Biol. 2017;46:17–25.

11. Eriksson M, Brown WT, Gordon LB, Glynn MW, Singer J, Scott L, et al. Recurrent de novo point mutations in lamin A cause Hutchinson-Gilford progeria syndrome. Nature. 2003;423(6937):293–8.
12. De Sandre-Giovannoli A, Bernard R, Cau P, Navarro C, Amiel J, Boccaccio I, et al. Lamin a truncation in Hutchinson-Gilford progeria. Science (New York, NY). 2055;300(5628):2003.
13. Ahmed MS, Ikram S, Bibi N, Mir A. Hutchinson-Gilford Progeria syndrome: a premature aging disease. Mol Neurobiol. 2018;55(5):4417–27.
14. Kubben N, Voncken JW, Demmers J, Calis C, van Almen G, Pinto Y, et al. Identification of differential protein interactors of lamin A and progerin. Nucleus (Austin, Tex). 2010;1(6):513–25.
15. Snow CJ, Dar A, Dutta A, Kehlenbach RH, Paschal BM. Defective nuclear import of Tpr in Progeria reflects the Ran sensitivity of large cargo transport. J Cell Biol. 2013;201(4):541–57.
16. Larrieu D, Vire E, Robson S, Breusegem SY, Kouzarides T, Jackson SP. Inhibition of the acetyltransferase NAT10 normalizes progeric and aging cells by rebalancing the Transportin-1 nuclear import pathway. Sci Signal. 2018;11(537):eaar5401.
17. Garcia-Aguirre I, Alamillo-Iniesta A, Rodriguez-Perez R, Velez-Aguilera G, Amaro-Encarnacion E, Jimenez-Gutierrez E, et al. Enhanced nuclear protein export in premature aging and rescue of the progeria phenotype by modulation of CRM1 activity. Aging Cell. 2019;18:e13002.
18. Tariq Z, Zhang H, Chia-Liu A, Shen Y, Gete Y, Xiong ZM, et al. Lamin A and microtubules collaborate to maintain nuclear morphology. Nucleus (Austin, Tex). 2017;8(4):433–46.
19. Novelli G, Muchir A, Sangiuolo F, Helbling-Leclerc A, D'Apice MR, Massart C, et al. Mandibuloacral dysplasia is caused by a mutation in LMNA-encoding lamin A/C. Am J Hum Genet. 2002;71(2):426–31.
20. Cenni V, D'Apice MR, Garagnani P, Columbaro M, Novelli G, Franceschi C, et al. Mandibuloacral dysplasia: A premature ageing disease with aspects of physiological ageing. Ageing Res Rev. 2018;42:1–13.
21. Bai S, Lozada A, Jones MC, Dietz HC, Dempsey M, Das S. Mandibuloacral dysplasia caused by LMNA mutations and uniparental disomy. Case reports in genetics. 2014;2014:508231.
22. Navarro CL, Cadinanos J, De Sandre-Giovannoli A, Bernard R, Courrier S, Boccaccio I, et al. Loss of ZMPSTE24 (FACE-1) causes autosomal recessive restrictive dermopathy and accumulation of Lamin A precursors. Hum Mol Genet. 2005;14(11):1503–13.
23. Capanni C, Mattioli E, Columbaro M, Lucarelli E, Parnaik VK, Novelli G, et al. Altered pre-lamin A processing is a common mechanism leading to lipodystrophy. Hum Mol Genet. 2005;14(11):1489–502.
24. Thill M, Nguyen TD, Wehnert M, Fischer D, Hausser I, Braun S, et al. Restrictive dermopathy: a rare laminopathy. Arch Gynecol Obstet. 2008;278(3):201–8.
25. Cabanillas R, Cadinanos J, Villameytide JA, Perez M, Longo J, Richard JM, et al. Nestor-Guillermo progeria syndrome: a novel premature aging condition with early onset and chronic development caused by BANF1 mutations. Am J Med Genet A. 2011;155a(11):2617–25.
26. Hutchison CJ. Lamins: building blocks or regulators of gene expression? Nat Rev Mol Cell Biol. 2002;3(11):848–58.
27. Mekhail K, Moazed D. The nuclear envelope in genome organization, expression and stability. Nat Rev Mol Cell Biol. 2010;11(5):317–28.
28. Loi M, Cenni V, Duchi S, Squarzoni S, Lopez-Otin C, Foisner R, et al. Barrier-to-autointegration factor (BAF) involvement in prelamin A-related chromatin organization changes. Oncotarget. 2016;7(13):15662–77.
29. Paquet N, Box JK, Ashton NW, Suraweera A, Croft LV, Urquhart AJ, et al. Nestor-Guillermo Progeria Syndrome: a biochemical insight into Barrier-to-Autointegration Factor 1, alanine 12 threonine mutation. BMC Mol Biol. 2014;15:27.
30. Guo H, Luo N, Hao F, Bai Y. p.Pro4Arg mutation in LMNA gene: a new atypical progeria phenotype without metabolism abnormalities. Gene. 2014;546(1):35–9.
31. Al-Haggar M, Madej-Pilarczyk A, Kozlowski L, Bujnicki JM, Yahia S, Abdel-Hadi D, et al. A novel homozygous p.Arg527Leu LMNA mutation in two unrelated Egyptian families

causes overlapping mandibuloacral dysplasia and progeria syndrome. Eur J Human Genet. 2012;20(11):1134–40.
32. Liang L, Zhang H, Gu X. Homozygous LMNA mutation R527C in atypical Hutchinson-Gilford progeria syndrome: evidence for autosomal recessive inheritance. Acta Paediatr (Oslo, Norway: 1992). 2009;98(8):1365–8.
33. Zirn B, Kress W, Grimm T, Berthold LD, Neubauer B, Kuchelmeister K, et al. Association of homozygous LMNA mutation R471C with new phenotype: mandibuloacral dysplasia, progeria, and rigid spine muscular dystrophy. Am J Med Genet A. 2008;146a(8):1049–54.
34. Lombardi F, Gullotta F, Columbaro M, Filareto A, D'Adamo M, Vielle A, et al. Compound heterozygosity for mutations in LMNA in a patient with a myopathic and lipodystrophic mandibuloacral dysplasia type A phenotype. J Clin Endocrinol Metab. 2007;92(11):4467–71.
35. Dittmer TA, Sahni N, Kubben N, Hill DE, Vidal M, Burgess RC, et al. Systematic identification of pathological lamin A interactors. Mol Biol Cell. 2014;25(9):1493–510.
36. Chu WK, Hickson ID. RecQ helicases: multifunctional genome caretakers. Nat Rev Cancer. 2009;9(9):644–54.
37. de Renty C, Ellis NA. Bloom's syndrome: why not premature aging?: a comparison of the BLM and WRN helicases. Ageing Res Rev. 2017;33:36–51.
38. Huang S, Lee L, Hanson NB, Lenaerts C, Hoehn H, Poot M, et al. The spectrum of WRN mutations in Werner syndrome patients. Hum Mutat. 2006;27(6):558–67.
39. Takemoto M, Mori S, Kuzuya M, Yoshimoto S, Shimamoto A, Igarashi M, et al. Diagnostic criteria for Werner syndrome based on Japanese nationwide epidemiological survey. Geriatr Gerontol Int. 2013;13(2):475–81.
40. Oshima J, Sidorova JM, Monnat RJ Jr. Werner syndrome: clinical features, pathogenesis and potential therapeutic interventions. Ageing Res Rev. 2017;33:105–14.
41. Yu CE, Oshima J, Fu YH, Wijsman EM, Hisama F, Alisch R, et al. Positional cloning of the Werner's syndrome gene. Science (New York, NY). 1996;272(5259):258–62.
42. Bernstein KA, Gangloff S, Rothstein R. The RecQ DNA helicases in DNA repair. Annu Rev Genet. 2010;44:393–417.
43. Oshima J, Martin GM, Hisama FM. Werner syndrome. In: Adam MP, Ardinger HH, Pagon RA, Wallace SE, Bean LJH, Stephens K, et al., editors. GeneReviews((R)). Seattle: University of Washington, Seattle University of Washington; 1993. GeneReviews is a registered trademark of the University of Washington, Seattle. All rights reserved.
44. Melcher R, von Golitschek R, Steinlein C, Schindler D, Neitzel H, Kainer K, et al. Spectral karyotyping of Werner syndrome fibroblast cultures. Cytogenet Cell Genet. 2000;91(1-4):180–5.
45. Brosh RM Jr, Opresko PL, Bohr VA. Enzymatic mechanism of the WRN helicase/nuclease. Methods Enzymol. 2006;409:52–85.
46. Cunniff C, Bassetti JA, Ellis NA. Bloom's syndrome: clinical spectrum, molecular pathogenesis, and cancer predisposition. Mol Syndromol. 2017;8(1):4–23.
47. Hickson ID, Mankouri HW. Processing of homologous recombination repair intermediates by the Sgs1-Top3-Rmi1 and Mus81-Mms4 complexes. Cell Cycle (Georgetown, Tex). 2011;10(18):3078–85.
48. Tikoo S, Sengupta S. Time to bloom. Genome Integrity. 2010;1(1):14.
49. Wang LL, Plon SE. Rothmund-Thomson syndrome. In: Adam MP, Ardinger HH, Pagon RA, Wallace SE, LJH B, Stephens K, et al., editors. GeneReviews((R)). Seattle: University of Washington; 1993. GeneReviews is a registered trademark of the University of Washington, Seattle. All rights reserved.
50. Wang LL, Gannavarapu A, Kozinetz CA, Levy ML, Lewis RA, Chintagumpala MM, et al. Association between osteosarcoma and deleterious mutations in the RECQL4 gene in Rothmund-Thomson syndrome. J Natl Cancer Inst. 2003;95(9):669–74.
51. Wang LL, Worley K, Gannavarapu A, Chintagumpala MM, Levy ML, Plon SE. Intron-size constraint as a mutational mechanism in Rothmund-Thomson syndrome. Am J Hum Genet. 2002;71(1):165–7.

52. Larizza L, Roversi G, Volpi L. Rothmund-Thomson syndrome. Orphanet J Rare Dis. 2010;5:2.
53. Gupta S, De S, Srivastava V, Hussain M, Kumari J, Muniyappa K, et al. RECQL4 and p53 potentiate the activity of polymerase gamma and maintain the integrity of the human mitochondrial genome. Carcinogenesis. 2014;35(1):34–45.
54. Croteau DL, Singh DK, Hoh Ferrarelli L, Lu H, Bohr VA. RECQL4 in genomic instability and aging. Trends Genet. 2012;28(12):624–31.
55. Lu L, Jin W, Wang LL. Aging in Rothmund-Thomson syndrome and related RECQL4 genetic disorders. Ageing Res Rev. 2017;33:30–5.
56. Mann MB, Hodges CA, Barnes E, Vogel H, Hassold TJ, Luo G. Defective sister-chromatid cohesion, aneuploidy and cancer predisposition in a mouse model of type II Rothmund-Thomson syndrome. Hum Mol Genet. 2005;14(6):813–25.
57. Karikkineth AC, Scheibye-Knudsen M, Fivenson E, Croteau DL, Bohr VA. Cockayne syndrome: clinical features, model systems and pathways. Ageing Res Rev. 2017;33:3–17.
58. Scheibye-Knudsen M, Croteau DL, Bohr VA. Mitochondrial deficiency in Cockayne syndrome. Mech Ageing Dev. 2013;134(5-6):275–83.
59. Tan WH, Baris H, Robson CD, Kimonis VE. Cockayne syndrome: the developing phenotype. Am J Med Genet A. 2005;135(2):214–6.
60. Cleaver JE. Cancer in xeroderma pigmentosum and related disorders of DNA repair. Nat Rev Cancer. 2005;5(7):564–73.
61. Velez-Cruz R, Zadorin AS, Coin F, Egly JM. Sirt1 suppresses RNA synthesis after UV irradiation in combined xeroderma pigmentosum group D/Cockayne syndrome (XP-D/CS) cells. Proc Natl Acad Sci U S A. 2013;110(3):E212–20.
62. Hebra F. On diseases of the skin, including the exanthemata. London: The New Sydenham Society; 1868. p. 399.
63. Black JO. Xeroderma Pigmentosum. Head Neck Pathol. 2016;10(2):139–44.
64. de Boer J, Hoeijmakers JH. Nucleotide excision repair and human syndromes. Carcinogenesis. 2000;21(3):453–60.
65. Lambert WC, Gagna CE, Lambert MW. Trichothiodystrophy: photosensitive, TTD-P, TTD, Tay syndrome. Adv Exp Med Biol. 2010;685:106–10.
66. Ahmed A, Almohanna H, Griggs J, Tosti A. Genetic hair disorders: a review. Dermatol Ther (Heidelb). 2019;9(3):421–48.
67. Mitchell SJ, Scheibye-Knudsen M, Longo DL, de Cabo R. Animal models of aging research: implications for human aging and age-related diseases. Ann Rev Anim Biosci. 2015;3:283–303.
68. Tigges J, Krutmann J, Fritsche E, Haendeler J, Schaal H, Fischer JW, et al. The hallmarks of fibroblast ageing. Mech Ageing Dev. 2014;138:26–44.
69. Goldman RD, Shumaker DK, Erdos MR, Eriksson M, Goldman AE, Gordon LB, et al. Accumulation of mutant lamin A causes progressive changes in nuclear architecture in Hutchinson-Gilford progeria syndrome. Proc Natl Acad Sci U S A. 2004;101(24):8963–8.
70. Liu Y, Rusinol A, Sinensky M, Wang Y, Zou Y. DNA damage responses in progeroid syndromes arise from defective maturation of prelamin A. J Cell Sci. 2006;119(Pt 22):4644–9.
71. Scaffidi P, Misteli T. Lamin A-dependent nuclear defects in human aging. Science (New York, NY). 2006;312(5776):1059–63.
72. Liu GH, Barkho BZ, Ruiz S, Diep D, Qu J, Yang SL, et al. Recapitulation of premature ageing with iPSCs from Hutchinson-Gilford progeria syndrome. Nature. 2011;472(7342):221–5.
73. Bergo MO, Gavino B, Ross J, Schmidt WK, Hong C, Kendall LV, et al. Zmpste24 deficiency in mice causes spontaneous bone fractures, muscle weakness, and a prelamin A processing defect. Proc Natl Acad Sci USA. 2002;99(20):13049–54.
74. Pendas AM, Zhou Z, Cadinanos J, Freije JM, Wang J, Hultenby K, et al. Defective prelamin A processing and muscular and adipocyte alterations in Zmpste24 metalloproteinase-deficient mice. Nat Genet. 2002;31(1):94–9.
75. Capell BC, Collins FS. Human laminopathies: nuclei gone genetically awry. Nat Rev Genet. 2006;7(12):940–52.

76. Liu B, Wang J, Chan KM, Tjia WM, Deng W, Guan X, et al. Genomic instability in laminopathy-based premature aging. Nat Med. 2005;11(7):780–5.
77. Yang SH, Bergo MO, Toth JI, Qiao X, Hu Y, Sandoval S, et al. Blocking protein farnesyltransferase improves nuclear blebbing in mouse fibroblasts with a targeted Hutchinson-Gilford progeria syndrome mutation. Proc Natl Acad Sci U S A. 2005;102(29):10291–6.
78. Varga R, Eriksson M, Erdos MR, Olive M, Harten I, Kolodgie F, et al. Progressive vascular smooth muscle cell defects in a mouse model of Hutchinson-Gilford progeria syndrome. Proc Natl Acad Sci U S A. 2006;103(9):3250–5.
79. Hernandez L, Roux KJ, Wong ES, Mounkes LC, Mutalif R, Navasankari R, et al. Functional coupling between the extracellular matrix and nuclear lamina by Wnt signaling in progeria. Dev Cell. 2010;19(3):413–25.
80. Yang SH, Meta M, Qiao X, Frost D, Bauch J, Coffinier C, et al. A farnesyltransferase inhibitor improves disease phenotypes in mice with a Hutchinson-Gilford progeria syndrome mutation. J Clin Invest. 2006;116(8):2115–21.
81. Mounkes LC, Kozlov S, Hernandez L, Sullivan T, Stewart CL. A progeroid syndrome in mice is caused by defects in A-type lamins. Nature. 2003;423(6937):298–301.
82. Osorio FG, Barcena C, Soria-Valles C, Ramsay AJ, de Carlos F, Cobo J, et al. Nuclear lamina defects cause ATM-dependent NF-kappaB activation and link accelerated aging to a systemic inflammatory response. Genes Dev. 2012;26(20):2311–24.
83. Zhang H, Kieckhaefer JE, Cao K. Mouse models of laminopathies. Aging Cell. 2013;12(1):2–10.
84. Osorio FG, Navarro CL, Cadiñanos J, López-Mejía IC, Quirós PM, Bartoli C, et al. Splicing-directed therapy in a new mouse model of human accelerated aging. Sci Transl Med. 2011;3(106):106ra7.
85. Villa-Bellosta R, Rivera-Torres J, Osorio FG, Acin-Perez R, Enriquez JA, Lopez-Otin C, et al. Defective extracellular pyrophosphate metabolism promotes vascular calcification in a mouse model of Hutchinson-Gilford progeria syndrome that is ameliorated on pyrophosphate treatment. Circulation. 2013;127(24):2442–51.
86. Lebel M, Leder P. A deletion within the murine Werner syndrome helicase induces sensitivity to inhibitors of topoisomerase and loss of cellular proliferative capacity. Proc Natl Acad Sci U S A. 1998;95(22):13097–102.
87. Massip L, Garand C, Turaga RV, Deschênes F, Thorin E, Lebel M. Increased insulin, triglycerides, reactive oxygen species, and cardiac fibrosis in mice with a mutation in the helicase domain of the Werner syndrome gene homologue. Exp Gerontol. 2006;41(2):157–68.
88. Chang S, Multani AS, Cabrera NG, Naylor ML, Laud P, Lombard D, et al. Essential role of limiting telomeres in the pathogenesis of Werner syndrome. Nat Genet. 2004;36(8):877–82.
89. van der Pluijm I, Garinis GA, Brandt RM, Gorgels TG, Wijnhoven SW, Diderich KE, et al. Impaired genome maintenance suppresses the growth hormone--insulin-like growth factor 1 axis in mice with Cockayne syndrome. PLoS Biol. 2007;5(1):e2.
90. Gorgels TG, van der Pluijm I, Brandt RM, Garinis GA, van Steeg H, van den Aardweg G, et al. Retinal degeneration and ionizing radiation hypersensitivity in a mouse model for Cockayne syndrome. Mol Cell Biol. 2007;27(4):1433–41.
91. Jaarsma D, van der Pluijm I, de Waard MC, Haasdijk ED, Brandt R, Vermeij M, et al. Age-related neuronal degeneration: complementary roles of nucleotide excision repair and transcription-coupled repair in preventing neuropathology. PLoS Genet. 2011;7(12):e1002405.
92. van der Horst GT, Meira L, Gorgels TG, de Wit J, Velasco-Miguel S, Richardson JA, et al. UVB radiation-induced cancer predisposition in Cockayne syndrome group A (Csa) mutant mice. DNA Repair (Amst). 2002;1(2):143–57.
93. van der Horst GT, van Steeg H, Berg RJ, van Gool AJ, de Wit J, Weeda G, et al. Defective transcription-coupled repair in Cockayne syndrome B mice is associated with skin cancer predisposition. Cell. 1997;89(3):425–35.
94. Chester N, Babbe H, Pinkas J, Manning C, Leder P. Mutation of the murine Bloom's syndrome gene produces global genome destabilization. Mol Cell Biol. 2006;26(17):6713–26.

95. Pickar-Oliver A, Gersbach CA. The next generation of CRISPR-Cas technologies and applications. Nat Rev Mol Cell Biol. 2019;20(8):490–507.
96. Crunkhorn S. Muscular dystrophy: new exon-skipping strategy rescues dystrophin. Nat Rev Drug Discov. 2015;14(4):236.
97. Lee JM, Nobumori C, Tu Y, Choi C, Yang SH, Jung HJ, et al. Modulation of LMNA splicing as a strategy to treat prelamin A diseases. J Clin Invest. 2016;126(4):1592–602.
98. McNally EM, Wyatt EJ. Welcome to the splice age: antisense oligonucleotide-mediated exon skipping gains wider applicability. J Clin Invest. 2016;126(4):1236–8.
99. Cao K, Blair CD, Faddah DA, Kieckhaefer JE, Olive M, Erdos MR, et al. Progerin and telomere dysfunction collaborate to trigger cellular senescence in normal human fibroblasts. J Clin Invest. 2011;121(7):2833–44.
100. Graziotto JJ, Cao K, Collins FS, Krainc D. Rapamycin activates autophagy in Hutchinson-Gilford progeria syndrome: implications for normal aging and age-dependent neurodegenerative disorders. Autophagy. 2012;8(1):147–51.
101. Ramos FJ, Chen SC, Garelick MG, Dai DF, Liao CY, Schreiber KH, et al. Rapamycin reverses elevated mTORC1 signaling in lamin A/C-deficient mice, rescues cardiac and skeletal muscle function, and extends survival. Sci Transl Med. 2012;4(144):144ra03.
102. Liao CY, Anderson SS, Chicoine NH, Mayfield JR, Academia EC, Wilson JA, et al. Rapamycin reverses metabolic deficits in lamin A/C-deficient mice. Cell Rep. 2016;17(10):2542–52.
103. Harhouri K, Navarro C, Depetris D, Mattei MG, Nissan X, Cau P, et al. MG132-induced progerin clearance is mediated by autophagy activation and splicing regulation. EMBO Mol Med. 2017;9(9):1294–313.
104. Basso AD, Kirschmeier P, Bishop WR. Lipid posttranslational modifications. Farnesyl transferase inhibitors. J Lipid Res. 2006;47(1):15–31.
105. Toth JI, Yang SH, Qiao X, Beigneux AP, Gelb MH, Moulson CL, et al. Blocking protein farnesyltransferase improves nuclear shape in fibroblasts from humans with progeroid syndromes. Proc Natl Acad Sci U S A. 2005;102(36):12873–8.
106. Harhouri K, Frankel D, Bartoli C, Roll P, De Sandre-Giovannoli A, Levy N. An overview of treatment strategies for Hutchinson-Gilford Progeria syndrome. Nucleus (Austin, Tex). 2018;9(1):246–57.
107. Christie M, Chang CW, Rona G, Smith KM, Stewart AG, Takeda AA, et al. Structural biology and regulation of protein import into the nucleus. J Mol Biol. 2016;428(10 Pt A):2060–90.
108. Cobb AM, Larrieu D, Warren DT, Liu Y, Srivastava S, Smith AJ, et al. Prelamin A impairs 53BP1 nuclear entry by mislocalizing NUP153 and disrupting the Ran gradient. Aging Cell. 2016;15(6):1039–50.
109. Ishizawa J, Kojima K, Hail N Jr, Tabe Y, Andreeff M. Expression, function, and targeting of the nuclear exporter chromosome region maintenance 1 (CRM1) protein. Pharmacol Ther. 2015;153:25–35.
110. Kirkinezos IG, Moraes CT. Reactive oxygen species and mitochondrial diseases. Semin Cell Dev Biol. 2001;12(6):449–57.
111. Xiong ZM, Choi JY, Wang K, Zhang H, Tariq Z, Wu D, et al. Methylene blue alleviates nuclear and mitochondrial abnormalities in progeria. Aging Cell. 2016;15(2):279–90.
112. Wang T, Kang W, Du L, Ge S. Rho-kinase inhibitor Y-27632 facilitates the proliferation, migration and pluripotency of human periodontal ligament stem cells. J Cell Mol Med. 2017;21(11):3100–12.
113. Kubben N, Zhang W, Wang L, Voss TC, Yang J, Qu J, et al. Repression of the antioxidant NRF2 pathway in premature aging. Cell. 2016;165(6):1361–74.
114. Gordon LB, Kleinman ME, Miller DT, Neuberg DS, Giobbie-Hurder A, Gerhard-Herman M, et al. Clinical trial of a farnesyltransferase inhibitor in children with Hutchinson-Gilford progeria syndrome. Proc Natl Acad Sci U S A. 2012;109(41):16666–71.
115. Capell BC, Erdos MR, Madigan JP, Fiordalisi JJ, Varga R, Conneely KN, et al. Inhibiting farnesylation of progerin prevents the characteristic nuclear blebbing of Hutchinson-Gilford progeria syndrome. Proc Natl Acad Sci U S A. 2005;102(36):12879–84.

116. Mehta IS, Bridger JM, Kill IR. Progeria, the nucleolus and farnesyltransferase inhibitors. Biochem Soc Trans. 2010;38(Pt 1):287–91.
117. Yang SH, Qiao X, Fong LG, Young SG. Treatment with a farnesyltransferase inhibitor improves survival in mice with a Hutchinson-Gilford progeria syndrome mutation. Biochim Biophys Acta. 2008;1781(1-2):36–9.
118. Larrieu D, Britton S, Demir M, Rodriguez R, Jackson SP. Chemical inhibition of NAT10 corrects defects of laminopathic cells. Science. 2014;344(6183):527–32.
119. Larrieu D, Viré E, Robson S, Breusegem SY, Kouzarides T, Jackson SP. Inhibition of the acetyltransferase NAT10 normalizes progeric and aging cells by rebalancing the Transportin-1 nuclear import pathway. Sci Signal. 2018;11(537):eaar5401.
120. Balmus G, Larrieu D, Barros AC, Collins C, Abrudan M, Demir M, et al. Targeting of NAT10 enhances healthspan in a mouse model of human accelerated aging syndrome. Nat Commun. 2018;9(1):1700.
121. Lee SJ, Jung YS, Yoon MH, Kang SM, Oh AY, Lee JH, et al. Interruption of progerin-lamin A/C binding ameliorates Hutchinson-Gilford progeria syndrome phenotype. J Clin Invest. 2016;126(10):3879–93.
122. Cao K, Graziotto JJ, Blair CD, Mazzulli JR, Erdos MR, Krainc D, et al. Rapamycin reverses cellular phenotypes and enhances mutant protein clearance in Hutchinson-Gilford progeria syndrome cells. Sci Transl Med. 2011;3(89):89ra58.

# Applications of CRISPR-Cas in Ageing Research

11

Scott Haston, Sara Pozzi, and Jose Mario Gonzalez-Meljem

## Abbreviations

| | |
|---|---|
| AAV | Adeno-associated virus |
| AD | Alzheimer's disease |
| Cas9 | CRISPR-associated protein 9 |
| CRISPR | Clustered regularly interspaced short palindromic repeat |
| CRISPRi | CRISPR interference |
| dCas9 | Nuclease-deficient Cas9 |
| DSB | Double-strand break |
| ES | Embryonic stem |
| gRNA | Guide RNA |
| HDR | Homology-directed repair |
| HGPS | Hutchinson-Gilford progeria syndrome |
| iPSC | Induced pluripotent stem cell |
| *Lmna* | Lamin A gene |
| lncRNA | Long non-coding RNA |
| miRNA | MicroRNA |

S. Haston
Developmental Biology and Cancer Research Programme, Birth Defects Research Centre, UCL Great Ormond Street Institute of Child Health, London, UK
e-mail: scott.haston.13@ucl.ac.uk

S. Pozzi
The Novo Nordisk Foundation Center for Stem Cell Biology, University of Copenhagen, Copenhagen, Denmark
e-mail: sara.pozzi@sund.ku.dk

J. M. Gonzalez-Meljem (✉)
Bioengineering Department, School of Engineering and Science, Tecnologico de Monterrey, Mexico City, Mexico
e-mail: jmgonzalezmeljem@tec.mx



J. C. Gomez-Verjan, N. A. Rivero-Segura (eds.), *Clinical Genetics and Genomics of Aging*, https://doi.org/10.1007/978-3-030-40955-5_11

| | |
|---|---|
| ncRNA | Non-coding RNA |
| PAM | Protospacer adjacent motif |
| PD | Parkinson's disease |
| SASP | Senescence-associated secretory phenotype |
| TALEN | Transcription activator-like effector nuclease |
| TERT | Telomerase reverse transcriptase |
| ZNF | Zinc finger nuclease |

## Introduction

Research into the underlying mechanisms of organismal ageing has advanced at a tremendous rate over the past decade. Studying the ageing process presents a significant challenge as it is a systemic phenomenon that affects numerous organs and tissue systems in humans. Due to the complex nature of the ageing process, it has been most extensively modelled using short-lived non-vertebrate systems such as nematode worms (*C. elegans*), yeast (*C. cerevisiae*) and flies (*D. melanogaster*), as well as longer-lived vertebrate models, such as the mouse (*M. musculus*) and zebrafish (*D. rerio*) [1]. Importantly, research using these model organisms alongside both traditional and novel genetic manipulation techniques has delineated nine hallmarks of ageing that are common across various species, including humans [2]. Tremendous effort is now being expended into understanding the relationship between these different hallmarks and how their interactions impact on the ageing process. This has created a constant necessity for studying multiple interactions between complex genetic pathways, sometimes under the influence of fluctuating factors, such as epigenetic mechanisms, and especially in vertebrate models where traditional genetic engineering techniques are less efficient or involve higher costs due to longer lifespans (the maximal lifespan of mice is around 3–4 years and 5 years for zebrafish). It has therefore become of great interest for the ageing research community to develop new in vivo and in vitro genetically engineered models capable of addressing complex research questions in a time-cost efficient manner.

Since its discovery, CRISPR-Cas technology has ignited a biological revolution by providing a highly versatile platform that allows fast and efficient genome editing in an ever-growing list of organisms. In this chapter we will first describe the most recent advances in the development and application of the CRISPR-Cas platform in biomedical research. Then we will discuss the most recent and notable basic research applications of this technology in the study of the molecular causes of ageing. Finally, we will review how CRISPR-Cas has been used for creating new models for the study of age-related diseases, as well as for manipulating disease-associated gene pathways.

## The CRISPR-Cas System

### Genome-Editing Technologies and Their Development

The development of the first genetic engineering techniques began in the late 1960s, when, for the first time, scientists modified an organism's DNA in a test tube [3]. However, several years had to pass for the development of the molecular methods necessary to conduct precise genetic and genomic modifications (i.e. targeting of an exact genomic location(s) or even defined regions within a gene with precisely the desired modification). These are collectively known as genome-editing (or gene-editing) technologies, and they were only but a dream for molecular biologists until the end of the last century. The first issue for precise genome editing required knowing the DNA sequence of the gene or region to be targeted, this information not being fully available in the case of human cells until completion of the Human Genome Project in 2003. The second issue involves modifying exactly an intended region with exactly the desired alteration, something that was impossible using early genome-engineering methods as they involved random mutagenesis across the genome.

Precise targeting of a defined genomic locus was only achieved when scientists harnessed a process known as *homologous recombination* in order to genetically modify mouse embryonic stem (ES) cells [4]. Homologous recombination mediates a highly precise DNA repair process known as homology-directed repair (HDR), which is mainly involved in repairing double-strand breaks (DSBs) that spontaneously occur in the cell's DNA. The resulting technology is known as *HDR-directed gene targeting*, and its true potential was demonstrated when the targeted ES cells were injected into blastocyst-stage embryos, which then generated living mice carrying the mutation. The description of the first gene-targeted mouse paved the way for scientists to be able to probe the function of thousands of genes by producing all kinds of gene knockouts and knock-ins in mice and other species. However, gene targeting via HDR displayed several caveats. The largest by far was a significantly low rate of integration success into the target genome, which, together with the long time required to breed fully mutant mice when using the ES cell approach, constantly led projects to become unsustainably long and costly. Additionally, many cell types were found not to be amenable to HDR-mediated gene targeting, as homologous recombination is mostly restricted to the S and G2 phases of the cell cycle in replicating cells [5]. Finally, experimental design was restricted to limits in the number and size of mutations that could be introduced into the genome.

In order to overcome these limitations, scientists sought to develop a tool that allowed them to control exactly where in the genome a DSB was to be introduced. If a DSB was targeted to an important functional region within a gene, then it could be repaired by the cell in a random fashion, leading to insertion or deletion mutations that abolished gene function. Alternatively, if an exogenous DNA template was provided, the DSB would then be repaired by HDR and the exogenous DNA sequence would be incorporated into the genome. The first of these gene-editing technologies to be successfully applied were eukaryotic zinc finger nucleases (ZNFs), which consist of several zinc finger DNA-binding domains that are artificially fused to a DNA-cleavage domain. Each finger domain recognises a 3 base pair (bp) sequence, and cutting requires dimerisation of a pair of ZNFs recognising adjacent sequences to the cut site. Therefore, a pair of 3-finger ZFNs determines an 18 bp sequence, which would be theoretically unique within a genome [6, 7]. Another successful genome-editing technology relies on the use of transcription activator-like effector nucleases (TALENs), which take advantage of the ability of TALE proteins to specifically recognise a single DNA base pair instead of three [8]. Then, similarly to ZFNs, an appropriate combination of TALEs could be fused to a nuclease domain and be designed to target any desired sequenced in the genome. Unfortunately, the design and engineering of target-specific fusion proteins (both ZNFs and TALENs) resulted very time-consuming and not trivial at all, which has greatly restricted their widespread usage.

## The Molecular Basis of CRISPR-Cas Technology and Its Variants

During the last decade, a more robust system in terms of targeting efficiency and ease of design was developed and rapidly became the most widely used gene-editing technique in the life sciences. CRISPR stands for *c*lustered *r*egularly *i*nterspaced *s*hort *p*alindromic *r*epeat DNA sequences. These short repeat elements were first observed in *E. coli* in 1987 and were later determined to be part of the bacterial adaptive immune system [9]. However, the first concrete experimental evidence of the potential widespread application of CRISPR came with the demonstration that following viral infection, bacteria could integrate specific sequences of the viral genome into their own. These sequences would then be used by bacteria to produce short RNAs able to recognise the viral DNA in subsequent infections and guide the Cas9 nuclease to it. The RNA/Cas9 complex would then induce a DSB in the viral DNA, disabling it [10]. This defence mechanism can be easily exploited in an experimental set-up, where short RNA sequences (around 20 base pairs), named gRNA (guide RNA), can be designed to bind any determined DNA sequence in virtually any kind of cell. gRNAs then become complexed to the Cas9 enzyme and will dictate the specificity of its enzymatic action, which in turn will lead to the generation of a DSB in the targeted genome.

The specificity of the DSB operated by the Cas9 enzyme is not exclusively dictated by the complementarity between the target sequence and the gRNA but involves the presence of a 2–6 bp PAM (protospacer adjacent motif) sequence adjacent to the target DNA sequence. Although the requirement of a specific PAM sequence in proximity to the target region by the Cas9 nuclease might be considered a limiting factor to its application, the discovery of Cas variants from other species or the development of artificial Cas nucleases targeting alternative PAM sequences is continuously expanding the capabilities of this already versatile system [11–13].

Another interesting example of the applications of variants of the system is shown by Cas proteins engineered to lose their nuclease activity but to retain their ability to target specific genomic loci. By conjugating these nuclease-deficient Cas9 proteins (dCas9) to a variety of fluorescent reporters or other functional molecules, these can now be delivered to define genomic loci in order to visualise them or to functionally interrogate their significance [14].

## Applications of CRISPR-Cas in Basic and Translational Biomedical Research

The advent of CRISPR-Cas has dramatically changed the way in which researchers generate animal models of human diseases. In fact, compared to other techniques discussed earlier in this chapter, CRISPR-Cas can now be used to generate mouse models carrying multiple genomic alterations in a single step [15]. Furthermore, injection or electroporation of CRISPR-Cas targeting constructs into early mouse zygotes allows skipping the tedious and time-consuming processes of generating mutant ES cell lines and then breeding several generations of mice. Therefore, CRISPR enables the straightforward generation of animals carrying multiple mutations by greatly increasing the success rate for producing genetically engineered mouse models from ~50% to 95% and reducing the time necessary from +1.5 years to 6–8 months [16, 17]. Moreover, the ability to rapidly generate animal models using CRISPR-Cas has expanded in recent years to a variety of species besides rodents, such as pigs, zebrafish, Xenopus and humans [18–21].

The notable accuracy and versatility of CRISPR-Cas for genome editing also opened the door to its use in preclinical and translational settings. In the latter case, CRISPR in vivo gene editing has led to several proof-of-concept studies that would have been unachievable without it, as in the first ever correction of inherited pathogenic mutations linked to degenerative disease in a living organism [22] and even shown to be possible in human embryos [23, 24]. It also has great potential in the field of precision medicine as large-scale population DNA sequencing studies have provided vast amounts of information linking particular diseases with specific genetic mutations which could, in theory, be targeted through CRISPR [25, 26]. This could be used during the identification and validation of potential DNA targets during the development of personalised drug or cell therapies, which will require the generation of engineered cell lines and/or animal models. Techniques such as HDR-mediated gene targeting are too labour intensive, with low targeting efficiencies and long times necessary for their establishment, and consequently are not ideally suited for drug discovery purposes. Conversely, CRISPR-Cas has been proven to be efficient for editing virtually any kind of cell line, from primary immune cells to induced pluripotent stem cells (iPSCs) [27, 28]. Additionally, CRISPR can also be used for functional screening in the development of combined inhibitory therapy aimed at strengthening the efficiency of targeted therapeutics. An example of the latter is shown in a study where a variation of the technology known as CRISPR interference (CRISPRi) was used in genome-wide scale to identify different survival pathways used by cancer cells after oncogene inactivation and allowing the identification of successful combination therapies [29]. In terms of translational applications, the overall safety of CRISPR genome editing in humans will require long-term scrutiny before its adoption in the clinic. Nonetheless, a number of CRISPR-based clinical trials are currently in progress, including studies focused on targeting patients' own T cells in order to improve the immune response towards some forms of malignant cancer [30, 31], and others aimed at correcting pathogenic mutations in the hematopoietic cells of patients with beta-thalassemia and sickle cell disease [32].

## Caveats and Ethical Concerns of CRISPR-Cas Applications

Despite the presence of both a PAM sequence and a specific gRNA, the CRISPR-Cas9 system is not infallible. In fact, DSBs can occur at different sites in the genome, potentially causing so-called "off-target" effects. This eventuality remains to date the biggest concern in the field, as possible undesirable modifications must be properly identified and followed in order to guarantee safety for medical purposes. Nevertheless, there is still little evidence of the biological consequence of Cas9 off-target effects. Two recent studies describe new methods to investigate potential off-target effects in both mammals and plants [33, 34]. In both cases, whole-genome sequencing revealed that selective nucleotide changes, such as conversion of an adenine to a guanine, caused off-target occurrence very rarely, with a frequency comparable to the one of spontaneous mutations. However, substitution of a cytosine with a thymidine was linked to a sizable number of off-target mutations. This newly acquired information adds to the plethora of studies conducted on the safety of CRISPR, which altogether highlight the need for the establishment of clinical standards for the future use of genome-editing techniques in the clinic. Despite this and other technical challenges still ahead for CRISPR genome editing, the pace at which this technology has developed in recent years suggests many of these concerns could be addressed soon, as long as proper ethical guidelines and regulatory mechanisms are established.

In December 2015, the National Academy of Science (NAS) and the National Academy of Medicine (NAM) joined forces to establish an international group aimed at the evaluation of all the ethical concerns raised by human genome editing. Their first report highlights a list of strict measures to be adopted in this area, such as a complete ban on gene editing with purposes different from the prevention and treatment of severe human conditions [35]. More recently, the Association for Responsible Research and Innovation in Genome Editing (ARRIGE) was founded in order to provide guidance on ethical protocols to be adopted when dealing with human genome engineering. The combined effort of these platforms will guarantee a solid base for future discussions on the subject. However, as an increasing number of diverse disciplines keep bringing together the world of CRISPR, it is likely that the implementation of ethical and research laws on genome editing will require the involvement of individual governments.

## Applications of CRISPR-Cas in Basic Research of the Molecular Causes of Ageing

### Investigating the Mechanisms of Longevity

Currently there have been no studies exploring the utility of the CRISPR-Cas system on experimentally extending the lifespan of physiologically aged laboratory animals. A main issue in this regard is that established vertebrate models already possess relatively long lifespans that make longevity extension studies economically unviable. One approach to circumvent this is to use laboratory animals which show accelerated ageing phenotypes, such as progeroid mice. Progeroid syndromes are rare congenital disorders that mimic physiological ageing but in a significantly accelerated manner, severely reducing the lifespan of affected individuals [36].

Genomic instability and increasing levels of DNA damage are thought to be causal factors during physiological ageing and a hallmark of the process [2]. These cellular stresses are also frequently observed in human progeroid syndromes and mouse models. In human HGPS the major genetic defect found (~90% of cases) is a substitution mutation in the gene encoding lamin A, an important constituent of the nuclear lamina, which results in the production of a toxic isoform known as progerin [37–39]. Generation of progerin results in deformation of the nuclear lamina leading to genomic instability, increased DNA damage and disruption to other cellular processes such as epigenetic control of gene regulation, cellular metabolism and nucleocytoplasmic transport [40–43]. Remarkably, two recent studies, published back to back, found that systemically administered CRISPR-Cas9, delivered by adeno-associated virus (AAV), and that targeted lamin A gene (*Lmna*) in a mouse model of HGPS were able to suppress the premature ageing phenotype and significantly increase survival [44, 45]. While the production of progerin from mutant *Lmna* alleles can drive accelerated ageing in HGPS patients, progerin is also found to be produced in healthy (wild-type *Lmna*) cells as a consequence of ageing, suggesting a role for the progerin isoform of lamin A during physiological ageing [46]. The success of this CRISPR-Cas-based approach in the alleviation of HGPS phenotypes in mice holds promise for future therapeutic interventions in human HGPS patients. Furthermore, this CRISPR-Cas system could be used for basic research into the role of progerin in genomic stability during normal ageing.

While progeroid syndromes recapitulate many of the hallmarks of physiological ageing, they are congenital disease states and the insight gained from such models may not be fully representative of the molecular changes that occur during the normal ageing process. Fortunately, ageing researchers have described a new model organism, the African turquoise killifish. This species may be of significant research value by lowering the time-cost requirements of physiological ageing studies in comparison to standard model organisms while being more relevant in terms of molecular biology than accelerated ageing syndromes such as progeria. The African turquoise killifish is a naturally short-lived vertebrate with a remarkably short lifespan of around 4–6 months [47, 48]. Importantly, killifish display canonical age-associated defects, including sarcopenia, reduced fertility, cognitive impairment and the development of cancer [47–49]. Furthermore, like other well-studied animal models of ageing, killifish show improved longevity when subjected to dietary restriction. [50] Killifish also possess telomeres that are approximately the same length as those found in humans (around 6–8 kb) [51], unlike mice which possess much longer telomeric repeats (around 50–150 kb) [52]. Together these observations suggest that killifish may be an excellent new model organism for elucidating the ageing process in vertebrates.

Recently, the sequenced reference genome of the killifish was generated alongside RNA-sequencing datasets for several organs and H3K4me3 chromatin immunoprecipitation sequencing to define transcriptional start sites [53]. Moreover, the authors of this study also demonstrated that the killifish is amenable to CRISPR-Cas9-mediated genome editing by generating killifish lines that were edited to carry mutated alleles in a suite of genes comprising the hallmarks of ageing [53]. These recently described genomic datasets, combined with the utility of CRISPR-Cas9, allow the killifish to be used as a powerful platform to rapidly explore the genetics underlying vertebrate ageing in rapid and scalable manner.

## Targeting of Telomeres and Telomerase

Telomeres are arrays of linked nucleotide hexamer repeats that are found at the ends of chromosomes in a vast clade of organisms [14]. While the sequence of these telomeric repeats can vary between organisms, their biological function is highly conserved, which is to limit damage inflicted on genes during the replication of chromosomes. Telomere length is progressively shortened with each round of genomic replication, unless it is restored through the action of a ribonucleoprotein termed telomerase, which consists of two molecules of telomerase reverse transcriptase (TERT), telomere RNA and dyskerin [54–56]. Therefore, over the life of an organism, telomeres gradually become shorter, until they reach a critical length, forcing cells into a state of permanent absence of proliferation termed replicative senescence. Importantly, the association of telomere length with ageing is not simply correlative [57, 58]. Studies in which telomeres are ablated result in the development of age-associated damage and reduction of proliferative ability [58–60]. This effect is most prominent in stem cell compartments, where elevated telomerase activity is normally observed [61, 62], as loss of telomerase in stem cells results in decreased replicative capacity and an impairment of their differentiation potential [62].

Due to the evidence shown above, telomere attrition is considered a hallmark of the ageing process [14, 63]; and while significant advances have been made in understating the basic biology of telomere function through in vitro research, the translation of this research to an in vivo context has been severely limited. The reason is that although numerous techniques exist to label telomeres and genomic regions, most of these are toxic to cells, can result in the induction of DNA damage or are non-compatible for in vivo applications. The CRISPR-Cas system has facilitated the refinement of these techniques by utilising dCas9 fused to a fluorescent protein, allowing telomeres to be visualised in living mice [64]. This work was also combined with CRISPR-Cas9-mediated disruption of the *TRF1* gene, which allowed for the real-time observation of the fusion and aggregation of telomeres. This technique can easily be expanded to look at the effects of various genetic manipulations on telomere dynamics in vivo.

As mentioned previously, damage to telomeres results in an assortment of cellular defects. The ability of the CRISPR-Cas system to delete defined genomic regions or to introduce precise mutations or new genetic elements provides an excellent tool to study telomere damage in living organisms. For example, studies introducing DSBs in telomeres have found that activation of the telomeric repair system is regulated by the *Rad51* gene. However, the findings from previous experiments were obscured by confounding factors such as the induction of apoptotic or senescence pathways [14]. These caveats were shown to be avoided by the use of CRISPR-Cas9 in order to greatly increase the precision of DSB induction in telomeres [65]. In another study, investigators used CRISPR-Cas9 to completely delete the telomeres from neuroblastoma cells and interrogated its effects on cellular function and the induction of senescence [66]. This analysis revealed that the complete loss of telomeres in these cells resulted in a loss of mitochondrial function and the aggregation of Parkinson's disease-associated proteins, allowing for the study of cellular ageing. CRISPR-Cas can also be used to introduce more precise mutations in telomeres, such as at the level of a single nucleotide. As an example, a mutation was introduced to the subtelomeric CTCF binding site known as TERRA, resulting in the loss of sister telomeres and impairing replicative potential. This work implicated CTCF and TERRA as being of significant importance for telomere maintenance and replication [67]. Further studies utilising the ability of the CRISPR-Cas9 system to remove telomeres in living organisms and in a cell-type-specific manner will allow for a greater understanding of the role that telomere attrition plays during the ageing process and in the development of age-associated diseases.

Investigations into the biological activity of telomerase have also been performed using CRISPR-Cas tools. As an example of this, a loss-of-function mutation was introduced by CRISPR in killifish telomerase, which resulted in the recapitulation of human pathologies seen with telomerase deficiency [53]. In another study, CRISPR-Cas9 was used to introduce a fluorescent marker into the *TERT* locus, allowing the dynamic visualisation of telomerase movement in living cells. This approach revealed that there are three stages of telomerase movement: a fast diffusion stage, a frequent but transient telomere association stage and a rarer but stable association stage that mediates telomere extension [68]. Moreover, CRISPR editing revealed that telomerase can bind to single-strand DNA telomere overhangs to catalyse the addition of multiple hexamer repeats in tandem [69]. These CRISPR-Cas-based studies provide important insights into the interplay of different molecular mechanisms involved in telomere maintenance during the ageing process and set the basis for future investigations into the spatio-temporal dynamics of the telomerase protein in vivo.

## Elucidation of Epigenetic Alterations

Research into the ageing process has revealed that genetic variation and somatic mutations can have profound effects on the longevity of an organism. However, it is appreciated that non-genetic variables also contribute heavily to the ageing process. Examples of these include calorie restriction, upregulated stress responses, lowered metabolic rate and decreased fertility [70–73]. It is suspected that these processes have an impact at the level of epigenetics, which encompass changes in heritable phenotypic traits without altering underlying genomic sequences. Core epigenetic mechanisms include the methylation, hydroxyl-methylation and demethylation of DNA sequences, as well as chromatin remodelling, histone modification, regulation by non-coding RNAs and gene imprinting [74]. Epigenetic mechanisms are vital players in the regulation of a myriad of biological processes including embryonic development, cellular reprogramming, gene regulation, X-chromosome inactivation, genomic imprinting, neurodegeneration, autoimmune response modulation, tumorigenesis and ageing [75–77]. For a detailed discussion of the epigenetic mechanisms regulating longevity, we refer readers to a comprehensive review on the subject [78].

While the CRISPR-Cas system has been typically used for genome editing, the technique has recently been expanded to allow epigenome editing by fusing dCas9 to an epigenetic modifying enzyme or a transcription factor. This allows to alter gene regulation within a region of choice by directing a dCas9/epigenetic modifier with specific gRNA sequences. [79, 80] This approach has been successfully employed by multiple groups to experimentally induce different types of epigenetic modifications such as histone methylation or acetylation, as well as DNA methylation or demethylation [79–82]. In the case of chromatin, which is the highest-order structure of genomic DNA and whose organisation has an important influence over gene expression, researchers have shown that fusions of Cas9 with fluorescent reporters can allow live imaging of discrete chromatin regions in order to study their state dynamics in respect to gene expression [83, 84]. Finally, non-coding RNAs (ncRNAs) such as microRNAs (miRNAs) and long non-coding RNAs (lncRNAs) have been shown to be amenable to modulation by the classic CRISPR-Cas mechanism of DSB generation [85, 86]. For example, specific miRNAs can be downregulated through the Cas9-mediated induction of DSBs in their Drosha and Dicer sites, which are essential for miRNA biogenesis, leading to downstream epigenetic effects [87].

The application of CRISPR-Cas in epigenome editing is currently in its infancy. However, the technique holds significant promise for providing clarity to the myriad of epigenetic mechanisms that may impact on the ageing process. In this regard, it must be noted that in comparison to other hallmarks of ageing, the range of discrepancies observed across model species is the broadest in the case of some epigenetic alterations. This prevents the use of many of the most time-cost efficient in vivo models of ageing such as yeast, worms and flies, as they can even lack some of those alterations. Therefore, the use of CRISPR-Cas for the fast and efficient generation of in vitro and in vivo models of higher species will prove invaluable for studying epigenetic mechanisms of ageing that are of relevance to humans.

## Dissecting the Role of Cellular Senescence

Another hallmark of the ageing process is the induction and accumulation of cells in a senescent state [2]. Cellular senescence is characterised by a stable arrest of the cell cycle while maintaining viability and metabolic activity. Senescent cells are also known to activate what is known as the senescence-associated secretory phenotype (SASP), which is a plethora of secreted factors comprising pro-inflammatory cytokines, chemokines, growth factors and matrix remodelling enzymes [88, 89]. Beyond telomere attrition in the case of replicative senescence, cellular senescence can be induced by many other cellular stresses like oncogene activation, loss of tumour suppressors, oxidative stress, persistent DNA damage response, ionising radiation and cytotoxic chemicals [88, 89]. Cellular senescence is thought to primarily act as a potent cell-autonomous tumour-suppressive mechanism by preventing the expansion of pre-malignant cells. However, research over the past decade has revealed that cellular senescence is a pleiotropic phenotype that has many context-dependent paracrine effects mediated by the SASP, such as aiding in tissue regeneration or, paradoxically, promoting tumorigenesis and the acquisition of malignancy [88–90].

While cellular senescence is appreciated as a hallmark of physiological ageing, it is not simply its consequence as the pharmacological or genetic removal of senescent cells can ameliorate ageing phenotypes in mice [91]. Therefore, a more detailed understanding of the induction and maintenance mechanisms of the senescent state will be advantageous in fully dissecting its relation to organismal ageing. To this end, the CRISPR-Cas system has been utilised for performing high-throughput genetic screens of genes and genetic pathways involved such processes. Some identified events include loss of *MTOR*, *CRISPLD2* or *MORF4L1*, which prevent both senescence and SASP induction, or *CHEK2*, *HAS1* or *MDK* loss, which promote the bypass of cellular senescence while retaining production of the SASP [92]. Conversely, CRISPR-Cas9 functional genetic screens have also identified genes whose deficiency is sufficient to promote the senescent state, such as the SWI/SNF component *SMARCB1* in melanoma cells [93]. Furthermore, CRISPR-Cas genome editing has been utilised in order to characterise enhancer elements in the genome that are essential for maintaining the senescent state. For example, a CRISPR-Cas9-based screen showed that the transcription factor AP-1 is a major regulator of the senescent state following oncogenic stress by interacting with a *FOXF1* enhancer, which is hyper-activated in senescent cells and necessary to maintain the cells in senescence [94].

Cellular senescence is an extremely complex and highly context-dependent cellular phenotype that poses great challenges to scientists aiming to understand its impact in all kinds of biological processes. Some difficulties include the absence of a single robust molecular marker able to identify senescent cells, the pleiotropic and dynamic nature of the SASP, the wide variety of different senescence-inducing stimuli and a high degree of phenotypic heterogeneity even among senescent cells belonging to the same population [95, 96]. In this regard, CRISPR-Cas genome-editing tools will provide feasible implementation of high-throughput assays able to further delineate important molecular pathways involved in inducing and maintaining cellular senescence in both physiological ageing and age-associated diseases.

## Applications of CRISPR-Cas in the Study of Ageing-Related Disease

### Cardiovascular Disease

One of the most notable contributions of CRISPR-Cas to ageing research is its ability to target non-proliferating cells (contrary to HDR-directed gene targeting), which comprise most cells in adult tissues. Therefore, it can be used both in vitro and in vivo for cell types of great relevance to age-related disease such cardiomyocytes and neurons [97, 98]. In the heart, the ability to target cardiomyocytes is of great importance, as this organ does not harbour a typical stem cell population. In order to address this issue, a mouse model expressing Cas9 specifically in cardiomyocytes was developed, which allows cardiac-specific targeting of any gene just by injecting the mice with AAVs carrying gene-specific gRNAS [99]. Additionally, a number of proof-of-concept studies have shown that CRISPR-Cas can be used to correct in vivo pathogenic mutations present within this cell population [97, 98, 100]

The application of CRISPR-Cas in the study of cardiovascular disease during physiological ageing has yet to be reported. It has, however, been used to rescue the alterations resembling cardiovascular disease observed in mouse models of Hutchinson-Gilford progeria syndrome (HGPS) [44, 45]. Also worth noting is the recent generation by CRISPR-Cas9 gene editing of the first minipig model of HGPS, which has a cardiovascular system similar to that of humans and was shown to recapitulate the cardiovascular alterations found in human HGPS patients [101].

### Neurodegenerative Diseases

In recent years, CRISPR-Cas technologies have significantly contributed to studies addressing the molecular pathogenesis of age-related neurodegenerative conditions such as Alzheimer's disease (AD) and Parkinson's disease (PD). Currently, it has mostly been utilised for developing new or improved tools in which to study the molecular mechanisms underlying these diseases, such as in patient-derived cell lines carrying pathogenic mutations.

In a notable study, researchers showed that the frequency of incorporation of a mutation could be predicted according to its distance to the site where a DSB was generated by the Cas9 nuclease. Using this information, they described the efficient generation of homozygous and heterozygous mutations in the amyloid precursor protein (APP) and presenilin 1 (PSEN1) genes in human iPSC lines, which were then differentiated into neurons that displayed AD-associated phenotypes, such as increased amyloid-β (Aβ) production [102]. In another study, patient-derived human iPSCs carrying a mutation in the presenilin 2 (PSEN2) were derived into basal forebrain cholinergic neurons, which were then targeted by CRISPR-Cas in order to correct the mutation, leading to decreased Aβ production and the recovery of normal electrophysiological functions [103]. The feasibility of correcting AD-causing mutations in the postmitotic neurons of living mice by CRISPR-Cas has also been shown in studies where the targeting constructs were delivered to their brains by AAVs or nanocomplexes [104, 105]. However, the genetic strategy used in these studies is only applicable for hereditary AD, which encompasses a minority of cases. This motivated a recent proof-of-concept study where a specific region of the APP gene was targeted by CRISPR (without ablating gene function) in order to diminish Aβ production in human iPSC-derived neurons as well as in the dentate gyrus of adult mice [106].

Similar applications of CRISPR-Cas have been conducted for the study of PD pathogenesis. It has been recently used, for example, to develop heterozygotic and homozygotic mutations in the synuclein A gene (SNCA) in human iPSCs, which were then differentiated into midbrain dopaminergic neurons displaying resistance to synuclein protein aggregation, a pathological hallmark of PD [107]. Notably, CRISPR-Cas has also been used to develop novel PD models by allowing the generation of minipigs carrying multiple mutations in PD-associated genes such as SNCA, parkin, DJ-1 and PINK1 [108–110].

Finally, CRISPR-based functional screening can also be used for discovering novel regulators of genes, pathways or cellular processes of importance to brain ageing or neurodegenerative disease. One study described a CRISPR screening method that led to the identification of two genes that conferred resistance to alpha-synuclein toxicity in human neurons [111], while more recently, CRISPR-Cas9 knockout screen revealed the role of CD22 in preventing microglial phagocytosis during aging. Notably, when researchers delivered a CD22-blocking antibody to the brains of ageing mice, they observed a restoration of microglial activity and cognitive function [112].

## Conclusions

There is no reason to doubt that the development of CRISPR-Cas genome editing represents an unprecedented breakthrough in modern science, as it has potential applications in a wide array of disciplines ranging from agriculture, zoology and renewable energy to biomedicine and synthetic biology. This powerful tool holds promise for further elucidating the molecular causes of ageing by allowing scientists to probe genetic and epigenetic pathways with a level of sophistication that was unattainable just a few years ago. It will allow so in traditional animal and cell models of ageing, but it will also drastically accelerate the generation of refined versions of those models or even allow the development of new research approaches in non-model organisms. Moreover, CRISPR-based genome editing is already having a significant impact in research aiming to understand the cellular and molecular origins of age-related diseases, as well as developing potential treatments against them. The application of CRISPR-Cas gene editing for the treatment of age-related diseases is not over the horizon yet, as it will require the identification of causative genes and their role under a variety of contexts that could be as diverse as the ageing process is across individuals. However, CRISPR-Cas might also hold the key for solving such conundrum, as it has opened the way for achieving true personalised medicine by providing both the precision and scalability required for conducting genome-wide functional screens during the refinement of drug- and cell-based therapies for age-related diseases.

**Acknowledgements** JMGM is part of the Translational OMICS Strategic Focus Group at Tecnologico de Monterrey.

## References

1. Tacutu R, et al. Human Ageing Genomic Resources: integrated databases and tools for the biology and genetics of ageing. Nucleic Acids Res. 2013;41:D1027–33.
2. López-Otín C, Blasco MA, Partridge L, Serrano M, Kroemer G. The hallmarks of aging. Cell. 2013;153:1194–217.
3. Danna K, Nathans D. Specific cleavage of simian virus 40 DNA by restriction endonuclease of Haemophilus influenzae. Proc Natl Acad Sci. 2006;68:2913–7.
4. Thomas KR, Capecchi MR. Site-directed mutagenesis by gene targeting in mouse embryo-derived stem cells: a general strategy for targeting mutations to non-selectable genes. Cell. 1987;53:503–8.
5. Orthwein A, et al. A mechanism for the suppression of homologous recombination in G1 cells. Nature. 2015;528:422–6.
6. Smith J. Requirements for double-strand cleavage by chimeric restriction enzymes with zinc finger DNA-recognition domains. Nucleic Acids Res. 2000;28:3361–9.
7. Carroll D. Genome engineering with zinc-finger nucleases. Genetics. 2011;188:773–82.
8. Christian M, et al. Targeting DNA double-strand breaks with TAL effector nucleases. Genetics. 2010;186:756–61.
9. Makino K, Nakata A, Ishino Y, Amemura M, Shinagawa H. Nucleotide sequence of the iap gene, responsible for alkaline phosphatase isozyme conversion in Escherichia coli, and identification of the gene product. J Bacteriol. 2016;169:5429–33.
10. Boyaval P, Moineau S, Romero DA, Horvath P. Against Viruses in Prokaryotes. Science. 2007;315:1709–12.
11. Hu JH, et al. Evolved Cas9 variants with broad PAM compatibility and high DNA specificity. Nature. 2018;556:57–63.
12. Kleinstiver BP, et al. Engineered CRISPR-Cas9 nucleases with altered PAM specificities. Nature. 2015;523:481–5.
13. Kleinstiver BP, et al. High-fidelity CRISPR–Cas9 nucleases with no detectable genome-wide off-target effects. Nature. 2016;529:490–5.
14. Brane A, Tollefsbol T. Targeting telomeres and telomerase: studies in aging and disease utilizing CRISPR/Cas9 technology. Cells. 2019;8:186.
15. Wang H, et al. One-step generation of mice carrying mutations in multiple genes by CRISPR/Cas-mediated genome engineering. Cell. 2013;153:910–8.
16. Yang H, et al. One-step generation of mice carrying reporter and conditional alleles by CRISPR/cas-mediated genome engineering. Cell. 2013;154:1370.
17. Cohen J. 'Any idiot can do it.' Genome editor CRISPR could put mutant mice in everyone's reach. Science (80). 2016; https://doi.org/10.1126/science.aal0334.

18. Voets O, et al. Highly efficient gene inactivation by adenoviral CRISPR/Cas9 in human primary cells. PLoS One. 2017;12:1–20.
19. Sudou N, Taira M, Horb ME, Miller RK. Tissue-specific gene inactivation in xenopus. Genetics. 2018;208:673–86.
20. Tessadori F, et al. Effective CRISPR/Cas9-based nucleotide editing in zebrafish to model human genetic cardiovascular disorders. Dis Model Mech. 2018;11:dmm035469.
21. Liu Q, et al. A Huntingtin Knockin Pig model recapitulates features of selective neurodegeneration in Huntington's disease. Cell. 2018;173:989–1002.e13.
22. Tabebordbar M, et al. 483. In vivo DMD gene editing in muscles and muscle stem cells of dystrophic mice. Mol Ther. 2016;24:S191–2.
23. Liang P, et al. CRISPR/Cas9-mediated gene editing in human tripronuclear zygotes. Protein Cell. 2015;6:363–72.
24. Ma H, et al. Correction of a pathogenic gene mutation in human embryos. Nature. 2017;548:413–9.
25. Weinstein JN, et al. The Cancer Genome Atlas Pan-Cancer analysis project. Nat Genet. 2013;45:1113–20.
26. Barretina J, et al. NIH Public Access of anticancer drug sensitivity. Nature. 2012;483:603–7.
27. Grobarczyk B, Franco B, Hanon K, Malgrange B. Generation of isogenic human iPS cell line precisely corrected by genome editing using the CRISPR/Cas9 system. Stem Cell Rev Rep. 2015;11:774–87.
28. Schumann K, et al. Generation of knock-in primary human T cells using Cas9 ribonucleoproteins. Proc Natl Acad Sci. 2015;112:10437–42.
29. Lou K, et al. KRASG12C inhibition produces a driver-limited state revealing collateral dependencies. Sci Signal. 2019;12:eaaw9450.
30. Su S, et al. CRISPR-Cas9 mediated efficient PD-1 disruption on human primary T cells from cancer patients. Sci Rep. 2016;6:1–14.
31. Cyranoski D. CRISPR gene editing tested in a person. Nature. 2016;539:479.
32. Vertex Pharmaceuticals Incorporated. CRISPR therapeutics and vertex announce FDA fast track designation for CTX001 for the treatment of beta thalassemia. Press Release. 2019.
33. Erwei Z, et al. Cytosine base editor generates substantial off-target single-nucleotide variants in mouse embryos. Science. 2019;126:21.
34. Pavlov YI, et al. Cytosine, but not adenine, base editors induce genome-wide off-target mutations in rice. Science. 2019;8:647–56.
35. The National Academies of Sciences Engineering and Medicine. Committee on Human Gene Editing: scientific, medical, and ethical considerations. 2017. https://doi.org/10.17226/24623
36. Burtner CR, Kennedy BK. Progeria syndromes and ageing: what is the connection? Nat Rev Mol Cell Biol. 2010;11:567–78.
37. Vidak S, Foisner R. Molecular insights into the premature aging disease progeria. Histochem Cell Biol. 2016;145:401–17.
38. Osorio FG, et al. Splicing-directed therapy in a new mouse model of human accelerated aging. Sci Transl Med. 2011;3:106ra107.
39. Eriksson M, et al. Recurrent de novo point mutations in lamin A cause Hutchinson-Gilford progeria syndrome. Nature. 2003;423:293–8.
40. Kubben N, Misteli T. Shared molecular and cellular mechanisms of premature ageing and ageing-associated diseases. Nat Rev Mol Cell Biol. 2017;18:595–609.
41. Gordon LB, Rothman FG, López-Otín C, Misteli T. Progeria: a paradigm for translational medicine. Cell. 2014;156:400–7.
42. Gonzalo S, Kreienkamp R, Askjaer P. Hutchinson-Gilford Progeria Syndrome: a premature aging disease caused by LMNA gene mutations. Ageing Res Rev. 2017;33:18–29.
43. Buchwalter A, Hetzer MW. Nucleolar expansion and elevated protein translation in premature aging. Nat Commun. 2017;8:328.
44. Beyret E, et al. Single-dose CRISPR–Cas9 therapy extends lifespan of mice with Hutchinson–Gilford progeria syndrome. Nat Med. 2019;25:419–22.

45. Santiago-Fernández O, et al. Development of a CRISPR/Cas9-based therapy for Hutchinson–Gilford progeria syndrome. Nat Med. 2019;25:423–6.
46. Scaffidi P, Misteli T. Lamin A-dependent nuclear defects in human aging. Science (80). 2006;312:1059–63.
47. Genade T, et al. Annual fishes of the genus Nothobranchius as a model system for aging research. Aging Cell. 2005;4:223–33.
48. Valenzano DR, Terzibasi E, Cattaneo A, Domenici L, Cellerino A. Temperature affects longevity and age-related locomotor and cognitive decay in the short-lived fish: Nothobranchius furzeri. Aging Cell. 2006;5:275–8.
49. Di Cicco E, Tozzini ET, Rossi G, Cellerino A. The short-lived annual fish Nothobranchius furzeri shows a typical teleost aging process reinforced by high incidence of age-dependent neoplasias. Exp Gerontol. 2011;46:249–56.
50. Terzibasi E, et al. Effects of dietary restriction on mortality and age-related phenotypes in the short-lived fish Nothobranchius furzeri. Aging Cell. 2009;8:88–99.
51. Hartmann N, et al. Telomeres shorten while Tert expression increases during ageing of the short-lived fish Nothobranchius furzeri. Mech Ageing Dev. 2009;130:290–6.
52. Lee HW, Gottlieb GJ, Horner JW, Greider CW, DePinho RA. Essential role of mouse telomerase in highly proliferative organs. Nature. 1998;392:569–74.
53. Harel I, et al. A platform for rapid exploration of aging and diseases in a naturally short-lived vertebrate. Cell. 2015;160:1013–26.
54. Nugent CI, Lundblad V. The telomerase reverse transcriptase: components and regulation. Genes Dev. 1998;12:1073–85.
55. Nguyen THD, et al. Cryo-EM structure of substrate-bound human telomerase holoenzyme. Nature. 2018;557:190–5.
56. Cohen SB, et al. Protein composition of catalytically active human telomerase from immortal cells. Science. 2007;315:1850–3.
57. Martínez P, Blasco MA. Telomere-driven diseases and telomere-targeting therapies. J Cell Biol. 2017;216:875–87.
58. Carneiro MC, et al. Short telomeres in key tissues initiate local and systemic aging in Zebrafish. PLoS Genet. 2016;12:e1005798.
59. Bernadotte A, Mikhelson VM, Spivak IM. Markers of cellular senescence. Telomere shortening as a marker of cellular senescence. Aging (Albany. NY). 2016;8:3–11.
60. Flores I, Cayuela ML, Blasco MA. Molecular biology: effects of telomerase and telomere length on epidermal stem cell behavior. Science (80). 2005;309:1253–6.
61. Sharpless NE, DePinho RA. How stem cells age and why this makes us grow old. Nat Rev Mol Cell Biol. 2007;8:703–13.
62. Ullah M, Sun Z. Klotho deficiency accelerates stem cells aging by impairing telomerase activity. J Gerontol Ser A. 2018; https://doi.org/10.1093/gerona/gly261.
63. Harley CB, Vaziri H, Counter CM, Allsopp RC. The telomere hypothesis of cellular aging. Exp Gerontol. 1992;27:375–82.
64. Duan J, et al. Live imaging and tracking of genome regions in CRISPR/dCas9 knock-in mice. Genome Biol. 2018;19:192.
65. Mao P, et al. Homologous recombination-dependent repair of telomeric DSBs in proliferating human cells. Nat Commun. 2016;7:12154.
66. Kim H, et al. CRISPR-Cas9 mediated telomere removal leads to mitochondrial stress and protein aggregation. Int J Mol Sci. 2017;18:2093.
67. Beishline K, et al. CTCF driven TERRA transcription facilitates completion of telomere DNA replication. Nat Commun. 2017;8:2114.
68. Schmidt JC, Zaug AJ, Cech TR. Live cell imaging reveals the dynamics of telomerase recruitment to telomeres. Cell. 2016;166:1188–1197.e9.
69. Schmidt JC, Zaug AJ, Kufer R, Cech TR. Dynamics of human telomerase recruitment depend on template- telomere base pairing. Mol. Biol. Cell. 2018;29:mbc.E17-11-0637.

70. Bordone L, Guarente L. Calorie restriction, SIRT1 and metabolism: understanding longevity. Nat Rev Mol Cell Biol. 2005;6:298–305.
71. Migliaccio E, et al. The p66(shc) adaptor protein controls oxidative stress response and life span in mammals. Nature. 1999;402:309–13.
72. Ruggiero C, et al. High basal metabolic rate is a risk factor for mortality: the Baltimore Longitudinal Study of Aging. J Gerontol – Ser A Biol Sci Med Sci. 2008;63:698–706.
73. Westendorp RGJ, Kirkwood TBL. Human longevity at the cost of reproductive success. Nature. 1998;396:743–6.
74. Xie N, Zhou Y, Sun Q, Tang B. Novel epigenetic techniques provided by the CRISPR/Cas9 system. Stem Cells Int. 2018;2018:7834175.
75. Voigt P, Reinberg D. Epigenome editing. Nat Biotechnol. 2013;31:1097–9.
76. Cheng Y, Xie N, Jin P, Wang T. DNA methylation and hydroxymethylation in stem cells. Cell Biochem Funct. 2015;33:161–73.
77. Fu S, Wu H, Zhang H, Lian CG, Lu Q. DNA methylation/hydroxymethylation in melanoma. Oncotarget. 2017;8:78163–73.
78. Sen P, Shah PP, Nativio R, Berger SL. Epigenetic mechanisms of longevity and aging. Cell. 2016;166:822–39.
79. Enríquez P. Focus: epigenetics: CRISPR-mediated epigenome editing. Yale J Biol Med. 2016;89:471.
80. Hu J, et al. Direct activation of human and mouse Oct4 genes using engineered TALE and Cas9 transcription factors. Nucleic Acids Res. 2014;42:4375–90.
81. Hilton IB, et al. Epigenome editing by a CRISPR-Cas9-based acetyltransferase activates genes from promoters and enhancers. Nat Biotechnol. 2015;33:510–7.
82. Amabile A, et al. Inheritable silencing of endogenous genes by hit-and-run targeted epigenetic editing. Cell. 2016;167:219–232.e14.
83. Fu Y, et al. CRISPR-dCas9 and sgRNA scaffolds enable dual-colour live imaging of satellite sequences and repeat-enriched individual loci. Nat Commun. 2016;7:11707.
84. Chen B, et al. Expanding the CRISPR imaging toolset with Staphylococcus aureus Cas9 for simultaneous imaging of multiple genomic loci. Nucleic Acids Res. 2016;44:e75.
85. Xiao A, et al. Chromosomal deletions and inversions mediated by TALENs and CRISPR/Cas in zebrafish. Nucleic Acids Res. 2013;41:e141.
86. Ho TT, et al. Targeting non-coding RNAs with the CRISPR/Cas9 system in human cell lines. Nucleic Acids Res. 2015;43:e17.
87. Chang H, et al. CRISPR/cas9, a novel genomic tool to knock down microRNA in vitro and in vivo. Sci Rep. 2016;6:22312.
88. Coppé J-P, Desprez P-Y, Krtolica A, Campisi J. The senescence-associated secretory phenotype: the dark side of tumor suppression. Ann Rev Pathol. 2010;5:99–118.
89. Faget DV, Ren Q, Stewart SA. Unmasking senescence: context-dependent effects of SASP in cancer. Nat Rev Cancer. 2019;19:439–53.
90. Gonzalez-Meljem JM, et al. Stem cell senescence drives age-attenuated induction of pituitary tumours in mouse models of paediatric craniopharyngioma. Nat Commun. 2017; https://doi.org/10.1038/s41467-017-01992-5.
91. Baker DJ, et al. Naturally occurring p16(Ink4a)-positive cells shorten healthy lifespan. Nature. 2016;530:184–9.
92. Liu X, et al. A large-scale CRISPR screen and identification of essential genes in cellular senescence bypass. Aging (Albany, NY). 2019;11:4011–31.
93. Wang L, et al. High-throughput functional genetic and compound screens identify targets for senescence induction in cancer. Cell Rep. 2017;21:773–83.
94. Han R, et al. Functional CRISPR screen identifies AP1-associated enhancer regulating FOXF1 to modulate oncogene-induced senescence. Genome Biol. 2018;19:118.
95. Tang H, et al. Single senescent cell sequencing reveals heterogeneity in senescent cells induced by telomere erosion. Protein Cell. 2019;10:370–5.

96. Hernandez-Segura A, et al. Unmasking transcriptional heterogeneity in senescent cells. Curr Biol. 2017;27:2652–2660.e4.
97. Xu L, Lau YS, Gao Y, Li H, Han R. Life-long {AAV}-Mediated {CRISPR} genome editing in dystrophic heart improves cardiomyopathy without causing serious lesions in mdx mice. Mol Ther. 2019; https://doi.org/10.1016/j.ymthe.2019.05.001.
98. Suzuki K, et al. In vivo genome editing via {CRISPR}/Cas9 mediated homology-independent targeted integration. Nature. 2016;540:144–9.
99. Carroll KJ, et al. A mouse model for adult cardiac-specific gene deletion with {CRISPR}/Cas9. Proc Natl Acad Sci USA. 2016;113:338–43.
100. Ishizu T, et al. Targeted genome replacement via homology-directed repair in non-dividing cardiomyocytes. Sci Rep. 2017;7:9363.
101. Dorado B, et al. Generation and characterization of a novel knockin minipig model of Hutchinson-Gilford progeria syndrome. Cell Discov. 2019;5:16.
102. Paquet D, et al. Efficient introduction of specific homozygous and heterozygous mutations using {CRISPR}/Cas9. Nature. 2016;533:125–9.
103. Ortiz-Virumbrales M, et al. {CRISPR}/Cas9-Correctable mutation-related molecular and physiological phenotypes in {iPSC}-derived Alzheimer's {PSEN2} {N141I} neurons. Acta Neuropathol. Commun. 2017;5:77.
104. György B, et al. {CRISPR}/Cas9 mediated disruption of the Swedish {APP} allele as a therapeutic approach for early-onset Alzheimer's disease. Mol Ther Nucleic Acids. 2018;11:429–40.
105. Park H, et al. In vivo neuronal gene editing via {CRISPR}-Cas9 amphiphilic nanocomplexes alleviates deficits in mouse models of Alzheimer's disease. Nat Neurosci. 2019;22:524–8.
106. Sun J, et al. {CRISPR}/Cas9 editing of {APP} C-terminus attenuates β-cleavage and promotes α-cleavage. Nat Commun. 2019;10:53.
107. Chen Y, et al. Engineering synucleinopathy-resistant human dopaminergic neurons by {CRISPR}-mediated deletion of the {SNCA} gene. Eur J Neurosci. 2019;49:510–24.
108. Zhou X, Xin J, Fan N, et al. Generation of CRISPR/Cas9-mediated gene-targeted pigs via somatic cell nuclear transfer. Cell. Mol. Life Sci. 2015;72:1175–84. https://doi.org/10.1007/s00018-014-1744-7.
109. Wang X, Cao C, Huang J, et al. One-step generation of triple gene-targeted pigs using CRISPR/Cas9 system. Sci Rep. 2016;6:20620. https://doi.org/10.1038/srep20620.
110. Zhu X, Zhong Y, Ge Y, et al. CRISPR/Cas9-Mediated Generation of Guangxi Bama Minipigs Harboring Three Mutations in α-Synuclein Causing Parkinson's Disease. Sci Rep. 2018;8:12420. https://doi.org/10.1038/s41598-018-30436-3.
111. Chen YC, Farzadfard F, Gharaei N, Chen WCW, Cao J, Lu TK. Randomized CRISPR-Cas Transcriptional Perturbation Screening Reveals Protective Genes against Alpha-Synuclein Toxicity. Mol Cell. 2017;68(1):247–57.e5. https://doi.org/10.1016/j.molcel.2017.09.014.
112. Pluvinage JV, et al. {CD22} blockade restores homeostatic microglial phagocytosis in ageing brains. Nature. 2019;568:187–92.

# Pharmacological Treatment for Aging: Are We There?

# 12

O. S. Barrera-Vázquez and Juan Carlos Gomez-Verjan

## Abbreviations

| | |
|---|---|
| 5hmC | 5-hydroxymethylcytosine |
| AA | Ascorbic acid |
| AD | Alzheimer disease |
| AMD: | Age-related macular degeneration |
| AMPK | 5′ adenosine monophosphate-activated protein kinase |
| ATG-13 | Autophagy-related gen 13 |
| CD36 | Cluster of differentiation 36 |
| COX-2 | Cyclooxygenase-2 |
| CR | Calorie restriction |
| CRM | Calorie restriction mimetic |
| DNA | Deoxyribonucleic acid (DNA) |
| Elk-1 | ETS Like-1 protein Elk-1 (Elk-1) |
| GSH | Glutathione |
| H3K27m3 | Histone H3 trimethylation at amino acid position 27 |
| HDCA | Histone deacetylase |
| IL-1α | Interleukin 1 alpha |
| Jmjd3 | Jumonji domain containing-3 |
| LMWA | Low molecular weight antioxidants |
| MAPK | Mitogen-activated protein kinase |
| mTOR | mammalian target of rapamycin |
| mTORC1 | mechanistic target of rapamycin complex 1 |
| NAD | Nicotinamide adenine dinucleotide |
| NADPH | Nicotinamide Adenine Dinucleotide Phosphate Hydrogen |

O. S. Barrera-Vázquez · J. C. Gomez-Verjan (✉)
División de Ciencias Básicas, Instituto Nacional de Geriatría (INGER), Mexico City, Mexico
e-mail: jverjan@inger.gob.mx



J. C. Gomez-Verjan, N. A. Rivero-Segura (eds.), *Clinical Genetics and Genomics of Aging*, https://doi.org/10.1007/978-3-030-40955-5_12

| | |
|---|---|
| NF-κB | Nuclear factor kappa-light-chain-enhancer of activated B cells |
| Nrf2/ARE | Nuclear factor erythroid 2 (NFE2)-related factor 2/ antioxidant responsive element |
| PD | Parkinson's disease |
| Raf1-MEK-MAPK | Raf-1- mitogen-induced extracellular kinase- mitogen-activated protein kinase |
| RONS | Reactive Oxygen and Nitrogen Species |
| ROS | Reactive species of oxygen |
| SASP | Senescence-associated secretory phenotype |
| TET | Ten-eleven translocation methylcytosine dioxygenase |
| ULK | Unc-51 like autophagy activating kinase |
| UQ | Ubiquinone |
| μM | Micromolar |

## Introduction

Human aging is known as a decline in the homeostatic reserve, leading to an accumulation of damage and therefore to the loss of several physiological functions, inducing an increase in the probabilities of death [1]. In addition, it is well known that this process has a strong correlation with the development of several age-related changes affecting appearance (like wrinkled skin and grey hair) and the organ functions, such as decreased kidney filtration rate and decreased muscular strength. On the other hand, the average lifespan has increased approximately by 3 months per year in both males and females since 1840, probably by the improvements in public health, education, and medicine. However, this increase in life expectancy is not accompanied by the same increase in healthspan [1], since aging is the leading risk factor for chronic pathologies and prevalence of age-related diseases, including, diabetes, arthritis, cancer, neurodegenerative diseases, among others.

On the other side, since the times of alchemy, humans have tried to expand lifespan through several methods with no or very few successes. However, until very recently, our knowledge of the main biological mechanisms involved in aging (refer to Chap. 1) have increased, and this has led to the development of several compounds focused on the regulation and manipulation of such. In this chapter, we focus on the main studies involved in the pharmacological test of both natural and synthetic compounds, due to their increasing use within the pharmacological research.

## Antioxidant Compounds

The oxidative stress theory of aging proposes that age-associated losses are due to the accumulation of oxidative damage to macromolecules such as lipids, DNA, and proteins by reactive oxygen and nitrogen species (RONS) [2]. An increase in

RONS levels generates damage and cellular senescence [2]. Moreover, senescent cells acquire an irreversible senescence-associated secretory phenotype (SASP), which promotes the secretion of soluble factors, such as interleukins and chemokines, growth factors, degradative enzymes, such as matrix metalloproteases, and insoluble proteins/extracellular matrix components [2]. Most of these SASP components are highly related to the regulation of mTOR, the production of IL-1α, an increase in NF-κB activity, epithelial-mesenchymal transition, and metastatic tumor progression, among others. Oxidative stress is also involved in chronic kidney malfunction, neurodegenerative diseases, and cancer [2]. In this context, research has been focused on the development of agents that could be useful for the treatment of the redox state and nutrient-rich antioxidants that mediate oxidative stress [3].

Antioxidants are essential for the antioxidative defense mechanisms of the body; some of them are small molecules (<900 Da) that regulate the physiological processes of the body [4]. Among them are minerals, vitamins, carotenoids, glutathione, and polyphenols [5]. These can be classified into molecules that cannot be synthesized by humans, such as vitamin C and vitamin E [4], and those that can be synthesized, such as glutathione, lipoic acid, uric acid, taurine, melatonin, and coenzyme Q [6].

## Glutathione

Glutathione (GSH) can be synthesized in the body from amino acids such as L-glutamic acid, L-cysteine, and glycine [7]. Interestingly, homeostasis of intracellular GSH is regulated by de novo synthesis [4]. Other properties of GSH are the metabolism of hormones, such as estrogens, leukotrienes, and prostaglandins, and signal transduction for transcription [8]. Alteration of GSH concentration is linked to dysregulation of cell proliferation, transcription of detoxification enzymes, and apoptosis [4].

Alteration in GSH-peroxidase and -reductase activity is found in diabetes [4]. In the brain, disruption in GSH homeostasis may induce oxidative stress and lead to neurodegenerative diseases, including Parkinson's disease (PD), Alzheimer's disease (AD), and dementia [4]. Studies show that a reduction in the levels of GSH is associated with AD [9]and cardiovascular diseases [10]. On the other hand, in PD exists an association with the depletion of GSH levels and an increase of ROS within the midbrain [11].

## Flavonoids

Flavonoids are the most studied class of polyphenols; there is information available on about 6000 flavonoids, isolated from pigments, fruits, and medicinal plants [12]. Several properties have been associated with these compounds, such as antioxidative, antimutagenic, anti-inflammatory, and anticarcinogenic [13]. Particularly, several reports show the antioxidant effects of flavonoids in oxidative stress induced by age-related diseases [4].

In older women, it was reported that high total flavonoids intake reduced the risk of cancer mortality compared to low total flavonoids consumption [14]. Also, a decrease in breast cancer risk among postmenopausal women was found to be associated with flavonoids intake [15]. Other reports showed that two flavonoid subclasses, namely procyanidins and isoflavones, exert preventive effects toward the risk of the development of colorectal cancer [4]. In this context, studies demonstrated that consuming a flavonoid-rich diet is associated with a lower risk of cardiovascular diseases since flavonoids can prevent cardiovascular diseases by their anti-inflammatory, antioxidant mechanisms and by increasing the high-density lipoprotein level [4]. Additionally, in diabetes, flavonoids from green tea and epicatechin induce the activation of the insulin receptor.

Flavonoids from cocoa, green tea, and citrus fruit exert beneficial effects on the brain [4]. Evidence suggests that flavonoids protect against neural injuries and degeneration in pathologies like AD and dementia. Flavonoids have also been reported to downregulate the development of AD-like pathophysiology and related neurodegenerative disorders by disrupting amyloid β protein production, activating α-secretase, and inhibiting β-secretase [16]. Together, this evidence showed that flavonoids have the potential to block the initiation and progression of age-related diseases. Thus, a high intake of flavonoids should be included in the diet of the elderly via supplementation or flavonoid-rich food.

## Carotenoids

Carotenoids are produced in the plastids of plants, algae, bacteria, and fungi [4]. There are approximately 600 carotenoids that have been discovered [17]. Two classes comprise the carotenoids: carotenes and xanthophylls [18]. They not only exert antioxidant properties but facilitate the modulation of the cell cycle, apoptosis, cell differentiation, and enhancement of the immune system and promote growth factors and adhesion molecules [4].

Carotenoids have a protective role in age-related macular degeneration (AMD), a leading cause of blindness in older adults. In the processes linked to AMD, it is described as the oxidative stress within the retina, besides the ROS generation [4]. However, it was found that individuals who consume a carotenoid-rich diet have a relatively low risk of age-related macular degeneration, indicating the positive effects of these molecules [19].

Other studies demonstrate that lutein may decrease the risk of cardiovascular diseases, coronary artery disease, and cancer [4]. It also inhibits breast cancer via modulation of NrF2/ARE and NF-κB pathways [20]. Another common carotenoid, lycopene, widely accepted as a potent antioxidant, reduces the risk of certain types of cancers, such as of the lung, prostate, and colon [4]. Lycopene suppresses the progression of carcinogenesis via its anti-inflammatory actions [21]. Interestingly, in a follow-up study conducted from 1986 to 2010 involving 49,898 males revealed that higher lycopene intake could prevent prostate cancer [22].

Studies in human and animal models suggested that carotenoids could reduce the risk of osteoporosis [23]. β-carotene significantly inhibited the viability of bone marrow–derived macrophages and decreased the NF-kB pathway [4]. A meta-analysis involving 140,265 participants and 4324 cases suggested that high dietary intake of total carotenoids reduced hip fracture risk by 28% [24] and bone density and fracture risk were inversely correlated with dietary intake of carotenoids [25].

Studies showed that high plasma levels of lutein reduced the risk of neural disorders [4]. Interestingly, a high level of lutein, zeaxanthin, and lycopene in serum has been associated with a lower risk of AD mortality [4].

## Dietary Minerals

The beneficial effect of mineral on aging is worth the attention; some minerals such as copper, magnesium, zinc, and selenium possess antioxidant properties. However, an overdose of mineral intake is not recommended and may cause a detrimental impact on health.

Zinc, an important mineral, that can be found in the retina and is implicated in the antioxidant defense system of the eye [26]. A study with 369 participants revealed that a low intake of zinc was associated with AMD [27]; additionally, a follow-up study for 6 years including 3640 participants revealed a significant role of zinc in AMD [28]. Similarly, a meta-analysis of 23,099 individuals demonstrated that dietary zinc blocks the progression of AMD and delays its progression [29].

Reports show, zinc supplementation may suppress oxidative stress induced by type 2 diabetes via insulin production and secretion processes [30]. Interestingly, zinc facilitates phosphorylation of the insulin receptor by allowing the transportation of more glucose into the cells. In this context, different studies showed that detection of thiobarbituric acid reactive substances in plasma was decreased in patients with type 2 diabetes treated with nutrimental supplements with zinc [30]. Evidence shows that zinc improves insulin sensitivity and reduces chronic hyperglycemia in type 2 diabetes [31]. Zinc suppresses the proliferation of cancerous cells by several mechanisms such as the inhibition of the mitochondrial terminal oxidation, electron transport and mitochondrial respiration, and the stimulation of the apoptogenic pathway [4]. Data from epidemiologic studies found that dietary zinc intake may reduce the risk of cancer [32]. In prostate cancer cells, zinc is accumulated in the expression of the zinc uptake transporter, ZIP1 [33]. The accumulated zinc exerts its antiproliferative activity toward the prostate cancer cells via activation of MAPK's [4]. In colorectal cancer, zinc was found to activate Raf-1-MEK-MAPK kinases, followed by the activation of Elk-1-dependent trans-reporter gene expression [4].

## Ascorbic Acid (Vitamin C)

Ascorbic acid or vitamin C (AA) is a cofactor for many enzyme-catalyzed reactions, such as maintaining connective and vascular tissue's integrity, enhancing the collagen biosynthesis and iron absorption, modulating the leukocyte and hematopoiesis functioning, neuroprotection, and hydroxylation of lysine and proline [4].

Data from population-based studies show a correlation between aging and reducing ascorbate levels in tissues [4]. AA level reduces for nearly 50% in leukocytes in individuals at the age of 85 and above compared to those at the age of 60 [34]. Despite the limited available evidence on ascorbate level in human brains, a previous study has reported that ascorbate level in the cerebral cortex declines for nearly 77% of individuals at age 80 and older compared to those at age 50 and younger [35]. A study showed that ascorbate shortage contributes to the dysregulation of 5hmC, which subsequently contributes to age-related neurodegenerative diseases [36]. Research evidence has demonstrated the potential protective function of ascorbate in neurodegenerative diseases [4]. Ascorbate supplementation markedly improves the differentiation of midbrain-derived neural stem cells against dopaminergic neurons, which is associated with TET-mediated 5hmC generation and Jmjd3-catalyzed loss of H3K27m3 [37]. In this regard, these findings imply that ascorbate plays a critical role in dopaminergic neuron differentiation [4]. Studies show, a high concentration of AA induces cytotoxicity against cancer cells in vitro and can delay tumor growth in xenograft models [4]. Notably, some research has emerged to suggest that AA improved endothelial function in diabetic patients [38].

## Vitamin E

Vitamin E usually, found in food, includes four tocopherols and four tocotrienols. Among all isoforms of vitamin E, $\gamma$-tocopherol is the primary form of vitamin E in the diet and exerts potent antioxidant properties [39].

An emerging role for tocopherols and tocotrienols in response to neuroinflammation has been demonstrated, and positive effects on oxidative damage and AD pathology have been proposed. The proposed aspects of the neuroinflammatory activity of this vitamin include the regulation of AD-associated enzymes, such as COX-2, 5-lipoxygenase, and NADPH oxidase [4]. Research evidence indicates that tocopherols and tocotrienols benefit in the stimulation of phosphoprotein phosphatase 2A, a phosphatase that plays a crucial role in tau homeostasis, which is lowered in human AD brains [40]. Moreover, data from clinical evidence showed that tocopherol and tocotrienol supplementation in AD patients reduces lipid peroxidation compared with the control [41].

Data from a cross-sectional study showed a positive relationship between bone mineral density and $\alpha$-tocopherol level in the elderly Chinese population [42]. A beneficial effect of tocopherol and tocotrienol supplementation has also been documented on the incidence of cardiovascular disease. On the other side, the decrease of CD36 scavenger receptor expression indicates the role of tocopherols and tocotrienols in the reduction of foam cell formation and atherosclerosis [43]. Another report showed that tocopherols and tocotrienols reduced pain-debilitating symptoms elicited by painful inflammation. The reduction of cytokine production has also been demonstrated in humans with arthritis [44]. Overall, tocopherols and tocotrienols might be promising tools for alleviating oxidative stress and preventing age-related diseases.

## Ubiquinone

Ubiquinone (UQ) or coenzyme Q10 is synthesized within the body cells or can be obtained from the diet [45]. Studies suggest, a reduction in the levels of UQ during aging may be involved in the predominant factors to develop age-related diseases [46]. Data from randomized controlled clinical trials demonstrated that supplementation with UQ induces an improvement in vascular dysfunction and decreases the glycemic response [47].

Another study reported that UQ enhances nerve conduction parameters of diabetic polyneuropathy and ameliorates oxidative stress without significant undesirable effects [4]. As well as evidence further supported that UQ increases insulin sensitivity and improves β cell function in diabetic patients [48].

In the case of neurodegenerative diseases, UQ plays a central role in the cellular dysfunction of PD since levels of UQ were relatively low in patients [4]. On the other hand, the treatment with UQ reduced the cellular pathophysiological alterations related to mitochondrial dysfunction in PD patients. These results show that a high concentration UQ administration may downregulate the functional decline experienced during the early stage of patients [4].

## Calorie Restriction and Its Effect on Aging

The reduction of calories by 10–30% compared to a typical diet prolongs the longevity of different species; moreover, it is known that several alchemists had long periods of fasting as a common practice [49]. Studies suggest that caloric restriction (CR) may decrease the levels of insulin and blood pressure in humans [50]. These findings support the hypothesis that CR could delay the effects of age [51].Thus, several compounds have calorie restriction mimetic (CRM) activities and have the ability to mimic the anti-aging effects of CR.

### Resveratrol

It is a polyphenol compound isolated from the skins of red grapes. Of all the most-studied CRM's, resveratrol ranks first. Resveratrol was published as CRM through the selection of small molecular libraries for compounds that activate sirtuins and extend the shelf life of different organisms (yeast, worms, flies, fish, and mice) [52, 53]. Resveratrol triggers the expression of antioxidant enzymes; additionally, it stimulates the activity of SIRT1 and AMPK and metabolic regulators of tissues [54]. The results of the research showed that it could mimic the benefits associated with caloric restriction. In this context, resveratrol was administered to 38 obese subjects and showed an increase in mitochondrial activity and fat oxidation [54]; on the other side, in another clinical study with 17 volunteers with type 2 diabetes, a decrease in systolic blood pressure and intrahepatic lipid content were observed after treatment [55]. Although the effect of extending the longevity of resveratrol has not been fully verified in humans, and clinical results of studies are quite promising, several works have shown contrasting effects of resveratrol due to the different conditions that are managed, such as the number of participants, their age, sex, health status, lifestyle, dose, environment (with or without food), and type of administration (capsule, tablet, powder, gel capsules, among others). So considering these aspects in future studies on the effects of resveratrol could help to study in greater depth the mechanisms of action of this compound [56].

## Rapamycin

Rapamycin is a macrolide isolated from *Streptomyces hygroscopicus*, a bacteria from Pascua Island (Rapa Nui). It has functions as an antibiotic, an immune suppressant drug, and it is also proposed as a CRM. After the first studies, it was found that rapamycin could induce the extension of the replicative life of yeast through the inhibition of TOR signaling [57]. This compound could extend the lifetime useful in 20-month-old mice in correlation with TOR activity [58]. These studies were the basis of the research to determine the function of rapamycin as a CRM, due to its modulating properties over proteostasis. In addition, studies suggest that rapamycin can be combined with other compounds (metformin, losartan, statins, propranolol, and aspirin among others) to potentiate their anti-aging activity [59].

## Metformin

Metformin has gained importance in gerontology since it has several functions, such as being a medication used for the treatment of type 2 diabetes by increasing insulin sensitivity and AMPK activity. Their CRM activity was assessed since metformin treatment enhances insulin sensitivity, glycolysis, and suppresses gluconeogenesis. Recently, it was proposed that metformin might increase the longevity of frailty patients [60]. In this context, several studies confirmed the longevity effect of metformin on worms, mice, flies, and rats [61]. Interestingly, in diabetic and cardiovascular disease patients treated with metformin, rates of survival have increased [62, 63]. Moreover, treatment with metformin among patients with diabetes reduces the risk of dementia [64].

## Inductors of Autophagy and its Impact on Aging

Autophagy has a role in homeostasis, which plays an essential role in the maintenance of cellular physiology and the prevention of cellular damage. Among the inducers of autophagy have been described the already-mentioned rapamycin, resveratrol, and polyamines; however, only polyamines have demonstrated results in clinical research in humans [65]. It is known that these compounds can induce the canonical autophagy pathway, which includes inactivation of the mammalian objective of the rapamycin complex 1 (mTORC1), allowing phosphorylation and activation of the Unc-51 complex (Ulk1/2), where the cascade of the other members of the complex is subsequently activated, ULK as FIP200 and ATG13 [65].

## Polyamines

Spermidine is a polyamine capable of inducing the macroautophagy of cells. It induces autophagy by inhibiting acetyltransferases, such as EP300 [66], one of the essential negative regulators of autophagy. Studies show that it has a potential for activity equivalent to that of rapamycin as an autophagy activator [67]. Spermidine prolongs the lifespan and duration of the health of various organisms, such as yeasts, nematodes, flies, and mice. In humans, spermidine levels reduced during aging, suggesting the association of the reduction of these levels with the deterioration associated with age. Epidemiological evidence supports that foods rich in spermidine counteract cardiovascular diseases and cancer [68].

## Senolytic Compounds

During aging, these senescence cells accumulate in many tissues and pathological sites in multiple chronic diseases. Senolytic compounds are agents that selectively induce death in senescent cells [69]. Studies showed that the treatment of senescent cells with genetic or pharmacological methods delays, prevents, or improves multiple phenotypes related to age [70]. So, it is important to expand the use of these compounds in clinical studies to be able to include the effects of testing on multiple morbidities. If the senolytics drugs or other interventions directed to the processes of fundamental aging happen to be effective and safe in the clinical tests, these could transform geriatric medicine, allowing the prevention or the treatment of multiple diseases and functional deficits [71].

Several compounds showed to be senolytic compounds: *Curcumin* (a constituent of the rhizome of turmeric, eliminated the senescent cells of the intervertebral disc obtained from patients, as well as reduced the SASP), *Quercetin* (a flavonoid, found in dietary plants; this compound was found in combination with the anti-cancer drug dasatinib and had efficacy as senolytic in several types of senescent cells), *Rapamycin* (a macrolide which inhibits mTOR, is shown to improve health, and inhibits cellular senescence in multiple cell types; it inhibits cellular senescence in vitro and increases longevity in several species), *Berberine* (an isoquinoline alkaloid that has the ability to modulate senescent cells so it can potentially be used as a senolytic drug), *Piperlongumine* (an alkaloid isolated from long pepper, has the ability to preferentially induce cell death in senescent WI-38 fibroblasts generated by both radiation and replication and induced by oncogenes), *Fisetin* (a flavonoid present in fruits and vegetables that induces apoptosis in senescent HUVEC cells), and *Phloretin* (a flavonoid that at a concentration of 50 μM reduces the viability of senescent lymphoma cells [71]).

Although these are preliminary results, the impact that the senolytics will have on human health and illnesses is still unknown. It is interesting to determine the phenomenon that would happen if the senescent cells were eliminated from organisms and if aging and dysfunction would be delayed or pathological processes would be triggered [72]. Studies in mice have found that senotherapy can prevent, stop, and reverse different age-related diseases [73]. Recently, in the first pilot study performed in humans (14 patients), senolytics drugs (dasatinib and quercetin) were used to treat Idiopathic Pulmonary Fibrosis; it was proved to be encouraging, since results showed that targeting senescent cells can alleviate the functional consequences of diseases in humans [74]. Later, a second preliminary study from a clinical trial of dasatinib plus quercetin in individuals with diabetic kidney disease showed important findings, which were verified not only in analysis of blood but also in changes in skin and fat tissue senescent cell abundance, with a decrease in circulating SASP factors [75].

## Activators of Telomerase

Telomerase is an enzyme with reverse transcriptase activity whose function is to replicate DNA at the ends of eukaryotic chromosomes, thus lengthening telomeres. However, telomerase is repressed after birth, resulting in a shortening of the telomere after each cell division. Evidence shows that a reduction in telomerase activity causes cells to bypass senescence [76].

The overexpression of telomerase in mice shows that it was sufficient to delay different pathologies associated with age as cognitive deterioration [77]. The activators of telomerase are important for the development of anti-aging compounds. The most studied activator low-power telomerase TA-65 (isolated from *Astragalus membranaceus*) was shown to induce a slight increase in telomere length in humans [78] as well as improve several age-related parameters.

## Drugs with Effects over Epigenetics and Aging

The epigenetic drugs have shown quite exciting results in the aging research field because they are capable of modulating the enzymes involved in gene-environmental mechanisms associated with age-related diseases. Drugs designed to modulate epigenetic targets, such as HDAC inhibitors, have been used in clinical trials. It is known that the therapeutic application of HDAC inhibitors resulted in the affectation of the transcription of several genes and processes, such as the suppression of tumors due to transcriptional reactivation of silent tumor suppressor genes and the transcriptional repression of proto-oncogenes [79]. Numerous studies have identified HDAC inhibitors as candidate drugs for the treatment of neurodegenerative disorders. Therefore, the development of specific drugs aimed at HDAC activity could be an anti-aging strategy with encouraging results.

On the other side, in recent years the therapeutic modulators of NAD-dependent class III histone deacetylases, so-called sirtuins, have caught attention for aging research since they seem to play a key role during cell response to a variety of stresses (oxidative or genotoxic) and are involved in senescence [80]. Evidence suggests that the activation or inhibition of sirtuins [81] may be useful to prevent or treat age-related diseases, where they showed protection against neurodegenerative diseases [82]. For instance, selective inhibitors of SIRT2 and AGK-2 has been reported to have protective effects against PD and in the treatment of AD [82]. Additionally, the inhibition of Sirt1 showed to sensitize cells for DNA-damaging cancer therapeutics and decrease tumor growth; some of them are already in clinical trials.

## Conclusions

As seen in this chapter, several compounds have anti-aging functions, such as antioxidants, CRM, autophagy inducers, senolytic compounds, among others, and may have the ability to possess anti-aging activity because they participate in the regulation of both the route and factors involved in aging. Although most of the results obtained from different investigations are still preliminary, it is worth mentioning that in recent years, clinical trials have begun in humans, with promising results; so more in-depth research should be carried out of these compounds, since the understanding and generation of molecular mechanisms generated using all these molecules could help us to develop new drugs for the treatment and prevention of chronic diseases associated with age.

## References

1. Hung WW, Ross JS, Boockvar KS, Siu AL. Recent trends in chronic disease, impairment and disability among older adults in the United States. BMC Geriatr. 2011;11:47.
2. Liguori I, Russo G, Curcio F, Bulli G, Aran L, Della-Morte D, et al. Oxidative stress, aging, and diseases. Clin Interv Aging. 2018;13:757–72.
3. Tan BL, Norhaizan ME. Nutrients and oxidative stress: friend or foe? Oxidative Med Cell Longev. 2018;2018:9719584.
4. Tan BL, Norhaizan ME, W-P-P L, Sulaiman Rahman H. Antioxidant and oxidative stress: a mutual interplay in age-related diseases. Front Pharmacol. 2018;9:1162.
5. Grune T, Schröder P, Biesalski HK. Low molecular weight antioxidants. Reactions, processes. Berlin: Springer; 2005. p. 77–90.
6. Sifuentes-Franco S, Pacheco-Moises FP. The role of oxidative stress, mitochondrial function, and autophagy in diabetic polyneuropathy. J Diabetes Res. 2017;2017:1673081.
7. Lu S, Wu D, Li G, Lv Z, Chen Z, Chen L, et al. Carbon dots-based ratiometric nanosensor for highly sensitive and selective detection of mercury (II) ions and glutathione. RSC Adv. 2016;6(105):103169–77.
8. Rotar O, Tenedja K, Arkhelyuk A, Rotar V, Davidencko I, Fediv V. Preparation of chitosan nanoparticles loaded with glutathione for diminishing tissue ischemia-reperfusion injury. Int J Adv Eng Nano Technol. 2014;1:19–23.

9. Peter C, Braidy N, Zarka M, Welch J, Bridge W. Therapeutic approaches to modulating glutathione levels as a pharmacological strategy in Alzheimer's disease. Curr Alzheimer Res. 2015;12(4):298–313.
10. Espinola-Klein C, Rupprecht HJ, Bickel C, Schnabel R, Genth-Zotz S, Torzewski M, et al. Glutathione peroxidase-1 activity, atherosclerotic burden, and cardiovascular prognosis. Am J Cardiol. 2007;99(6):808–12.
11. Mischley LK, Leverenz JB, Lau RC, Polissar NL, Neradilek MB, Samii A, et al. A randomized, double-blind phase I/IIa study of intranasal glutathione in Parkinson's disease. Mov Dis. 2015;30(12):1696–701.
12. Nascimento-Souza MA, de Paiva PG, Perez-Jimenez J, Do Carmo Castro Franceschini S, Ribeiro AQ. Estimated dietary intake and major food sources of polyphenols in elderly of Vicosa, Brazil: a population-based study. Eur J Nutr. 2018;57(2):617–27.
13. Panche AN, Diwan AD, Chandra SR. Flavonoids: an overview. J Nutr Sci. 2016;5:e47.
14. Ivey KL, Hodgson JM, Croft KD, Lewis JR, Prince RL. Flavonoid intake and all-cause mortality. Am J Clin Nutr. 2015;101(5):1012–20.
15. Fink BN, Steck SE, Wolff MS, Britton JA, Kabat GC, Schroeder JC, et al. Dietary flavonoid intake and breast cancer risk among women on Long Island. Am J Epidemiol. 2007;165(5):514–23.
16. Braidy N, Behzad S, Habtemariam S, Ahmed T, Daglia M, Nabavi SM, et al. Neuroprotective effects of Citrus fruit-derived flavonoids, Nobiletin and Tangeretin in Alzheimer's and Parkinson's disease. CNS Neurol Disord Drug Targets. 2017;16(4):387–97.
17. Paliwal C, Ghosh T, George B, Pancha I, Maurya R, Chokshi K, et al. Microalgal carotenoids: potential nutraceutical compounds with chemotaxonomic importance. Algal Res. 2016;15:24–31.
18. Yaroshevich IA, Krasilnikov PM, Rubin AB. Functional interpretation of the role of cyclic carotenoids in photosynthetic antennas via quantum chemical calculations. Comput Theor Chem. 2015;1070:27–32.
19. Eisenhauer B, Natoli S, Liew G, Flood VM. Lutein and zeaxanthin-food sources, bioavailability and dietary variety in age-related macular degeneration protection. Nutrients. 2017;9(2):120.
20. Chang J, Zhang Y, Li Y, Lu K, Shen Y, Guo Y, et al. NrF2/ARE and NF-kappaB pathway regulation may be the mechanism for lutein inhibition of human breast cancer cell. Future Oncol (London, England). 2018;14(8):719–26.
21. Carini F, David S, Tomasello G, Mazzola M, Damiani P, Rappa F, et al. Colorectal cancer: an update on the effects of lycopene on tumor progression and cell proliferation. J Biol Regul Homeost Agents. 2017;31(3):769–74.
22. Zu K, Mucci L, Rosner BA, Clinton SK, Loda M, Stampfer MJ, et al. Dietary lycopene, angiogenesis, and prostate cancer: a prospective study in the prostate-specific antigen era. J Natl Cancer Inst. 2014;106(2):djt430.
23. Rao L, Rao A. Oxidative stress and antioxidants in the risk of osteoporosis—role of the antioxidants lycopene and polyphenols. In: Topics in osteoporosis. Crotia: IntechOpen; 2013.
24. Xu J, Song C, Song X, Zhang X, Li X. Carotenoids and risk of fracture: a meta-analysis of observational studies. Oncotarget. 2017;8(2):2391–9.
25. Hayhoe RPG, Lentjes MAH, Mulligan AA, Luben RN, Khaw KT, Welch AA. Carotenoid dietary intakes and plasma concentrations are associated with heel bone ultrasound attenuation and osteoporotic fracture risk in the European Prospective Investigation into Cancer and Nutrition (EPIC)-Norfolk cohort. Br J Nutr. 2017;117(10):1439–53.
26. Ugarte M, Grime GW, Osborne NN. Distribution of trace elements in the mammalian retina and cornea by use of particle-induced X-ray emission (PIXE): localisation of zinc does not correlate with that of metallothioneins. Metallomics. 2014;6(2):274–8.
27. Aoki A, Inoue M, Nguyen E, Obata R, Kadonosono K, Shinkai S, et al. Dietary n-3 fatty acid, alpha-tocopherol, zinc, vitamin D, vitamin C, and beta-carotene are associated with age-related macular degeneration in Japan. Sci Rep. 2016;6:20723.
28. Age-Related Eye Disease Study Research Group. A randomized, placebo-controlled, clinical trial of high-dose supplementation with vitamins C and E, beta carotene, and zinc for

age-related macular degeneration and vision loss: AREDS report no. 8. Arch Ophthalmol (Chicago: 1960). 2001;119(10):1417–36.
29. Gorusupudi A, Nelson K, Bernstein PS. The age-related eye disease 2 study: micronutrients in the treatment of macular degeneration. Adv Nutr. 2017;8(1):40–53.
30. Anderson RA, Roussel AM, Zouari N, Mahjoub S, Matheau JM, Kerkeni A. Potential antioxidant effects of zinc and chromium supplementation in people with type 2 diabetes mellitus. J Am Coll Nutr. 2001;20(3):212–8.
31. Vashum KP, McEvoy M, Milton AH, Islam MR, Hancock S. Attia J. is serum zinc associated with pancreatic beta cell function and insulin sensitivity in pre-diabetic and normal individuals? Findings from the Hunter Community study. PLoS One. 2014;9(1):e83944.
32. Costello LC, Franklin RB. A comprehensive review of the role of zinc in normal prostate function and metabolism; and its implications in prostate cancer. Arch Biochem Biophys. 2016;611:100–12.
33. Franklin RB, Costello LC. Zinc as an anti-tumor agent in prostate cancer and in other cancers. Arch Biochem Biophys. 2007;463(2):211–7.
34. Attwood EC, Robey E, Kramer JJ, Ovenden N, Snape S, Ross J, et al. A survey of the haematological, nutritional and biochemical state of the rural elderly with particular reference to vitamin C. Age Ageing. 1978;7(1):46–56.
35. Schaus R. The ascorbic acid content of human pituitary, cerebral cortex, heart, and skeletal muscle and its relation to age. Am J Clin Nutr. 1957;5(1):39–41.
36. Al-Mahdawi S, Virmouni SA, Pook MA. The emerging role of 5-hydroxymethylcytosine in neurodegenerative diseases. Front Neurosci. 2014;8:397.
37. He XB, Kim M, Kim SY, Yi SH, Rhee YH, Kim T, et al. Vitamin C facilitates dopamine neuron differentiation in fetal midbrain through TET1- and JMJD3-dependent epigenetic control manner. Stem Cells. 2015;33(4):1320–32.
38. Ashor AW, Lara J, Mathers JC, Siervo M. Effect of vitamin C on endothelial function in health and disease: a systematic review and meta-analysis of randomised controlled trials. Atherosclerosis. 2014;235(1):9–20.
39. Joshi YB, Pratico D. Vitamin E in aging, dementia, and Alzheimer's disease. BioFactors (Oxford, England). 2012;38(2):90–7.
40. Voronkov M, Braithwaite SP, Stock JB. Phosphoprotein phosphatase 2A: a novel druggable target for Alzheimer's disease. Future Med Chem. 2011;3(7):821–33.
41. Morris MC, Evans DA, Tangney CC, Bienias JL, Wilson RS, Aggarwal NT, et al. Relation of the tocopherol forms to incident Alzheimer disease and to cognitive change. Am J Clin Nutr. 2005;81(2):508–14.
42. Shi WQ, Liu J, Cao Y, Zhu YY, Guan K, Chen YM. Association of dietary and serum vitamin E with bone mineral density in middle-aged and elderly Chinese adults: a cross-sectional study. Br J Nutr. 2016;115(1):113–20.
43. Ozer NK, Negis Y, Aytan N, Villacorta L, Ricciarelli R, Zingg JM, et al. Vitamin E inhibits CD36 scavenger receptor expression in hypercholesterolemic rabbits. Atherosclerosis. 2006;184(1):15–20.
44. Bhattacharya I, Saxena R, Gupta V. Efficacy of vitamin E in knee osteoarthritis management of north Indian geriatric population. Ther Adv Musculoskelet Dis. 2012;4(1):11–9.
45. Quinzii CM, DiMauro S, Hirano M. Human coenzyme Q10 deficiency. Neurochem Res. 2007;32(4–5):723–7.
46. Motohashi N, Gallagher R, Anuradha V, Gollapudi R. Co-enzyme Q10 (ubiquinone): it's implication in improving the life style of the elderly. Med Clin Rev. 2017;3(S1):10.
47. Mantle D. Coenzyme Q10 supplementation for diabetes and its complications: an overview. Br J Diabetes. 2017;17(4):145–8.
48. Raygan F, Rezavandi Z, Dadkhah Tehrani S, Farrokhian A, Asemi Z. The effects of coenzyme Q10 administration on glucose homeostasis parameters, lipid profiles, biomarkers of inflammation and oxidative stress in patients with metabolic syndrome. Eur J Nutr. 2016;55(8):2357–64.
49. Ribarič S. Diet and aging. Oxidative Med Cell Longev. 2012;2012:741468.

50. Spindler SR, Mote PL, Flegal JM, Teter B. Influence on longevity of blueberry, cinnamon, green and black tea, pomegranate, sesame, curcumin, morin, pycnogenol, quercetin, and taxifolin fed iso-calorically to long-lived, F1 hybrid mice. Rejuvenation Res. 2013;16(2):143–51.
51. Pallauf K, Chin D, Günther I, Birringer M, Lüersen K, Schultheiß G, et al. Resveratrol, lunularin and dihydroresveratrol do not act as caloric restriction mimetics when administered intraperitoneally in mice. Sci Rep. 2019;9(1):4445.
52. Wood JG, Rogina B, Lavu S, Howitz K, Helfand SL, Tatar M, et al. Sirtuin activators mimic caloric restriction and delay ageing in metazoans. Nature. 2004;430(7000):686–9.
53. Baur JA, Pearson KJ, Price NL, Jamieson HA, Lerin C, Kalra A, et al. Resveratrol improves health and survival of mice on a high-calorie diet. Nature. 2006;444(7117):337–42.
54. Crandall JP, Oram V, Trandafirescu G, Reid M, Kishore P, Hawkins M, et al. Pilot study of resveratrol in older adults with impaired glucose tolerance. J Gerontol Ser A Biol Sci Med Sci. 2012;67(12):1307–12.
55. Dash S, Xiao C, Morgantini C, Szeto L, Lewis GF. High-dose resveratrol treatment for 2 weeks inhibits intestinal and hepatic lipoprotein production in overweight/obese men. Arterioscler Thromb Vasc Biol. 2013;33(12):2895–901.
56. Ramírez-Garza SL, Laveriano-Santos EP, Marhuenda-Muñoz M, Storniolo CE, Tresserra-Rimbau A, Vallverdú-Queralt A, et al. Health effects of resveratrol: results from human intervention trials. Nutrients. 2018;10(12):1892.
57. Powers RW 3rd, Kaeberlein M, Caldwell SD, Kennedy BK, Fields S. Extension of chronological life span in yeast by decreased TOR pathway signaling. Genes Dev. 2006;20(2):174–84.
58. Harrison DE, Strong R, Sharp ZD, Nelson JF, Astle CM, Flurkey K, et al. Rapamycin fed late in life extends lifespan in genetically heterogeneous mice. Nature. 2009;460(7253):392–5.
59. Blagosklonny MV. Does rapamycin slow down time? Oncotarget. 2018;9(54):30210–2.
60. Wang CP, Lorenzo C, Espinoza SE. Frailty attenuates the impact of metformin on reducing mortality in older adults with type 2 diabetes. J Endocrinol Diabetes Obes. 2014;2(2):1031.
61. Novelle MG, Ali A, Dieguez C, Bernier M, de Cabo R. Metformin: a hopeful promise in aging research. Cold Spring Harb Perspect Med. 2016;6(3):a025932.
62. Scarpello JH. Improving survival with metformin: the evidence base today. Diabetes Metab. 2003;29(4 Pt 2):6s36–43.
63. Yin M, Zhou J, Gorak EJ, Quddus F. Metformin is associated with survival benefit in cancer patients with concurrent type 2 diabetes: a systematic review and meta-analysis. Oncologist. 2013;18(12):1248–55.
64. Patrone C, Eriksson O, Lindholm D. Diabetes drugs and neurological disorders: new views and therapeutic possibilities. Lancet Diabetes Endocrinol. 2014;2(3):256–62.
65. Barbosa MC, Grosso RA, Fader CM. Hallmarks of aging: an autophagic perspective. Front Endocrinol (Lausanne). 2019;9:790.
66. Sacitharan PK, Lwin S, Gharios GB, Edwards JR. Spermidine restores dysregulated autophagy and polyamine synthesis in aged and osteoarthritic chondrocytes via EP300. Exp Mol Med. 2018;50(9):123.
67. Du Toit A, De Wet S, Hofmeyr JHS, Müller-Nedebock KK, Loos B. The precision control of autophagic flux and vesicle dynamics—a micropattern Approach. Cells. 2018;7(8):94.
68. Madeo F, Bauer MA, Carmona-Gutierrez D, Kroemer G. Spermidine: a physiological autophagy inducer acting as an anti-aging vitamin in humans? Autophagy. 2018;15(1):165–8.
69. Kirkland JL, Tchkonia T, Zhu Y, Niedernhofer LJ, Robbins PD. The clinical potential of Senolytic drugs. J Am Geriatr Soc. 2017;65(10):2297–301.
70. Yousefzadeh MJ, Zhu Y, McGowan SJ, Angelini L, Fuhrmann-Stroissnigg H, Xu M, et al. Fisetin is a senotherapeutic that extends health and lifespan. EBioMedicine. 2018;36:18–28.
71. Malavolta M, Bracci M, Santarelli L, Sayeed MA, Pierpaoli E, Giacconi R, et al. Inducers of senescence, toxic compounds, and Senolytics: the multiple faces of Nrf2-activating phytochemicals in Cancer adjuvant therapy. Mediat Inflamm. 2018;2018:4159013.
72. Childs BG, Durik M, Baker DJ, van Deursen JM. Cellular senescence in aging and age-related disease: from mechanisms to therapy. Nat Med. 2015;21(12):1424–35.

73. Kang DH, Park YS, Lee DY. Senotherapy for attenuation of cellular senescence in aging and organ implantation. J Ind Eng Chem. 2018;60:1–8.
74. Justice JN, Nambiar AM, Tchkonia T, LeBrasseur NK, Pascual R, Hashmi SK, et al. Senolytics in idiopathic pulmonary fibrosis: results from a first-in-human, open-label, pilot study. EBioMedicine. 2019;40:554–63.
75. Hickson LJ, Langhi Prata LGP, Bobart SA, Evans TK, Giorgadze N, Hashmi SK, et al. Senolytics decrease senescent cells in humans: preliminary report from a clinical trial of Dasatinib plus quercetin in individuals with diabetic kidney disease. EBioMedicine. 2019;47:446–56.
76. Hornsby PJ. Telomerase and the aging process. Exp Gerontol. 2007;42(7):575–81.
77. Bär C, Blasco MA. Telomeres and telomerase as therapeutic targets to prevent and treat age-related diseases. F1000Res. 2016;5:F1000. Faculty Rev-89
78. Harley CB, Liu W, Blasco M, Vera E, Andrews WH, Briggs LA, et al. A natural product telomerase activator as part of a health maintenance program. Rejuvenation Res. 2011;14(1):45–56.
79. Boumber Y, Issa JP. Epigenetics in cancer: what's the future? Oncology (Williston Park). 2011;25(3):220–6. 8
80. Vaiserman AM, Pasyukova EG. Epigenetic drugs: a novel anti-aging strategy? Front Genet. 2012;3:224.
81. Carafa V, Nebbioso A, Altucci L. Sirtuins and disease: the road ahead. Front Pharmacol. 2012;3:4.
82. Mai A. Small-molecule chromatin-modifying agents: therapeutic applications. Epigenomics. 2010;2(2):307–24.

# Integrative Outlooks About Clinical and Biomedical Research in Ageing

13

C. García-Peña, Raúl Medina-Campos, E. Delgado-de Anda, and O. S. Barrera-Vázquez

## Abbreviations

| | |
|---|---|
| 3D | Three-dimensional |
| ADP | Adenosine diphosphate |
| AFAR | American Federation for Research on Ageing |
| AGE | Advanced Glycation End-products (AGE) |
| APOE | Apolipoprotein E |
| Asn297 | Asparagine 297 |
| BAT | Brown adipose tissue |
| BRCA1 | Breast Cancer 1 |
| BRCA2 | Breast Cancer 2 |
| CA-125 | Cancer Antigen 125 |
| CALERIE | Comprehensive Assessment of Long-term Effects of Reducing Intake of Energy |
| CpG | 5′—C—phosphate—G—3 |
| CR | Caloric restriction |
| CRAMP | Cathelicidin Related Antimicrobial Peptide |
| CRISPR-Cas9 | Clustered Regularly Interspaced Short Palindromic Repeats-Cas9 |
| CRON | Calorie Restriction with Optimum Nutrition |
| DAMPs | Damage-associated molecular pattern molecules |
| DNA | Deoxyribonucleic acid |
| EF-1α | Elongation Farctor 1 alpha |
| EGFR | Epidermal Growth Factor Receptor |
| FOXO3 | Forkhead box O3 |
| IGF-1 | Insulin/Insulin-like Growth Factor 1 |

C. García-Peña (✉) · R. Medina-Campos · E. Delgado-de Anda · O. S. Barrera-Vázquez
National Institute of Geriatrics, Mexico City, Mexico
e-mail: mcgarcia@inger.gob.mx; rmedina@inger.gob.mx



J. C. Gomez-Verjan, N. A. Rivero-Segura (eds.), *Clinical Genetics and Genomics of Aging*, https://doi.org/10.1007/978-3-030-40955-5_13

| | |
|---|---|
| IgG | Immunoglobulin G |
| IIS | Insulin/Insulin-like Growth Factor 1 Signalling |
| IL-6 | Interleukin 6 |
| lncRNA | long noncoding RNA |
| Meg3 | Maternally expressed 3 |
| miR-1248 | microRNA-1248 |
| miR-126-3p | miRNA-126-3p |
| miR-151a-3p | miRNA-151a-3p |
| miR-181a-5p | miRNA-181a-5p |
| miR-21 | microRNA-21 |
| miR-239 | microRNA-239 |
| miR-246 | miRNA-246 |
| MIR31HG | MIR31 Host Gene |
| MiR-34a | microRNA-34a |
| miR-71 | miRNA-71 |
| miRNA | microRNA |
| mTOR | mammalian target of rapamycin |
| NAD | Nicotinamide adenine dinucleotide |
| p-S6RP | phosphorylated S6 ribosomal protein |
| PTMs | Posttranslational modifications |
| RNA | ribonucleic acid |
| ROS | Reactive Oxygen Species |
| SASP | Senescence-associated with the secretory phenotype |
| SAβ-gal | Senescence-associated β-galactosidase |
| SIRT1 | Sirtuin 1 |
| SIRT2 | Sirtuin 2 |
| SIRT6 | Sirtuin 6 |
| TNFα | Tumor necrosis factor alpha |
| VSCFA-TG | Triacylglycerols containing very short chain fatty acids |
| γ-H2AX | Gamma-H2A histone family member X |

## Introduction

Ageing is a highly complex biological process that encompasses genetic, environmental, and evolutionary features [1]. The latest findings in the biology of ageing suggest that ageing is a plastic process and may be modified or even delayed [2–4], thus resulting in an increased lifespan [5]. Such a delay in ageing should also have the ability to postpone both physiological decline and age-related diseases across the life course, thus prolonging the healthy lifespan [4].

Advances in human genomics, proteomics, and pharmacogenomics have opened the path towards truly personalized medicine, with the identification of genes linked to diseases, the development of specifically targeted drugs, and the ability to associate specific genotypes with health conditions which can lead to a preventive or a predictive focus [6]. We are now able to understand the genetic basis of many diseases, which in turn allows for diverse applications in medical sciences [7], such as, the mutations in BRCA1 and BRCA2 and their relationship with susceptibility to breast cancer and ovarian cancer [8]; proteomics, on the other hand, allows the identification of proteins that intervene in physiological and pathological processes and act as biomarkers of specific conditions. Biomarkers have had an application for the early detection of certain types of cancer, such as the CA-125 biomarker for early-stage ovarian cancer [9], identification of phosphorylated proteins such as EGFR for colon cancer [10], c-Kit for gastrointestinal cancer [11], and Her2 for breast cancer [12].

Several genomics tools applied to geroscience have allowed a growing understanding of the biology of ageing. Several studies of the human genome by genetic, transcriptomic, and epigenomic methodologies have resulted in the identification of various positive linkage regions, genes, and pathways that are involved in the lifespan variation [13].

Although it is known that health and lifespan are heavily influenced by genetics [14], variations in the lifespan of different individuals within the same species seem to be more the result of the accumulation over time of molecular damage that compromises the function of the cells [15]. These molecular alterations can occur both at the genetic and epigenetic levels and depend on genetic, environmental, and stochastic factors [16]. This complex multifactorial mix determined characteristics, such as longevity and a healthy lifespan, which are central concerns of human existence (Fig. 13.1). This chapter describes different types of tools in genomics used in ageing research and their different applications in clinical scenarios.

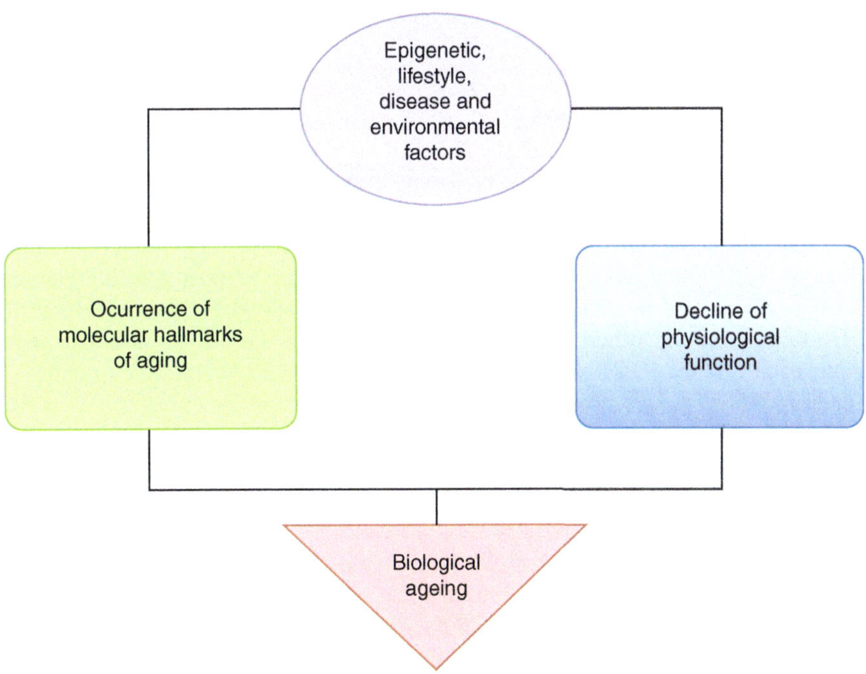


**Fig. 13.1** Biological ageing is a multifactorial process. The molecular hallmarks of ageing and physiological function are both influenced by genetic, epigenetic, and environmental factors

## Ageing Is Adjusted by Genetic, Environmental, and Stochastic Processes

Enough evidence suggests that ageing is the result of different events such as molecular damage, mutations, incomplete repair, genetic programs, and continued development, among others [16]. These events, in turn, are caused by genetic factors, environmental conditions, and even stochastic factors, which are mentioned below in this chapter.

## Influence of Genetic Factors in Ageing and Lifespan

Ageing is defined as the decline of physiological functions in several tissues and organs inducing an increasing probability of death [17]. The understanding of genetic factors involved in ageing has been limited due to the complexity of this process and the heterogeneity among individuals and even among tissues [18–20]. Tissue cells adopt a senescent phenotype as a consequence of multiple intrinsic, extrinsic, and stochastic factors [21]. The combination of these genetic factors is related to longevity and healthy ageing [22]. Although this decline is somewhat predictable, some individuals show a much slower decline and get to live past the age of 100. Studies in these individuals showed polymorphisms in some genes which are associated with long life, such as APOE and FOXO3. However, these associations have not been consistent across different populations, suggesting that ageing is rather polygenic [23].

## Environmental Conditions

Several studies show the influence of the environment on the ageing process [24]. Environmental factors may affect homeostasis and lead to the development of diseases, thus affecting the quality of life in older age [25]. They also produce cellular damage, which causes an accelerated shortening of the telomeres at the genetic level, accompanied by changes in DNA methylation, acetylation or deacetylation of histones, among others. Altogether, these changes induce an aberrant gene expression that may lead to physiological decline and cell, tissue, and organ dysfunction [26, 27].

Nutritional genomics studies the biologically active components of the diet and how they exert their functional effect [28, 29]. Dietary factors have a profound effect on many aspects of health and ageing. Behavior is another powerful modulator of health and ageing. Unhealthy lifestyles, such as the consumption of tobacco and alcohol [30], added to environmental pollution, and other factors such as oxidative stress, exposure to heavy metals, and endurance exercise are related to DNA damage, premature ageing, and age-related diseases such as cancer and atherosclerosis [31–34]. However, these factors are still studied to elucidate and have a deeper knowledge of these processes. On the other hand, healthy behaviors exert a positive effect on ageing. Regular exercise reduces psychological stress and oxidative stress and has an anti-inflammatory effect by reducing IL-6 and TNFα levels [35, 36].

## Individual Genotype

Individual differences in biological ageing may be due in part to the specific variations of the genotype but also genome-environment interactions [21, 37]. The maintenance of genomic stability and integrity is considered an essential factor required for cell viability and the overall longevity of an organism. The accumulation of physical damage is one of the leading causes of the ageing process. When considering oxidative damage as one of the causes of the damage of genetic material, these changes alter vital processes, such as replication, transcription, and translation, leading to genomic instability and personalized processes of ageing [38, 39].

There are three types of damage that DNA can suffer: mutations, epimutations, and changes induced by senescence [22]. Organisms have developed cellular mechanisms to repair damage to their genome, such as nucleotide and base cleavage system, repair coupled to transcription, and repair by homologous combination. However, as an organism ages, DNA-repairing mechanisms become increasingly ineffective; this leads to damage accumulation, which eventually leads to telomere shortening, age-related diseases, and ageing itself [21]. The response capacity of everyone to efficiently repair the cumulative DNA damage is strongly related to the exposure to the environment and stochastic factors. The contribution of each of these factors remains to be determined in future studies.

## Stochastic Factors

Ageing is no longer regarded as a programmed process, but rather the result of damage accumulation, which results from stochastic (i.e. random) events or exposures [40]. The variables that affect the ageing of an organism are the result of chance and must be studied from a probabilistic approach. According to the stochastic theories of ageing, random factors may induce ageing directly (by nonspecified mechanisms) and increase the probability of developing age-related diseases.

Different stochastic theories of ageing focus on specific mechanisms that may lead to ageing. The catastrophic error theory poses that the accumulation of errors in protein synthesis causes damage in cell function. The theory of cross-linking holds this process between proteins and other macromolecules responsible for ageing, while the theory of free radicals suggests that ageing is the result of inadequate protection against cell and tissue damage by free radicals and oxidative stress throughout life. Finally, the wear-and-tear theory poses that the cumulative damage that eventually leads to ageing and death is, in fact, the result of the continuous functioning of vital processes, during which stochastic errors gradually arise.

Thus, ageing and age-related diseases are probably not mediated by a single factor or primary mechanism, but rather their result of multiple mechanisms, some of which may be genetically determined, and others may be the result of environmental exposures or stochastic. However, not all these processes are currently accounted for, and their precise contribution to ageing remains unclear. It is, therefore, necessary to further aim research efforts at identifying these connections; this may eventually lead to the development of better treatments for age-related diseases and maybe even anti-ageing strategies.

## Biomarkers in Ageing

The heterogeneity of ageing is such that two individuals of the same age may exhibit substantial differences regarding ageing features. The rate of ageing seems to be relatively variable from one individual to the other and is not easy to measure. Biomarkers that accurately correlate with the rate of ageing are, therefore, highly desirable and would be of great clinical use. They would not only allow differentiating persons with the same age but different biological ageing rates, but would also provide a quantitative frame of reference to define healthy ageing and better predict the remaining life expectancy at any age.

Since 2013, the American Federation for Research on Ageing (AFAR) has proposed that an ageing biomarker must meet the following requirements: (1) It must be able to predict the rate of ageing; (2) it should not influence the effects of the disease; (3) it should be able to be tested on repeated occasions without harming the individual; (4) it must be valid in both humans and laboratory animals.

Unfortunately, biomarkers that meet all the criteria proposed by AFAR are still lacking [41]. However, some biomarkers are already available that meet the first two requirements. They will be reviewed in this section (for more details, see Chap. 5).

### DNA and Chromosomic Biomarkers

#### Telomeres

Telomeres are complexes of ribonucleoproteins located at the end of chromosomes that shorten their length with progressing age. This shortening of telomeres is the result of the absence of the activity of an enzyme called telomerase, and in turn it induces several processes, such as apoptosis, senescence, or oncogenic transformation of somatic cells, affecting the health and lifespan of an individual [42]. Human telomere shortening has been mostly studied in leukocytes and linked not only to ageing and life expectancy [43] but also to age-related diseases, including cardiovascular diseases, neurological disorders, and cancer [44].

#### DNA Damage and Repair Biomarkers

Recently, a correlation has been described between cellular senescence and DNA damage in the fashion of double-stranded breaks [45] and genomic rearrangements [46]. Furthermore, the controlled induction of double-stranded breaks in the DNA of the murine liver results in the induction of age-related pathology [47]. Protein γ-H2AX is a factor of the histone complex that quickly phosphorylates after a doubled strand break occurs in DNA. It is, therefore, an essential participant in DNA repair, which makes it a reliable marker of DNA damage and, potentially, a useful biomarker of ageing. Likewise, other markers as CRAMP, EF-1α, stathmin, N-acetyl-glucosaminidase, and chitinase have been founded in serum during DNA damage [47].

### DNA Methylation

Methylation is the most common form of epigenetic modification of the DNA. It occurs in distinct patterns according to age, thus providing a reasonably suitable biomarker for ageing [47]. Analysis of DNA methylation patterns in blood has identified three CpG sites capable of predicting age with an absolute mean deviation from the chronological age of fewer than 5 years [48]. Besides, this biomarker has been promising in the study of age-related diseases, such as diabetes [49] (for more details, see Chap. 7).

## RNA and Transcriptome

### Transcriptome Profiles

Single-cell RNA sequencing technology (RNA-seq) has advanced rapidly, and its application has now expanded to the study of biomarkers of ageing. There is a variation of cell-to-cell expression, measured by single-cell RNA-seq of high-dimensional flow cytometry sorted T-cells and that this variation is associated with ageing and susceptibility to diseases related to this process [47]. Also, a recent study using gene expression profiles of whole blood from 14,983 patients showed a differential expression of 1497 genes in an age-dependent manner [47]. They were later used to calculate the transcriptomic profile of an individual's age. These pieces of evidence suggest that the transcriptome can be used as a marker to evaluate ageing.

### Noncoding RNA

Two classes of noncoding RNAs are intensely studied concerning ageing: micro RNAs (miRNAs) and long noncoding RNAs (lncRNAs).

MiRNAs are a class of small noncoding RNAs (21 to 23 nucleotides in length) in charge of regulating a wide range of biological processes, including metabolism and ageing [47], through the mechanism of base pairing. MiRNAs can reside in exosomes or bind to proteins or circulating lipoprotein factors, which makes them stable in plasma and readily measurable as biomarkers. MiR-34a was found to correlate with age-related hearing loss in both the murine model and humans [47]. Besides, miR-21 was determined as an inflammatory-type biomarker in a study conducted on 365 miRNAs in the plasma of healthy and old humans [47]. MiR-151a-3p, miR-181a-5p, and miR-1248 were significantly decreased in old humans, where it was determined that there is an association of these miRNAs with inflammatory processes [50]. A study of the expression of green fluorescent protein (GFP) driven by miRNA promoters showed that miR-126-3p correlated positively with age in 136 healthy subjects from 20 to 90 years of age [47]. Likewise, the levels of mir-71, mir-246, and mir-239 vary in adulthood through different individuals, considering them as predictors for an individual's life expectancy [51].

The long noncoding RNA (lncRNAs) are a different class of noncoding RNAs of approximately 200 nucleotides in length and lacking open reading frames [52]. Recent studies show the role of lncRNAs during ageing [47]. It was identified that MIR31HG is positively regulated in oncogenes induced by senescence and required for the repression of the INK4A locus mediated by Polycomb groups [53]. Other studies showed that Meg3 is positively regulated both in cardiovascular ageing and in senescent human umbilical venous endothelial cells [47]. Although the majority of studies of lncRNAs have been anecdotal, it is worth mentioning that the use of the CRISPR-Cas9 technique of functional lncRNAs41 will allow future studies to understand the functions of lncRNA in the ageing process [54] (for more details, see Chap. 10).

## Metabolism

Studies show that calorie restriction is the most consistent means to prolong life expectancy and health across several experimental models [55], ranging from yeasts to primates. It not only increases life expectancy, but it also delays the onset of many features and hallmarks of ageing, including age-related diseases. Transcriptional profiles are currently being applied and investigated. One of them is a caloric restriction (CR), which increases the response to oxidative stress and reduces the shortening of telomeres in chromosomes; this has a direct intervention in the repair of DNA damage. Data from human trials (such as CALERIE, Biosphere-2 and CRON) indicate that moderate CR accompanied by adequate nutrition has positive effects on health and dramatically reduces the multiple metabolic factors involved in the pathogenesis of disease chronicles, including type 2 diabetes, heart and cerebrovascular diseases, and cancer [56].

### Sensing of Nutrients

One of the best-studied routes in the sensing of nutrients is the signaling pathway of the Insulin/Insulin-like Growth Factor 1 (IGF-1), also known as IIS, which has a role in the detection of glucose levels and has the potential to modulate longevity [57]. IGF-1 shows a decrease in either wild-type mice or murine models of premature ageing, whereas if IIS activity is attenuated by one of several mechanisms, it extends life expectancy [47]. These results may suggest that members of the IIS pathway, such as growth hormone and IGF-1, may be used as biomarkers of ageing.

One of the main functions of the mechanical target of the rapamycin protein (mTOR) is to check if the amino acids are in high concentrations. Studies indicate that the inhibition of mTOR generates a prolongation in life expectancy [47], and in contrast to the IIS pathway, it was determined in aged humans and mice that mTOR activity increases with age in the ovarian surface epithelium, favoring the appearance of pathological processes [47]. On the other hand, studies in mature ovaries showed that the phosphorylated S6 ribosomal protein (p-S6RP or pS6) is used both as a downstream target protein and as a marker of the active mTOR pathway [47], so these characteristics make p-S6RP a useful biomarker of aging [58].

Sirtuins are a class of proteins with mono-ADP-ribosyltransferase, deacetylase, desuccinylase, demalonylase, demyristoylase, and depalmitoylase activity. In the ageing processes, low levels of NAD+ seem to downregulate sirtuin levels in turn. In primary human dermal fibroblast cultures, consecutive cell passages are associated with a downregulation of the sirtuins SIRT1 and SIRT6 and SIRT2 is also reduced with age in human peripheral mononuclear blood cells [47]. These findings suggest that sirtuins may be suitable biomarkers for ageing.

#### Protein Metabolism

After synthesis, many proteins undergo posttranslational modifications (PTMs), which may or may not be enzyme mediated. Carbamylation is a form of nonenzymatic PTM which appears to be related to ageing, because carbamylated proteins tend to accumulate in aged tissues. This feature makes the carbamylated proteins as molecular markers of ageing and diseases related to this process, including cardiovascular and kidney diseases [47].

Advanced glycation end-products (AGE) are the result of nonenzymatic glycation, which produces heterogeneous bioactive molecules, such as lipids, proteins, and nucleic acids [59]. The accumulation of AGEs in aged tissues leads to several processes, such as inflammation, obesity, apoptosis, and other adverse processes related to ageing [47]. These AGEs are detected by various techniques, such as gas chromatography, high-performance liquid chromatography, spectrometry, and immunochemical technique [60], which make them robust biomarkers that can be analyzed by different methodologies.

Another type of AGEs with potential as biomarkers of ageing are N-glycans. These glycoproteins are highly conserved in eukaryotes and are characterized by sugar chains attached to the nitrogen of the amide of asparagine. One such example is N-linked glycation in Asn297 of the Fc portion of IgG (IgG-G0), which may contribute to the low-grade pro-inflammatory state during the ageing process [61].

#### Lipid Metabolism

Serum lipid analysis has found that phosphosphingolipids are putative markers and biological modulators of healthy ageing [62]. However, the design of these studies should be reconsidered because patients were used as "control of unhealthy ageing" and were compared with a group of centenarians of "successful ageing", having as disagreement the chronological age between both groups [47]. It is not clear whether it was the age difference or the healthy ageing condition that contributed to the differences in lipidomics. On the other hand, studies show that triacylglycerols containing very short-chain fatty acids (VSCFA-TG) are proposed as possible biomarkers of ageing of the brown adipose tissue (BAT), which has been shown to have a reduction during ageing, influencing thermogenesis [63].

### Mitochondria and Oxidative Stress

Another critical group of biomarkers of ageing is the marker of oxidative stress. These are byproducts of oxidative damage to proteins that accrue with age.

Examples include o-tyrosine, 3-chlorotyrosine, and 3-nitrotyrosine, which result from oxidative damage to proteins; 8-iso prostaglandin F2α, which is a marker of damage to phospholipids; and 8-hydroxy 2′-deoxyguanosine and 8-hydroxyguanosine, which result from oxidative damage to nucleic acids [47]. The concentration of these biomarkers in body fluids can be detected through high-performance liquid chromatography and mass spectrometry.

It should be noted that free radicals, the source of oxidative stress, are produced mainly in the mitochondria. However, it has been found that dysfunctional mitochondria can also contribute to ageing independently of reactive oxygen species (ROS) [64]. For those reasons, other alternative strategies have been designed to measure mitochondrial dysfunction in both blood and muscle [65], such as the respirometric profile, which has been of great help to study this process (for more details, see Chap. 3).

## Cellular Senescence

Cellular senescence refers to the response of mitotically competent cells (cells that are not terminally differentiated and therefore can divide) against stimuli that have the potential to cause neoplastic transformations and which present an arrest in their cycle [47]. It has been found that in mitotic tissues, there is a gradual accumulation of senescent cells, which may eventually be a causative factor of ageing. For this reason, markers of cellular senescence may also be used as biomarkers for ageing. One of them is senescence-associated β-galactosidase (SAβ-gal), which shows an age-related increase in lysosomal mass [66], but it has a low specificity rate, which can generate false positives [67]. On the other hand, p16INK4A is considered a permanent marker of the cell cycle [68]. Finally, the activated and persistent response to DNA damage, shortening of telomeres and senescence-associated with the secretory phenotype (SASP) are other markers of cellular senescence.

## Inflammation and Intercellular Communication

While senescent cells no longer replicate, they are still metabolically active and secrete proteins in a recognizable pattern known as SASP. This is a widely heterogeneous group of proteins with autocrine and paracrine effects [47], including soluble signaling factors, such as interleukins, chemokines, and growth factors, as well as proteins that are associated with sterile inflammation, such as interleukin-6, tumor necrosis factor-alpha, monocyte chemoattractant, protein-1, matrix metalloproteinases, and IGF-binding proteins [69].

Damage-associated molecular pattern molecules (DAMPs), such as heat shock proteins, histones, high mobility group 1, and S100 box, make up a class of molecules released after a cell injury or death and mediates the immune response [47]. Given that ageing and cancer share some common origins and hallmarks, such as genomic instability, epigenetic alteration, aberrant telomeres, inflammation and immune injury, reprogrammed metabolism, and degradation system impairment, DAMPs may be potential biomarkers for both processes [70].

## Phenotype Biomarkers

Although most studies focus on longevity alone as a primary phenotype, other phenotypes have been explored, such as the quantification of external human features [47], which uses three-dimensional (3D) facial images and analyzes facial components associated with age, such as mouth width, nose width, and eye corner droop. This type of bioimage analysis has rendered relatively accurate calculations of the actual age, although this accuracy tended to fall with increasing age after 40 years [71].

## Integration of Biomarkers of Ageing

Biomarkers of ageing allow estimating the biological age of an organism (Table 13.1) while providing information on their health status. Different studies are looking for the integrated use of multiple biomarkers, in order to make the estimation of health status more accurate. As we could see throughout this chapter, there are a large

**Table 13.1** Biomarkers of ageing

| Biomarker class | Biomarker subclass | Biomarker | Tendency during ageing | References |
|---|---|---|---|---|
| DNA and chromosome | Telomere | Leukocyte telomere length | Decrease | [75] |
| | DNA repair | γ-H2A.X immunohistochemistry | Increase | [76–79] |
| | Epigenetic modification | DNA methylation | Global hypomethylation and local hypermethylation | [79] |
| RNA and transcriptome | Transcriptome profiles | Heterogeneity of CD38 in CD4 + CD27+ T cells | Decrease | [80] |
| | | Heterogeneity of CD197 in CD4 + CD25+ T cells | Increase | [80] |
| | | miR-34a, miR-21, miR-126-3p | Increase | [81–83] |
| | Circulating microRNAs (miRNAs) | miR-151a-3p, miR-181a-5p, miR-1248 | Decrease | [50] |
| | | MIR31HG | Decrease in cell senescence | [53] |
| | Long noncoding RNAs | AK156230 | Increase in cell senescence | [84] |
| | | Meg3 | Decrease in cell senescence | [85] |

(continued)

**Table 13.1** (continued)

| Biomarker class | Biomarker subclass | Biomarker | Tendency during ageing | References |
|---|---|---|---|---|
| | Nutrient sensing | Growth hormone and insulin/insulin-like growth factor 1 (IGF-1) | Decrease | [86–88] |
| | | Mechanistic target of rapamycin (mTOR) and pS6RP | Increase | [58, 89] |
| Metabolism | | NAD+, SIRT1, SIRT2, SIRT3, SIRT6 | Decrease | [47] |
| | Protein metabolism | Protein carbamylation, such as homocitrulline rate | Increase | [90, 91] |
| | | Advanced glycation end products and N-glycans | Increase | [47] |
| | Lipid metabolism | Triglycerides | Increase | [92] |
| Oxidative stress and mitochondria | | o-tyrosine, 3-chlorotyrosine, 3-nitrotyrosine, 8-iso prostaglandin F2α, 8-hydroxy-2′-deoxyguanosine, 8-hydroxyguanosine | Increase | [47, 93] |
| Cell senescence | | Senescence-associated β-galactosidase | Increase in cell senescence | [47] |
| | | p16INK4A | Increase in cell senescence | [68, 94] |
| Inflammation and intercellular communication | | Senescence-associated secretory phenotype | Increase | [47] |
| Phenotype | Physical function and anthropometry | Walking speed, chair stand, standing balance, grip strength, muscle mass | Decrease | [95] |
| | | Body mass index, waist circumference | Increase | [95] |
| | Facial features | Mouth width | Increase | [71] |
| | | Nose width | Increase | [71] |
| | | Mouth-nose distance | Increase | [71] |
| | | Eye corner slope | Decrease | [71] |

Biomarkers classified according to their type and their modulation in ageing

number of biomarkers that are candidates to determine human ageing. However, these biomarkers have considerable variability among different individuals because the ageing process has an intrinsic multicausal nature. So, a multisystemic integration of biomarkers to determine biological age is still reliably found.

Currently, thanks to the different analyses performed using new technologies and new knowledge on the molecular basis, there are leading to the discovery of many novel molecular markers. Some of these technologies are the omics techniques, such as metabolomics, proteomics or genomics, also induces data generation, offering an overview of new biomarkers of ageing. However, it remains to be clarified which markers can be an accurate, reliable predictor of ageing.

Among the various studies carried out to solve these questions, the MARK-AGE study was a project supported by the European Commission. The main objective of this project was to carry out a population study of approximately 3200 subjects to identify a set of ageing biomarkers, which together with correctly established parameters, would measure the biology of an individual, compared to the result that would only have using a biomarker individually [72].

A recent study conducted in the Dunedin cohort [73] combined measurements of telomere lengths, epigenetic clocks and composite biomarkers and compared them to clinically relevant outcomes, such as health status, physical function, cognitive decline, and personal signs of ageing. The 71–cytosine-phosphate-guanine epigenetic clock and biomarker composites were consistently related to these outcomes. In another study, neural networks were applied to predict an age by using measurements from necessary blood tests, such as albumin, glucose, alkaline phosphatase, urea, and erythrocytes [74].

It should be mentioned that although the objectives of those researchers sound encouraging and ambitious, the search for biomarkers of ageing for their application in the improvement of human health, and prevention of diseases related to ageing, will only increase the generation of data. The great part of the search for biomarkers has been as a result of the extensive studies of human cohorts, resulting in genomic, functional, phenotypic, and lifestyle data of the individuals studied (Table 13.1). Thus, due to the generation of these data and technological advances, possibly in the future, artificial intelligence programs will be able to reliably forecast the life of an individual, as well as the possible diseases that he may suffer in ageing; so these advances and discoveries will allow us to achieve a "personalized medical treatment" as a result of to the integration of biomarkers of ageing.

## Ageing Is a Treatable Condition

The sharp increase in human life expectancy around the world in the past two centuries has resulted in the emergence of age-related diseases and disabilities as major public health concerns. In response, global efforts are now aimed at generating strategies to increase both the productive and healthy period of individuals. To this purpose, it is essential to develop better therapies for age-related diseases, such as cancer, cardiovascular diseases, neurodegenerative diseases, type 2 diabetes, chronic obstructive pulmonary disease, and even the age-related susceptibility to infectious diseases. Research, development, and distribution of these treatments or therapies should be done in a faster way. One controversial way to make this happen is to recognize ageing as a treatable condition [96], albeit not a disease in itself. This recognition could generate improvements in the treatment of ageing, such as:

1. The general public will be encouraged to request and apply preventive therapies to improve ageing.
2. The medical and technological pharmaceutical industry will be encouraged to develop and market better therapies and technologies for ageing.
3. Health, life insurance and health care systems will get a new area of reimbursement practices, which will stimulate them and their personnel to promote healthy ageing.
4. Regulators and policymakers will be stimulated to increase public funds for research and development related to ageing. Scientists and students will be encouraged to raise the problem of ageing scientifically and vital.

An extension of the health span has not entirely accompanied the extension of the human lifespan. Most people experience a variable period of poor health at the end of their lives [97, 98]. For these reasons, it is imperative to develop strategies that not only allow us to increase life expectancy but also to delay and better treat age-related diseases [69, 98, 99]. It should be mentioned that there is evidence that shows that nonpharmaceutical interventions are also effective, particularly exercise, dietary regimens and lifestyle modifications [98]. On the other hand, several pharmaceutical pipelines have shown promising results, such as the blocking of factors involved in cellular signaling relevant to ageing. In this regard, mTOR and AMPK are particularly relevant [97, 98].

## Conclusions

Ageing is a highly complex biological process with multiple features. Strongly influenced by metabolic, environmental and genetic factors, which have been seen to act concurrently. To this day, the understanding of the molecular mechanisms that involve the cellular and molecular damage responsible for biological ageing remains poor, so this high complexity of all these processes has been the reason of why no single biomarker has reliably and adequately captured the concept of biological ageing, at least of healthy ageing. Still, with the implementation of new technologies, more and more potentially useful biomarkers are emerging.

However, the validation of these results is still under development, so it remains to be clarified which markers will be able to show a reliable prediction of biological ageing and provide an optimal measure of ongoing health. On the other hand, it is also essential to carry out a massive consensus with the participation of scientists, policymakers, and other interested parties, in order to objectively establish the clinical criteria for healthy and "unhealthy" ageing, thus allowing a better assessment and better informed clinical decisions, while at the same time providing encouragement for further research and development of effective evidence-based therapies for the treatment of age-related diseases.

## References


1. McHugh D, Gil J. Senescence and aging: causes, consequences, and therapeutic avenues. J Cell Biol. 2018;217(1):65–77.
2. Kirkwood TB, Austad SN. Why do we age? Nature. 2000;408(6809):233–8.
3. Sierra F, et al. Prospects for life span extension. Annu Rev Med. 2009;60:457–69.
4. Miller RA. Genes against aging. J Gerontol A Biol Sci Med Sci. 2012;67(5):495–502.
5. Goldman DP, et al. Substantial health and economic returns from delayed aging may warrant a new focus for medical research. Health Aff (Millwood). 2013;32(10):1698–705.
6. Esplin ED, Oei L, Snyder MP. Personalized sequencing and the future of medicine: discovery, diagnosis and defeat of disease. Pharmacogenomics. 2014;15(14):1771–90.
7. Marian AJ. Clinical applications of molecular genetic discoveries. Transl Res. 2016;168:6–14.
8. Mersch J, et al. Cancers associated with BRCA1 and BRCA2 mutations other than breast and ovarian. Cancer. 2015;121(2):269–75.
9. Scholler N, Urban N. CA125 in ovarian cancer. Biomark Med. 2007;1(4):513–23.
10. Rego RL, et al. Prognostic effect of activated EGFR expression in human colon carcinomas: comparison with EGFR status. Br J Cancer. 2009;102:165.
11. Koch C, Trojan J. Established and potential predictive biomarkers in gastrointestinal cancer – c-kit, Her2, Ras and beyond. Digestion. 2015;91(4):294–302.
12. Perrier A, et al. The extracellular domain of Her2 in serum as a biomarker of breast cancer. Lab Investig. 2018;98(6):696–707.
13. Deelen J, et al. Identifying the genomic determinants of aging and longevity in human population studies: progress and challenges. Bioessays. 2013;35(4):386–96.
14. Martin GM, Bergman A, Barzilai N. Genetic determinants of human health span and life span: progress and new opportunities. PLoS Genet. 2007;3(7):e125.
15. Kirkwood TBL. Time of our lives. What controls the length of life? EMBO Rep. 2005;6 Spec No(Suppl 1):S4–8.
16. Gladyshev VN. Aging: progressive decline in fitness due to the rising deleteriome adjusted by genetic, environmental, and stochastic processes. Aging Cell. 2016;15(4):594–602.
17. Wheeler HE, Kim SK. Genetics and genomics of human ageing. Philos Trans R Soc Lond B Biol Sci. 2011;366(1561):43–50.
18. Mitnitski A, Howlett SE, Rockwood K. Heterogeneity of human aging and its assessment. J Gerontol A Biol Sci Med Sci. 2017;72(7):877–84.
19. Lowsky DJ, et al. Heterogeneity in healthy aging. J Gerontol A Biol Sci Med Sci. 2014;69(6):640–9.
20. Curtius K, et al. A molecular clock infers heterogeneous tissue age among patients with Barrett's esophagus. PLoS Comput Biol. 2016;12(5):e1004919.
21. Rodríguez-Rodero S, et al. Aging genetics and aging. Aging Dis. 2011;2(3):186–95.
22. Fraga MF. Genetic and epigenetic regulation of aging. Curr Opin Immunol. 2009;21(4):446–53.
23. Abondio P, et al. The genetic variability of APOE in different human populations and its implications for longevity. Genes. 2019;10(3):222.
24. de Magalhães JP, et al. Genome-environment interactions that modulate aging: powerful targets for drug discovery. Pharmacol Rev. 2012;64(1):88–101.
25. Farage MA, et al. Intrinsic and extrinsic factors in skin ageing: a review. Int J Cosmet Sci. 2008;30(2):87–95.
26. Nicolia V, Lucarelli M, Fuso A. Environment, epigenetics and neurodegeneration: focus on nutrition in Alzheimer's disease. Exp Gerontol. 2015;68:8–12.

27. Benayoun BA, Pollina EA, Brunet A. Epigenetic regulation of ageing: linking environmental inputs to genomic stability. Nature reviews. Mol Cell Biol. 2015;16(10):593–610.
28. Ordovas JM, Corella D. Nutritional genomics. Annu Rev Genomics Hum Genet. 2004;5:71–118.
29. Stover PJ, Caudill MA. Genetic and epigenetic contributions to human nutrition and health: managing genome-diet interactions. J Am Diet Assoc. 2008;108(9):1480–7.
30. Villiers-Tuthill A, et al. The relationship of tobacco and alcohol use with ageing self-perceptions in older people in Ireland. BMC Public Health. 2016;16:627.
31. Ward-Caviness CK, et al. Long-term exposure to air pollution is associated with biological aging. Oncotarget. 2016;7(46):74510–25.
32. Menck CF, Munford V. DNA repair diseases: what do they tell us about cancer and aging? Genet Mol Biol. 2014;37(1 Suppl):220–33.
33. Mastaloudis A, et al. Endurance exercise results in DNA damage as detected by the comet assay. Free Radic Biol Med. 2004;36(8):966–75.
34. Geller AM, Zenick H. Aging and the environment: a research framework. Environ Health Perspect. 2005;113(9):1257–62.
35. Woods JA, et al. Exercise, inflammation and aging. Aging Dis. 2011;3(1):130–40.
36. Chung HY, et al. Molecular inflammation: underpinnings of aging and age-related diseases. Ageing Res Rev. 2009;8(1):18–30.
37. Kent JW Jr, et al. Genotypexage interaction in human transcriptional ageing. Mech Ageing Dev. 2012;133(9–10):581–90.
38. Warburton DER, Nicol CW, Bredin SSD. Health benefits of physical activity: the evidence. CMAJ Can Med Assoc J. 2006;174(6):801–9.
39. Xie K, et al. Epigenetic alterations in longevity regulators, reduced life span, and exacerbated aging-related pathology in old father offspring mice. Proc Natl Acad Sci U S A. 2018;115(10):E2348–57.
40. Dictionary O. Oxford dictionaries. Lang Matters 2014.
41. Johnson TE. Recent results: biomarkers of aging. Exp Gerontol. 2006;41(12):1243–6.
42. Aubert G, Lansdorp PM. Telomeres and aging. Physiol Rev. 2008;88(2):557–79.
43. Kimura M, et al. Telomere length and mortality: a study of leukocytes in elderly Danish twins. Am J Epidemiol. 2008;167(7):799–806.
44. Lai T-P, Wright WE, Shay JW. Comparison of telomere length measurement methods. Philos Trans R Soc Lond Ser B Biol Sci. 2018;373(1741):20160451.
45. Sedelnikova OA, et al. Senescing human cells and ageing mice accumulate DNA lesions with unrepairable double-strand breaks. Nat Cell Biol. 2004;6(2):168–70.
46. Dolle ME, et al. Rapid accumulation of genome rearrangements in liver but not in brain of old mice. Nat Genet. 1997;17(4):431–4.
47. Xia X, et al. Molecular and phenotypic biomarkers of aging. F1000Research. 2017;6:860.
48. Weidner CI, et al. Aging of blood can be tracked by DNA methylation changes at just three CpG sites. Genome Biol. 2014;15(2):R24.
49. Bacos K, et al. Blood-based biomarkers of age-associated epigenetic changes in human islets associate with insulin secretion and diabetes. Nat Commun. 2016;7:11089.
50. Noren Hooten N, et al. Age-related changes in microRNA levels in serum. Aging (Albany NY). 2013;5(10):725–40.
51. Pincus Z, Smith-Vikos T, Slack FJ. MicroRNA predictors of longevity in Caenorhabditis elegans. PLoS Genet. 2011;7(9):e1002306.
52. Fatica A, Bozzoni I. Long non-coding RNAs: new players in cell differentiation and development. Nat Rev Genet. 2014;15(1):7–21.
53. Montes M, et al. The lncRNA MIR31HG regulates p16(INK4A) expression to modulate senescence. Nat Commun. 2015;6:6967.
54. Zhu S, et al. Genome-scale deletion screening of human long non-coding RNAs using a paired-guide RNA CRISPR-Cas9 library. Nat Biotechnol. 2016;34(12):1279–86.

55. Fontana L, Partridge L, Longo VD. Extending healthy life span–from yeast to humans. Science. 2010;328(5976):321–6.
56. Most J, et al. Calorie restriction in humans: an update. Ageing Res Rev. 2017;39:36–45.
57. Pan H, Finkel T. Key proteins and pathways that regulate lifespan. J Biol Chem. 2017;292(16):6452–60.
58. Bajwa P, et al. Age related increase in mTOR activity contributes to the pathological changes in ovarian surface epithelium. Oncotarget. 2016;7(15):19214–27.
59. Semba RD, Nicklett EJ, Ferrucci L. Does accumulation of advanced glycation end products contribute to the aging phenotype? J Gerontol A Biol Sci Med Sci. 2010;65(9):963–75.
60. Nagai R, et al. Antibody-based detection of advanced glycation end-products: promises vs. limitations. Glycoconj J. 2016;33(4):545–52.
61. Dall'Olio F, et al. N-glycomic biomarkers of biological aging and longevity: a link with inflammaging. Ageing Res Rev. 2013;12(2):685–98.
62. Montoliu I, et al. Serum profiling of healthy aging identifies phospho- and sphingolipid species as markers of human longevity. Aging (Albany NY). 2014;6(1):9–25.
63. Gohlke S, et al. Identification of functional lipid metabolism biomarkers of brown adipose tissue aging. Mol Metab. 2019;24:1–17.
64. Tyrrell DJ, et al. Blood cell respirometry is associated with skeletal and cardiac muscle bioenergetics: implications for a minimally invasive biomarker of mitochondrial health. Redox Biol. 2016;10:65–77.
65. Tyrrell DJ, et al. Respirometric profiling of muscle mitochondria and blood cells are associated with differences in gait speed among community-dwelling older adults. J Gerontol A Biol Sci Med Sci. 2015;70(11):1394–9.
66. Kurz DJ, et al. Senescence-associated (beta)-galactosidase reflects an increase in lysosomal mass during replicative ageing of human endothelial cells. J Cell Sci. 2000;113(Pt 20):3613–22.
67. Yang NC, Hu ML. The limitations and validities of senescence associated-beta-galactosidase activity as an aging marker for human foreskin fibroblast Hs68 cells. Exp Gerontol. 2005;40(10):813–9.
68. Vandenberk B, et al. p16INK4a: a central player in cellular senescence and a promising aging biomarker in elderly cancer patients. J Geriatr Oncol. 2011;2(4):259–69.
69. Tchkonia T, et al. Cellular senescence and the senescent secretory phenotype: therapeutic opportunities. J Clin Invest. 2013;123(3):966–72.
70. Huang J, et al. DAMPs, ageing, and cancer: the 'DAMP Hypothesis'. Ageing Res Rev. 2015;24(Pt A):3–16.
71. Chen W, et al. Three-dimensional human facial morphologies as robust aging markers. Cell Res. 2015;25(5):574–87.
72. Bürkle A, et al. MARK-AGE biomarkers of ageing. Mech Ageing Dev. 2015;151:2–12.
73. Belsky DW, et al. Eleven telomere, epigenetic clock, and biomarker-composite quantifications of biological aging: do they measure the same thing? Am J Epidemiol. 2018;187(6):1220–30.
74. Putin E, et al. Deep biomarkers of human aging: application of deep neural networks to biomarker development. Aging (Albany NY). 2016;8(5):1021–33.
75. Rehkopf DH, et al. Leukocyte telomere length in relation to 17 biomarkers of cardiovascular disease risk: a cross-sectional study of US adults. PLoS Med. 2016;13(11):e1002188.
76. Wang C, et al. DNA damage response and cellular senescence in tissues of aging mice. Aging Cell. 2009;8(3):311–23.
77. Rube CE, et al. Accumulation of DNA damage in hematopoietic stem and progenitor cells during human aging. PLoS One. 2011;6(3):e17487.
78. Kuo LJ, Yang LX. Gamma-H2AX – a novel biomarker for DNA double-strand breaks. In Vivo. 2008;22(3):305–9.
79. Pal S, Tyler JK. Epigenetics and aging. Sci Adv. 2016;2(7):e1600584.

80. Lu Y, et al. Systematic analysis of cell-to-cell expression variation of T lymphocytes in a human cohort identifies aging and genetic associations. Immunity. 2016;45(5):1162–75.
81. Olivieri F, et al. Age- and glycemia-related miR-126-3p levels in plasma and endothelial cells. Aging (Albany NY). 2014;6(9):771–87.
82. Olivieri F, et al. Age-related differences in the expression of circulating microRNAs: miR-21 as a new circulating marker of inflammaging. Mech Ageing Dev. 2012;133(11–12):675–85.
83. Li X, et al. Circulatory miR34a as an RNAbased, noninvasive biomarker for brain aging. Aging (Albany NY). 2011;3(10):985–1002.
84. Chen YN, et al. Identification of the lncRNA, AK156230, as a novel regulator of cellular senescence in mouse embryonic fibroblasts. Oncotarget. 2016;7(33):52673–84.
85. Boon RA, et al. Long noncoding RNA Meg3 controls endothelial cell aging and function: implications for regenerative angiogenesis. J Am Coll Cardiol. 2016;68(23):2589–91.
86. Schumacher B, et al. Delayed and accelerated aging share common longevity assurance mechanisms. PLoS Genet. 2016;4(8):e1000161.
87. Corpas E, Harman SM, Blackman MR. Human growth hormone and human aging. Endocr Rev. 1993;14(1):20–39.
88. Crimmins E, et al. Biomarkers related to aging in human populations. Adv Clin Chem. 2008;46:161–216.
89. Dieterlen MT, et al. Assay validation of phosphorylated S6 ribosomal protein for a pharmacodynamic monitoring of mTOR-inhibitors in peripheral human blood. Cytometry B Clin Cytom. 2012;82(3):151–7.
90. Verbrugge FH, Tang WH, Hazen SL. Protein carbamylation and cardiovascular disease. Kidney Int. 2015;88(3):474–8.
91. Gorisse L, et al. Protein carbamylation is a hallmark of aging. Proc Natl Acad Sci U S A. 2016;113(5):1191–6.
92. Glei DA, et al. Age-related changes in biomarkers: longitudinal data from a population-based sample. Res Aging. 2011;33(3):312–26.
93. Syslova K, Bohmova A, Mikoska M. Multimarker screening of oxidative stress in aging. Oxid Med Cell Longev. 2014;2014:562860.
94. Liu Y, et al. Expression of p16(INK4a) in peripheral blood T-cells is a biomarker of human aging. Aging Cell. 2009;8(4):439–48.
95. Wagner KH, et al. Biomarkers of aging: from function to molecular biology. Nutrients. 2016;8(6):E338.
96. Stambler I. Recognizing degenerative aging as a treatable medical condition: methodology and policy. Aging Dis. 2017;8(5):583–9.
97. Masoro EJ, Austad SN. Handbook of the biology of aging. San Diego: Academic; 2010.
98. de Cabo R, et al. The search for antiaging interventions: from elixirs to fasting regimens. Cell. 2014;157(7):1515–26.
99. Longo VD, et al. Interventions to slow aging in humans: are we ready? Aging Cell. 2015;14(4):497–510.

# Index





J. C. Gomez-Verjan, N. A. Rivero-Segura (eds.), *Clinical Genetics and Genomics of Aging*, https://doi.org/10.1007/978-3-030-40955-5

**D**

The manufacturer's authorised representative in the EU is Springer Nature Customer Service Centre GmbH, Europaplatz 3, 69115 Heidelberg, Germany. If you have any concerns regarding our products, please contact ProductSafety@springernature.com

Printed and bound by CPI Group (UK) Ltd, Croydon, CR0 4YY
30/07/2026
02181743-0001